Drug Hypersensitivity and Desensitizations

Editor

MARIANA C. CASTELLS

IMMUNOLOGY AND ALLERGY CLINICS OF NORTH AMERICA

www.immunology.theclinics.com

Consulting Editor
STEPHEN A. TILLES

November 2017 • Volume 37 • Number 4

ELSEVIER

1600 John F. Kennedy Boulevard • Suite 1800 • Philadelphia, Pennsylvania, 19103-2899

http://www.theclinics.com

IMMUNOLOGY AND ALLERGY CLINICS OF NORTH AMERICA Volume 37, Number 4

November 2017 ISSN 0889-8561, ISBN-13: 978-0-323-54883-0

Editor: Jessica McCool

Developmental Editor: Kristen Helm

Immunology and Allergy Clinics of North America (ISSN 0889–8561) is published quarterly by Elsevier Inc., 360 Park Avenue South, New York, NY 10010-1710. Months of issue are February, May, August, and November. Periodicals postage paid at New York, NY and additional mailing offices. Subscription prices are $320.00 per year for US individuals, $528.00 per year for US institutions, $100.00 per year for US students and residents, $395.00 per year for Canadian individuals, $220.00 per year for Canadian students, $670.00 per year for Canadian institutions, $445.00 per year for international individuals, $670.00 per year for international institutions, $220.00 per year for international students. To receive student/resident rate, orders must be accompanied by name of affiliated institution, date of term, and the *signature* of program/residency coordinator on institution letterhead. Orders will be billed at individual rate until proof of status is received. Foreign air speed delivery is included in all *Clinics* subscription prices. All prices are subject to change without notice. **POSTMASTER**: Send address changes to *Immunology and Allergy Clinics of North America,* Elsevier Health Sciences Division, Subscription Customer Service, 3251 Riverport Lane, Maryland Heights, MO 63043. **Customer Service: 1-800-654-2452 (U.S. and Canada); 314-447-8871 (outside U.S. and Canada). Fax: 314-447-8029. E-mail: journalscustomerservice-usa@elsevier.com (for print support); journalsonlinesupport-usa@elsevier.com (for online support).**

Reprints. For copies of 100 or more, of articles in this publication, please contact the Commercial Reprints Department, Elsevier Inc., 360 Park Avenue South, New York, New York 10010-1710. Tel. 212-633-3874, Fax: 212-633-3820, E-mail: reprints@elsevier.com.

Immunology and Allergy Clinics of North America is covered in MEDLINE/PubMed (Index Medicus), Current Contents/Life Sciences, Science Citation Index, ISI/BIOMED, Chemical Abstracts, and EMBASE/Excerpta Medica.

Contributors

CONSULTING EDITOR

STEPHEN A. TILLES, MD
Executive Director, ASTHMA Inc. Clinical Research Center, Partner, Northwest Asthma & Allergy Center, Clinical Professor of Medicine, University of Washington, Seattle, Washington, USA

EDITOR

MARIANA C. CASTELLS, MD, PhD
Director Drug Hypersensitivity and Desensitization Center, Mastocytosis Center Brigham and Women's Hospital/Dana Farber Cancer Institute, Professor in Medicine, Harvard Medical School, Boston, Massachusetts, USA

AUTHORS

MARCELO VIVOLO AUN, MD, PhD
Clinical Immunology and Allergy Division, University of Sao Paulo, School of Medicine, Sao Paulo, Brazil

ALEENA BANERJI, MD
Department of Medicine, Division of Rheumatology, Allergy, and Immunology, Massachusetts General Hospital, Boston, Massachusetts, USA

SEVIM BAVBEK, MD, Prof, FAAAAI
Full Time Professor, Division of Immunology and Allergy, Department of Chest Diseases, Ankara University School of Medicine, Ankara, Turkey

ANA DIOUN BROYLES, MD
Assistant Professor, Division of Allergy and Immunology, Boston Children's Hospital, Harvard Medical School, Boston, Massachusetts, USA

KATHLEEN M. BUCHHEIT, MD
Department of Medicine, Division of Rheumatology, Immunology and Allergy, Brigham and Women's Hospital, Harvard Medical School, Boston, Massachusetts, USA

DINAH FOER, MD
Department of Medicine, Division of Rheumatology, Immunology and Allergy, Brigham and Women's Hospital, Harvard Medical School, Boston, Massachusetts, USA

VIOLETA RÉGNIER GALVÃO, MD, PhD
Division of Clinical Immunology and Allergy, University of São Paulo, School of Medicine, São Paulo, São Paulo, Brazil

PEDRO GIAVINA-BIANCHI, MD, PhD
Clinical Immunology and Allergy Division, University of Sao Paulo, School of Medicine, Sao Paulo, Brazil

DANIEL HAR, MD
Division of Allergy and Immunology, The University of Texas Southwestern Medical Center, Dallas, Texas, USA

JORGE KALIL, MD, PhD
Clinical Immunology and Allergy Division, University of Sao Paulo, School of Medicine, Sao Paulo, Brazil

MIN JUNG LEE, MD
Assistant Professor of Pediatrics and Internal Medicine, Division of Allergy and Immunology, The University of Texas Southwestern Medical Center, Dallas, Texas, USA

SIMON A. MALLAL, MBBS, FRACP, FRCPA
Institute for Immunology and Infectious Diseases, Murdoch University, Murdoch, Western Australia; Departments of Medicine, and Pathology, Microbiology and Immunology, Vanderbilt University Medical Center, Nashville, Tennessee, USA

CAITLIN M.G. McNULTY, MD
Division of Allergic Diseases, Mayo Clinic, Rochester, Minnesota, USA

BRIAN MODENA, MD
Division of Allergy, Asthma and Immunology, Scripps Clinic, San Diego, California, USA

ALLISON EADDY NORTON, MD
Assistant Professor, Division of Pediatric Pulmonary, Allergy and Immunology, Vanderbilt University School of Medicine, Nashville, Tennessee, USA

IRIS M. OTANI, MD
Department of Medicine, Division of Pulmonary, Critical Care, Allergy, and Sleep Medicine, UCSF Medical Center, San Francisco, California, USA

MIGUEL A. PARK, MD
Assistant Professor of Medicine, Division of Allergic Diseases, Mayo Clinic, Rochester, Minnesota, USA

REBECCA PAVLOS, PhD
Institute for Immunology and Infectious Diseases, Murdoch University, Murdoch, Western Australia

ELIZABETH J. PHILLIPS, MD, FIDSA, FAAAAI
Institute for Immunology and Infectious Diseases, Murdoch University, Murdoch, Western Australia; Departments of Medicine, Pathology, Microbiology and Immunology, and Pharmacology, Vanderbilt University Medical Center, Nashville, Tennessee, USA

MATTHIEU PICARD, MD, FRCPC
Assistant Clinical Professor, Department of Medicine, Division of Allergy and Immunology, Hôpital Maisonneuve-Rosemont, Université de Montréal, Montréal, Québec, Canada

RAFAEL BONAMICHI SANTOS, MD
Division of Clinical Immunology and Allergy, University of São Paulo, School of Medicine, São Paulo, São Paulo, Brazil

ROLAND SOLENSKY, MD
Division of Allergy and Immunology, The Corvallis Clinic, Oregon State University, Oregon Health & Science University College of Pharmacy, Corvallis, Oregon, USA

CELESTINE WANJALLA, MD, PhD
Department of Medicine, Vanderbilt University Medical Center, Nashville, Tennessee, USA

ANDREW A. WHITE, MD
Division of Allergy, Asthma and Immunology, Scripps Clinic, San Diego, California, USA

KATIE D. WHITE, MD, PhD
Department of Medicine, Vanderbilt University Medical Center, Nashville, Tennessee, USA

KATHARINE M. WOESSNER, MD
Division of Allergy, Asthma and Immunology, Scripps Clinic, San Diego, California, USA

JOHNSON WONG, MD
Department of Medicine, Division of Rheumatology, Allergy, and Immunology, Massachusetts General Hospital, Boston, Massachusetts, USA

Contents

Drug-Induced Anaphylaxis　　　　　　　　　　　　　　**629**

Marcelo Vivolo Aun, Jorge Kalil, and Pedro Giavina-Bianchi

> Drugs are among the main triggers of anaphylaxis, but identification of the culprit drug is frequently difficult. To confirm diagnosis of the causative agent, medical records and clinical history are fundamental. There are a few in vitro tests available in clinical practice, such as serum-specific IgE and basophil activation test. Skin tests are often useful for the diagnosis, although drug challenge is indicated in patients with inconclusive clinical history or to provide safe alternatives. Treatment of anaphylaxis is standard and intramuscular epinephrine is the main agent to prevent morbidity and mortality. Rapid desensitization may be indicated in selected cases.

Penicillin and Beta-Lactam Hypersensitivity　　　　　　**643**

Daniel Har and Roland Solensky

> Ten percent of patients report penicillin allergy, but more than 90% of these individuals can tolerate penicillins. Skin testing remains the optimal method for evaluation of possible IgE-mediated penicillin allergy and is recommended by professional societies, as the harms for alternative antibiotics include antimicrobial resistance, prolonged hospitalizations, readmissions, and increased costs. Removal of penicillin allergy leads to decreased utilization of broad-spectrum antibiotics, such as fluoroquinolones and vancomycin. There is minimal allergic cross-reactivity between penicillins and cephalosporins. IgE-mediated allergy to cephalosporins is usually side-chain specific and may warrant graded challenge with cephalosporins containing dissimilar R1 or R2 group side chains.

Platinum Chemotherapy Hypersensitivity: Prevalence and Management　　**663**

Iris M. Otani, Johnson Wong, and Aleena Banerji

> Hypersensitivity reactions to platinum agents are common. For carboplatin and cisplatin, the first hypersensitivity reaction typically occurs around the second and third re-exposure during the second line of therapy (eighth and ninth courses overall). For oxaliplatin, the first hypersensitivity reaction can occur throughout the treatment course. Skin testing helps risk stratify patients to appropriate desensitization protocols and assess risk for breakthrough HSRs during desensitization. A risk-stratification protocol using

3 serial skin tests and desensitization protocols enables patients with platinum agent hypersensitivity to receive first-line chemotherapy treatment safely.

Taxanes are an important class of antineoplastic agents used in the treatment of a wide variety of cancers. However, paclitaxel and docetaxel, which are the most commonly used taxanes, elicit immediate hypersensitivity reactions (HSRs) in 5% to 10% of patients. Almost all patients that experience these reactions can be safely re-exposed to taxanes either through desensitization or challenge. This article describes the clinical presentation, diagnosis, and management of HSRs to taxanes and discusses the different options for their safe readministration.

The use of monoclonal antibodies (mAbs) has become broader because of their recognized effectiveness in the treatment of autoimmune, neoplastic, and inflammatory diseases. Consequently, hypersensitivity reactions (HSR) secondary to mAbs are being reported more often, and each mAb-related HSR presents specific features. This article discusses the main biological agents and associated HSR, the clinical presentation of such reactions, and the role of tryptase and skin testing in the diagnosis. Rapid drug desensitization procedures to mAbs enable selected allergic patients to receive full therapeutic doses in a safe manner and are also discussed.

Proper management of drug allergy in children is based on a thorough history, in vitro testing (if available), in vivo testing, and drug challenge. This approach has been well developed with beta-lactam drugs but not with non–beta-lactam drugs and monoclonal antibodies. Children commonly develop rashes during an antibiotic course, which can lead to misdiagnosis of drug allergy. Clinical reactions to monoclonal antibodies vary and are managed depending on the type. A better knowledge of drug reactions that can occur in antibiotic allergy and monoclonal allergy can aid a provider in better management of their drug-allergic pediatric patients.

Aspirin and nonsteroidal antiinflammatory drugs (NSAIDs) are widely used in the United States and throughout the world for a variety of indications. Several unique hypersensitivity syndromes exist to this class of medications, making them one of the common reasons for consultation to the allergist. The lack of any laboratory-based diagnostic studies to assist in identifying the culprits in these reactions make evaluation of aspirin and NSAID hypersensitivity challenging. Identifying patients appropriate for oral challenge and/or desensitization protocols is the standard pragmatic approach to this issue when it arises.

drug development. Up to 50% of such reactions are preventable. Although many ADRs can be predicted based on the on-target pharmacologic activity, ADRs arising from drug interactions with off-target receptors are recognized. Off-target ADRs include the immune-mediated ADRs (IM-ADRs) and pharmacologic drug effects. In this review, we discuss what is known about the immunogenetics and pathogenesis of IM-ADRs and the hypothesized role of heterologous immunity in the development of IM-ADRs.

IMMUNOLOGY AND ALLERGY
CLINICS OF NORTH AMERICA

FORTHCOMING ISSUES

February 2018
Food Allergy
J. Andrew Bird, *Editor*

May 2018
The Airway and Exercise
J. Tod Olin and James H. Hull, *Editors*

August 2018
Mastocytosis
Mariana C. Castells, *Editor*

RECENT ISSUES

August 2017
Angioedema
Marc A. Riedl, *Editor*

May 2017
Biologic Therapies of Immunologic Diseases
Bradley E. Chipps and Stephen P. Peters, *Editors*

February 2017
Allergic Skin Diseases
Peck Y. Ong and Peter Schmid-Grendelmeier, *Editors*

ISSUE OF RELATED INTEREST

Infectious Disease Clinics of North America, June 2016 (Vol. 30, No. 2)
Antibiotic Resistance: Challenges and Opportunities
Richard R. Watkins and Robert A. Bonomo, *Editors*
Available at: http://www.id.theclinics.com/

Erratum

An error was made in the August 2017 issue of *Immunology and Allergy Clinics of North America* (Volume 37, Issue 3) in the article, "Emerging Therapies in Hereditary Angioedema," by Meng Chen and Marc A. Riedl. It should be noted that this article was supported by the NIH Grant number T32 AI 007469. The online version of the article has been updated to include this note.

Foreword

Drug Hypersensitivity: Broadening Horizons

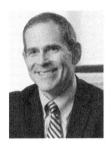

Stephen A. Tilles, MD
Consulting Editor

Historically, the focus of drug hypersensitivity research was penicillin and other beta-lactam antibiotics. In fact, a PubMed search for "drug hypersensitivity penicillin" yields nearly 4000 citations dating back to 1945, which is far more than any other drug category. This seemingly narrow emphasis was appropriate, given the astounding number of patients with "penicillin allergy" listed on their medical record, and the resultant availability of penicillin skin-testing reagents and desensitization protocols has made it possible to successfully and safely reintroduce penicillin to most of these patients. In contrast, the development of reliable diagnostic tests for most other agents has not panned out. Nevertheless, in recent years, the hard work of multiple investigators has led to the emergence of effective management strategies for a wide variety of drugs.

In this issue of *Immunology and Allergy Clinics of North America*, Editor Mariana C. Castells, herself one of the pioneers of desensitization to chemotherapeutic agents and biologics, has assembled a world class group of authors, covering a broad range of subjects related to drug hypersensitivity and desensitization. For example, there are separate articles reviewing hypersensitivity to platins, taxanes, monoclonal antibodies, progesterone, nonsteroidal anti-inflammatory drugs, and of course, beta-lactams. In addition, there is a review on drug reactions in children, another on drug-induced anaphylaxis, and another on severe delayed drug reactions.

This issue of the *Immunology and Allergy Clinics of North America* will serve as an essential reference for practicing allergists, physicians in training, and oncologists,

Immunol Allergy Clin N Am 37 (2017) xv–xvi
http://dx.doi.org/10.1016/j.iac.2017.08.003
0889-8561/17/© 2017 Published by Elsevier Inc.

immunology.theclinics.com

rheumatologists, and other specialists whose practice involves high-stakes decisions regarding alternatives when faced with a significant adverse drug reaction.

Stephen A. Tilles, MD
ASTHMA Inc Clinical Research Center
Northwest Asthma & Allergy Center
University of Washington
9725 3rd Avenue NE, Suite 500
Seattle, WA 98115, USA

E-mail address:
stilles@nwasthma.com

Preface

Drug Hypersensitivity and Desensitizations

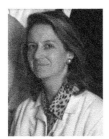

Mariana C. Castells, MD, PhD
Editor

Hypersensitivity to drugs has increased in the twenty-first century due to an explosion in new and targeted medications to address diseases through personalized and precision medicine. From 45 monoclonal antibodies in 2017, there will be 75 in 2020, with four US Food and Drug Administration approvals targeting allergic diseases in the last 6 months. Small molecules are the newest generation of drugs, and reactions to apparently poorly allergenic compounds are becoming more frequent. As I was working with the authors on their submissions for this issue, I was asked to consult for a pharmaceutical company whose star medication was found to have great efficacy against a rare and deadly cancer in early clinical trials, but several patients had presented unexpected hypotension and anaphylaxis, which raised concerns about public safety and potential clinical use. Reactions to drugs are the limiting step for their use, preventing patients from optimal treatment with first-line therapies. Most hypersensitivity reactions cannot be predicted in silico, in vitro, or in animal models, and health care providers and patients are unprepared for the reactions, their recognition and diagnosis, and their management and treatment. The groundbreaking therapeutic management of these reactions with desensitization is the next generation of personalized allergy treatments to provide patients with their best medication options.

This issue of the *Immunology and Allergy Clinics of North America* is entirely devoted to drug hypersensitivity and desensitizations to provide state-of-the-art understanding of the incidence, clinical presentation, mechanism, and diagnosis of hypersensitivity reactions to the most commonly used medications. From antibiotics, aspirin, and nonsteroidal anti-inflammatory drugs (NSAIDs) to cancer therapies and progesterone, the authors provide the phenotypes, endotypes, and biomarkers of the reactions and their management and treatment with desensitization, when indicated.

Aun, Kalil, and Giavina-Bianchi provide a new look at the drugs implicated in anaphylaxis in the emergency room. Penicillin allergy is claimed by 10% of the

Immunol Allergy Clin N Am 37 (2017) xvii–xviii
http://dx.doi.org/10.1016/j.iac.2017.08.002
0889-8561/17/© 2017 Published by Elsevier Inc. immunology.theclinics.com

population, but when appropriately tested, less than 1% of patients are truly allergic. Har and Solensky provide new insights into how to address, diagnose, and manage penicillin and beta-lactam allergy. Hypersensitivity to chemotherapy drugs limits first-line treatments in a substantial number of allergic patients. Otani, Wong, and Banerji provide an in-depth understanding of platins-mediated reactions, and Picard provides a new approach to taxanes reactions. New targeted human and humanized monoclonal antibodies used for cancer and chronic inflammatory diseases are thought to be less allergenic than chimeric antibodies, and yet, Bonamichi Santos and Régnier Galvão provide evidence of increasing hypersensitivity reactions and provide approaches to their diagnosis and management. Although children are less exposed to medications, there is a growing concern about reactions, which limit their use. Norton and Broyles provide an in-depth review of the management of reactions to antibiotics and monoclonal antibodies. Aspirin and NSAIDs can induce complex reactions that range from aspirin exacerbated respiratory disease to anaphylaxis. Modena, White, and Woessner provide a working classification of the reactions and their management. Whether delayed cutaneous hypersensitivity reactions can be treated with rapid desensitization is a novel concept explored by McNulty and Park. Subcutaneous administration of monoclonal antibodies and other medications is a convenient and safe delivery method that is gaining public acceptance. Bavbek and Lee provide a fresh look at subcutaneous reactions and their potential for desensitization. Progestogen hypersensitivity is a new entity recently described by Foer and Buchheit, which encompasses entities from catamenial anaphylaxis to infertility and can be treated with desensitization. In the last article, Pavlos, White, Wanjalla, Mallal, and Phillips provide a state-of-the-art understanding of the role of genetics and viral infections for Stevens Johnson Syndrome and severe cutaneous adverse reactions to drugs.

Bringing new understanding of the phenotypes, endotypes, and biomarkers of hypersensitivity drug reactions should create new standards and platforms for allergists and clinical immunologists regarding management and treatment options. Patient-centered and -personalized desensitizations are high-risk, sophisticated, and standardized approaches, only to be enforced by trained allergists with a deep understanding of the underlying mechanisms and the potential benefits of the reintroduction of the medication. Research is needed to unravel more specific and sensitive diagnostic tools for drug hypersensitivity reactions and to provide personalized management options based on precision medicine.

Mariana C. Castells, MD, PhD
Drug Hypersensitivity and Desensitization Center
Mastocytosis Center Brigham and Women's Hospital/
Dana Farber Cancer Institute
Harvard Medical School
60 Fenwood Road, Room 5002
Boston, MA 02115, USA

850 Boylston Street
Brookline, MA 02445, USA

E-mail addresses:
mcastells@partners.org
mcastells@bwh.harvard.edu

Drug-Induced Anaphylaxis

Marcelo Vivolo Aun, MD, PhD*, Jorge Kalil, MD, PhD,
Pedro Giavina-Bianchi, MD, PhD

KEYWORDS

- Anaphylaxis • Drug allergy • Adverse drug reactions • Hypersensitivity
- Nonsteroidal anti-inflammatory drugs • Epinephrine

KEY POINTS

- Drugs are among the main triggers of anaphylaxis.
- Diagnosis of the causative agent is difficult, and includes clinical history and in vitro and in vivo tests.
- Skin tests are useful only for IgE-mediated anaphylaxis.
- Drug challenge is indicated in doubtful clinical history and to provide safe drug options.
- Rapid desensitization is indicated in selected cases when no cost-effective option is available.

INTRODUCTION

Hypersensitivity reactions (HSRs) induced by drugs are a subgroup of adverse drug reactions that are unexpected and characterized by objectively reproducible symptoms or signs initiated by exposure to a drug at a dose tolerated by normal individuals.[1] As defined by the International Consensus on Drug Allergy, immediate HSRs, which occur within the first few hours after drug exposure, are characterized by urticaria, angioedema, rhinoconjunctivitis, bronchospasm, and anaphylaxis.[2] Anaphylaxis is defined as a serious, generalized, or systemic HSR that can be life-threatening or fatal.[3]

Along with food and hymenoptera venom allergy, drugs are among the leading causes of anaphylaxis, particularly in adults.[4,5] HSRs to drugs are a serious public health problem in inpatient and outpatient settings, because of high morbidity and socioeconomic costs, and they are potentially fatal.[4]

In accordance with international guidelines, the diagnosis of anaphylaxis is based on clinical findings (**Box 1**).[6] It relies on recognition of characteristic signs and

Disclosure Statement: Authors declare they have nothing to disclose about this entire article.
Avenida Eneas de Carvalho Aguiar 155, 8th Floor, Prédio dos Ambulatórios, Bloco 03, 05403-900, Sao Paulo, Brasil
* Corresponding author.
E-mail address: marcelovivoloaun@gmail.com

Immunol Allergy Clin N Am 37 (2017) 629–641
http://dx.doi.org/10.1016/j.iac.2017.06.002
0889-8561/17/© 2017 Elsevier Inc. All rights reserved.
immunology.theclinics.com

Box 1
Clinical criteria for the diagnosis of anaphylaxis

Anaphylaxis is highly likely when any one of the following three criteria is fulfilled:

1. Acute onset of an illness with skin-mucosal involvement and at least one of the following:
   A. Respiratory compromise
   B. Decreased blood pressure, syncope, or collapse OR

2. Two or more of the following that occur rapidly after exposure to a likely allergen for that patient
   A. Skin-mucosal involvement
   B. Respiratory compromise
   C. Decreased blood pressure, syncope, or collapse
   D. Gastrointestinal symptoms OR

3. Decreased blood pressure after exposure to a known allergen for that patient

Adapted from Simons FER, Ardusso LRF, Bilò MB, et al. World Allergy Organization guidelines for the assessment and management of anaphylaxis. World Allergy Organ J 2011;4(2):15; with permission.

---

symptoms, which occur minutes to a few hours after exposure to a known or potential trigger, often presenting rapid progression.

The target organs involved are variable. Typically, symptoms occur in two or more body systems: skin and mucosa, upper and lower respiratory tract, gastrointestinal tract, cardiovascular system, and central nervous system. In certain circumstances, anaphylaxis is diagnosed when only one body system is involved (eg, after an insect sting, sudden onset of cardiovascular symptoms may be the only manifestation). Skin manifestations are present in 80% to 90% of all patients, and anaphylaxis is harder to recognize when they are absent. The pattern of symptoms and signs differ from one patient to another, and even in the same patient from one anaphylactic reaction to another. At the beginning of an episode, it is difficult to predict the rate of progression or the ultimate severity.[6–8] Misdiagnosis or overdiagnosis of anaphylaxis can occur, as described in patients with acute multisystem symptoms after ingestion of caustic substances, foreign body inhalation, acute urticaria, or angioedema.[6]

Anaphylaxis is a common manifestation in patients with systemic mastocytosis, particularly in adults with indolent systemic mastocytosis without skin involvement. Systemic mastocytosis is a disorder characterized by the abnormal proliferation and accumulation of clonal mast cells in tissues, generally harboring the KIT D816 V mutation and showing aberrant CD25 expression, accompanied by increased baseline tryptase levels.[9] It is well defined that patients with hymenoptera venom–induced anaphylaxis who present severe reactions, including hypotension, are at high risk of having systemic mastocytosis, but this is not so clear in the case of drug reactions.[10] To exclude mastocytosis, patients presenting a drug-induced anaphylactic reaction should undergo measurement of basal serum tryptase.[10]

EPIDEMIOLOGY

The prevalence of anaphylaxis is not well known, with an estimated overall incidence that ranges from 3 to 50 per 100,000 person-years, with a lifetime prevalence of 0.05% to 2%.[11] Incidence and mortality associated with anaphylaxis have been increasing, possibly because of food and drug allergy, respectively.[12–14] The main causes of anaphylaxis in epidemiologic studies are drugs, food, and hymenoptera venom.[6] Furthermore, excluding pediatric cohorts (wherein foods are the most common trigger), medications are the most frequent cause of fatal anaphylaxis in reports from the United States, United Kingdom, Australia, and New Zealand.[15]

Epidemiologic studies regarding drug-induced anaphylaxis (DIA) have increased in the last 5 years. Until 2005, few studies evaluated drugs as triggers of systemic HSRs. Classes of drugs most commonly cited as triggers of anaphylaxis were antibiotics, mainly β-lactams; dextrans; radioiodinated contrast media; allergen extracts; and analgesics, particularly diclofenac.[16–18] However, the rate of anaphylaxis induced by different classes of drugs is widely variable around the world.

Since 2013, new studies, with different methodologic designs, showed different results regarding culprit medications in DIA.[4,19–26] Two of them, performed in France and Portugal, observed that antibiotics are still the main cause of DIA, followed by anesthesia agents, nonsteroidal anti-inflammatory drugs (NSAIDs), radiocontrast media, vaccines, immunotherapy, and chemotherapeutic and biologic agents.[20,21] However, some other case series reported NSAIDs as the major cause of DIA, particularly in Latin American populations.[4,19,21–23] Finally, a recent study from Korea assessing in-hospital DIA showed that platinum compounds are a major causative agent.[26]

Several factors may explain such discrepancies between different populations. First, anaphylaxis definition and methods differ between the case series. In the Taiwan study, for example, International Classification of Diseases-9 was used to define anaphylaxis.[25] However, even International Classification of Diseases-10 is inadequate and led to undernotification of anaphylaxis in epidemiologic studies.[27] Second, genetic background, which is associated with higher risk to develop reaction to a specific drug, varies from one population to another. Finally, drugs are used differently in distinct regions. In Latin America, particularly in Brazil, NSAIDs are used indiscriminately. Dipyrone (metamizole) is available and it has been reported to be the main cause of anaphylaxis among all NSAIDs.[4,19,21]

In the first Portuguese casuistry based on a national pharmacovigilance system, NSAIDs were not included between the major causes of anaphylaxis.[21] However, a second Portuguese case series was published by allergists one year later based on spontaneous notification in allergy units.[4] In that study, NSAIDs were among the main causes of DIA, in accordance with Latin-American publications.[4,19,22,24] Confirming the diagnosis of anaphylaxis caused by NSAIDs may be difficult if European Network for Drug Allergy (ENDA) classification of NSAID HSR is used (discussed later).[28] For example, many cases, particularly less severe ones, may have been lost in the French and Portuguese pharmacovigilance studies published in 2013.[20,21]

MECHANISMS INVOLVED IN DRUG-INDUCED ANAPHYLAXIS

DIA may occur by immune-mediated (allergic, mainly IgE-dependent) and nonimmune-mediated (nonallergic) mechanisms.[29–31] Regarding IgE-mediated reactions, most drugs have low molecular weight and are not able to directly elicit an immune response. In these cases, they act as haptens or prohaptens to become immunogenic.[29] However, IgG-mediated anaphylaxis was only documented in animal models.[32]

Several nonimmune-mediated mechanisms of anaphylaxis have been described, such as direct degranulation of mast cell/basophil, complement activation, adenosine, and cyclooxygenase metabolism interferences, and contact system activation.[32] These reactions can be clinically indistinguishable from IgE-mediated anaphylaxis. Moreover, DIA can also occur because of contaminants.[29] In 2007, there were about

80 deaths in the United States and Germany caused by anaphylactic reactions to heparin contaminated with oversulfated chondroitin.[33]

Particularly in hypersensitivity to NSAIDs, nonallergic reactions are more frequent than IgE-mediated reactions. These idiosyncratic reactions seem to occur based on an imbalance of cyclooxygenase metabolism, with overproduction of leukotrienes and underproduction of prostaglandins.[28] NSAID HSR has been classified in five different endotypes/phenotypes based on mechanisms involved and clinical presentation.[28] Nevertheless, this classification is not able to include all patients with HSR to NSAIDs. One specific phenotype that is not cited in the ENDA classification[28] is the designated "blended reaction"[34] These reactions are "mixed" reactions, when patients have immediate skin plus respiratory symptoms induced by different classes of NSAIDs, characterizing a nonallergic anaphylaxis. In the European classification, anaphylaxis triggered by NSAIDs is mainly considered IgE-mediated. In two recent articles, these blended reactions are better discussed, and two new classification proposals are described.[35,36]

In our experience, nonallergic HSR to NSAIDs, including anaphylaxis, is much more frequent that IgE-mediated HSR.[19] However, NSAID nonallergic anaphylaxis tends to be less severe than IgE-mediated anaphylaxis. In a previous study published by our group, we showed that nonallergic NSAID-induced anaphylaxis rarely causes hypotension, and our patients had a higher frequency of urticarial, angioedema, and bronchospasm, compatible with a blended reaction. However, IgE-mediated anaphylaxis to other drugs was associated with higher rates of hospitalization, intensive care unit admission, and intubation (**Table 1**).[19]

A novel mechanism was recently proposed to explain some nonallergic ("pseudoallergic") reactions induced by drugs. It has been recently described that basic secretagogues activate mouse mast cells in vitro and in vivo through a single receptor, the Mrgprb2, which is orthologue of the human G-protein-coupled receptor MRGPRX2.[37] It has been shown in mice that quinolones, neuromuscular blocking agents, and icatibant activate mast cells through Mrgprb2. Some non-IgE

Table 1
Comparison between IgE-mediated drug-induced anaphylaxis and nonallergic-induced anaphylaxis induced by nonsteroidal anti-inflammatory drugs in terms of clinical features and severity

Total N = 77	IgE-Mediated DIA, % N = 20	NSAIDs-Induced Anaphylaxis (Nonallergic), % N = 57	P Value (Chi-Square Test)
Signs and symptoms			
Urticaria and angioedema	70	91.2	.020
Bronchospasm	65	86	.042
Hypotension	75	22.8	.001
Severity criteria			
Hospitalization	80	22.8	.001
ICU admission	50	17.5	.004
Intubation and/or tracheostomy	45	14	.004

Abbreviation: ICU, intensive care unit.
Adapted from Aun MV, Blanca M, Garro LS, et al. Nonsteroidal anti-inflammatory drugs are major causes of drug-induced anaphylaxis. J Allergy Clin Immunol Pract 2014;2(4):419; with permission.

mediated "anaphylactoid" reactions in humans triggered by quinolones and neuro-muscular blocking agents could be explained by this mechanism.[37,38]

Lastly, some drugs can act as a "cofactor" to elicit an anaphylactic reaction. The most commonly cited drugs in this category are NSAIDs. Other drugs turn mild reactions into life-threatening and treatment refractory anaphylaxis, such as angiotensin-converting enzyme inhibitors, angiotensin receptor blockers, and β-blockers.[6,29,32]

Table 2 summarizes the main triggers of DIA, possible mechanisms involved, and possible in vitro and in vivo tests available.

Table 2
Drugs and/or agents mostly cited in case series as causes of drug-induced anaphylaxis, probable mechanisms involved, and evidence of IgE participation for allergic reactions

Drug/Agent	Type of HSR	Evidence of IgE-Mediated Reaction	References
Antibiotics			
β-Lactams	IgE-mediated	Skin tests Serum sIgE BAT	Decuyper et al,[39] 2017
Quinolones	IgE-mediated and nonallergic (mast cell degranulation through MRGPRX2 pathway?)	Serum IgE BAT	McNeil et al,[37] 2015; Aranda et al,[40] 2011
NSAIDs			
Pyrazolones	IgE-mediated and nonallergic	Skin tests BAT	Decuyper et al,[39] 2017
Other groups	Nonallergic IgE-mediated?	BAT ?	Kowalski et al,[28] 2011; Ayso et al,[41] 2013
Chemotherapeutic agents			
Platinum salts	IgE-mediated	Skin tests Serum sIgE BAT	Giavina-Bianchi et al,[42] 2017; Caiado and Castells,[43] 2015; Giavina-Bianchi et al,[44] 2017
Taxanes	IgE-mediated and nonallergic	Skin tests	Picard et al,[45] 2016; Prieto Garcia and Pineda de la Losa,[46] 2010
Biologic agents	IgE-mediated, cytokine storm, or mixed reactions	Skin tests for a few agents	Galvão and Castells,[47] 2015; Brennan et al,[48] 2009; Picard and Galvão,[49] 2017
Intraoperative agents			
NMBAs	IgE-mediated and nonallergic (mast cell degranulation through MRGPRX2 pathway?)	Skin tests Serum sIgE	McNeil et al,[37] 2015; Decuyper et al,[39] 2017
Latex	IgE-mediated	Skin tests Serum sIgE	Gaspar and Faria,[50] 2012
Radioiodinated contrast media	IgE-mediated and nonallergic	Skin tests BAT	Decuyper et al,[39] 2017

Abbreviations: BAT, basophil activation test; NMBAs, neuromuscular blocking agents; sIgE, serum-specific IgE.

DIAGNOSIS
Anaphylaxis

Physicians must be prepared and well trained to confirm the diagnosis of anaphylaxis. Diagnosis is essentially clinical and based on signs and symptoms presented during the reaction (see **Box 1**).[6] Underdiagnosis is more common when there is no mucocutaneous involvement.[6]

Particularly in perioperative anaphylaxis, surgeons and anesthesiologists should be aware of this uncommon condition. There are several differential diagnoses of respiratory and cardiovascular dysfunction during surgeries, and skin involvement that is observed in more than 90% of patients with anaphylaxis may be less frequent in perioperative reactions, making the diagnosis more difficult. In addition, skin manifestations are also not easily recognized when present, because the patient is covered and sedated, being unable to report pruritus.[51] Anesthesiologists should not underestimate immediate isolated skin manifestations. Although these reactions are not anaphylactic, they are considered grade I systemic reactions and they may predict a more severe reaction in a subsequent re-exposure to the culprit agent.[52]

In systemic acute reactions after NSAID exposure, clinical diagnosis of anaphylaxis based on the current ENDA classification in five endotypes/phenotypes of reactions is difficult.[28] Using this classification, anaphylaxis is restricted to those IgE-mediated severe reactions induced by one group of NSAIDs in patients who tolerate other groups. These patients are considered selective responders.

However, many patients cross-intolerant to different groups of NSAIDs may present skin (urticaria/angioedema) plus respiratory compromise (rhinosinusitis and bronchospasm), in an acute basis, which is compatible with anaphylaxis.[19] These blended reactions seem to be non-IgE-mediated and nonallergic, resulting from the inhibition of cyclooxygenase-1 and prominently cysteinyl leukotriene overproduction.[28,34,53] They are frequently less severe than IgE-mediated anaphylaxis (see **Table 1**).[19] However, clinicians should keep in mind that these reactions should be considered anaphylactic and patients must not take any NSAID until evaluation by the allergist.

Serum tryptase levels measured 30 to 180 minutes after symptoms onset may support the clinical diagnosis of anaphylaxis in some but not all patients.[6] If possible, the test should be done after intraoperative reactions, and an elevated "acute" serum tryptase level is highly predictive of IgE-mediated reaction.[54] If a high level of tryptase is found after an anaphylactic reaction, it should be measured again within a few weeks to exclude the diagnosis of mast cell disorders. Other mediators and their metabolites are potential biomarkers and can be measured in serum and/or 24-hour urine, although most of them are not available in clinical practice. The most studied are histamine, N-methylhistamine, N-methylimidazole acetic acid, methylimidazole acetic acid, carboxypeptidase, platelet aggregation factor (PAF), prostaglandin D2 (PGD2), prostaglandin F alfa (PGFalfa), and leukotriene E4 (LTE4).

Etiologic Agent

Clinicians should initiate investigation just after the acute reaction. Detailed analysis of patient clinical history is the primary and most important tool available for diagnosis of DIA. Even if the physician has confirmed the diagnosis of DIA and has identified the culprit agent, the patient should undergo evaluation by an allergist, bringing the initial medical report. Follow-up is essential because education regarding anaphylaxis is important to prevent potential future events.[29]

When many drugs are suspected to cause the anaphylactic reaction, a copy of the medical record, particularly in the perioperative reactions, is crucial. Then the allergist should draw a "time line" to identify which agents should be considered as real suspects and to define the investigation algorithm. History of prior HSRs to any drug should be taken into consideration, because it is not uncommon to see patients who present severe reactions after re-exposure to unrecognized culprit drugs or to drugs with high risk of cross-reactivity or cross-intolerance.

After a detailed clinical history, in vitro or in vivo tests are used to complete the investigation. Because anaphylaxis is a typical immediate reaction, according to the mechanisms involved, investigation should concentrate on specific IgE and/or basophil and mast cell activation.

In terms of laboratory tests to diagnose the culprit agent, few options are available in clinical practice. Serum-specific IgE assays are available for few drugs and, particularly for β-lactam antibiotics, its sensitivity is low.[6] Basophil activation tests may help in diagnosing IgE-mediated or non-IgE-mediated hypersensitivity. However, commercially available basophil activation tests do not have their accuracy established.[29]

Thus, in vivo tests are the best option to help allergists to confirm or exclude different drugs as the causative agent of an HSR. Either skin and drug provocation tests (DPT) are important options to diagnose HSRs. As suggested by international guidelines, drug allergy is an HSR involving a specific immunologic mechanism.[2] In drug allergy, skin testing is the method most widely used to determine sensitization, because other tests are less sensitive (in vitro tests) and specific, or potentially harmful (DPT). When facing a potential allergic reaction, the recommendation is to perform skin tests before DPT, because they allow one to define the mechanism involved in the reaction and they are safer than DPT.[2] It is recommended to perform skin prick tests and, if they are negative, intradermal tests. Some of the main triggers of DIA and the indications of in vitro and in vivo tests are summarized in **Table 2**. Although there is no international consensus on how skin tests with drugs should be performed and interpreted, there are many drugs for which nonirritating concentrations have been shown to be reliable.[55]

When clinical history and skin testing are not enough to confirm the diagnosis, DPT may be recommended.[2] DPT is the controlled administration of a specific drug with the purpose of diagnosing HSR. They are considered the gold standard for establishing or excluding the diagnosis of hypersensitivity to a given drug. In addition to reproducing the allergic symptoms, DPTs reproduce any clinical manifestation of hypersensitivity, regardless of the mechanism involved (immune- or nonimmune-mediated).[56] However, in a patient with a likely diagnosis of DIA, drug challenge to the culprit drug should not be performed. Negative skin tests to most implicated drugs lack the negative predictive value to recommend drug challenges in the setting of a reliable history.[29]

In DIA, allergists should keep DPT for specific situations, such as to find a safe therapeutic alternative to an implicated drug (eg, another β-lactam antibiotic for a patient with penicillin-induced anaphylaxis). In our experience, finding an alternative to the culprit drug is safe and is the major indication to perform a DPT.[57] Another indication to perform DPT is in "allergic" patients who had reactions not suggestive of anaphylaxis. In a previous review of DIA published in this journal,[29] Kuruvilla and Khan described that vocal cord dysfunction is an important differential diagnosis of anaphylaxis, particularly when the reaction is recurrent with many unrelated drugs. In these patients, DPT with the suspect agent is indicated in conjunction with laryngoscopy.[29]

When a drug is excluded as the cause of an HSR, it is important to rewrite a new medical record, changing the previous status.[29] Obviously, if DPT was performed with an alternative drug, this report should describe the tolerance to the drug tested, but maintaining the status of hypersensitive to the drug probably implicated in the reaction.

In **Fig. 1** we propose a diagnostic algorithm for DIA.

MANAGEMENT
Anaphylactic Reaction

Anaphylaxis is a life-threatening medical emergency in which prompt intervention is critical. During an acute reaction, the patient should be placed on the back with their lower extremities elevated. Epinephrine (adrenaline) is the first-line drug to treat anaphylaxis because it is the only medication proven to reduce hospitalization and death. It should be injected by the intramuscular (IM) route in a dose of 0.01 mg/kg of a 1:1000 (1 mg/mL) solution, to a maximum of 0.5 mg in adults and 0.3 mg in children. The dose is repeated every 5 to 15 minutes, as needed.[6,8,58]

The route of epinephrine administration for anaphylaxis should be IM, instead of subcutaneous or intravenous (IV) routes. Particularly for DIA in hospitalized patients, during intraoperative immediate HSR or while administering antibiotics, chemotherapy, or monoclonal antibodies, physicians tend to use IV adrenaline, because venous access is already available. However, there are limited data on the effective and safe dose of IV epinephrine to anaphylaxis. In a recent study, the IV route of epinephrine for anaphylaxis was associated with a higher frequency of overdoses and more adverse events, inducing 10% of cardiac ischemia.[59] In conclusion,

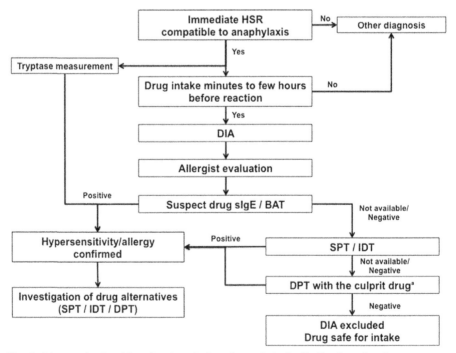

Fig. 1. Diagnostic algorithm for drug-induced anaphylaxis. [a]Indications for drug provocation test with the suspect drug include unreliable clinical history (reaction was not truly anaphylaxis), such as drug-induced vocal cord dysfunction. BAT, basophil activation test; IDT, intradermal test; sIgE, serum-specific IgE; SPT, skin prick test.

IM epinephrine, preferably applied into the thigh, is the proper route to treat anaphylaxis.[6]

Large volumes of fluids should be administered as soon as hypotension and shock are recognized.[60] Second-line medications, such as antihistamines, β_2-adrenergic agonists, and glucocorticoids, must not delay adrenaline administration. Glucocorticoids are typically used to prevent biphasic episodes of anaphylaxis and have little or no effect on initial symptoms and signs.[6,8]

Patients who present anaphylaxis while under treatment with β-blockers may benefit from glucagon administration. Moreover, physicians should pay special attention in patients under angiotensin-converting enzyme inhibitor treatment, because they frequently present prolonged hypotension with poor prognosis.[6,8]

Follow-up

After the initial HSR, prevention of new episodes is crucial. Once the diagnosis of DIA has been established, the mainstay of treatment is avoidance of the drug involved and those chemically related, which could potentially lead to cross-intolerance or cross-reactivity. Patients must avoid drugs related to the culprit one until an appointment with the allergist, who will evaluate the clinical history and perform in vivo and/or in vitro testing if necessary. As soon as investigation is complete, a final medical report should be written by the allergist to allow patients and their physicians' orientation.[6] However, even patients with clear medical reports are not totally free of a recurrent anaphylactic reaction. Epinephrine auto-injectors should be prescribed aiming to decrease morbidity and mortality associated with a future inadvertent reaction.[6]

In case of radiocontrast media hypersensitivity, patients with a history of immediate reactions should receive corticosteroid and antihistamine premedication before re-exposure. Because IgE-mediated anaphylaxis to radiocontrast media is rare, there is a universal consensus that routinely skin testing for all patients with a past reaction is not effective.[60]

In some cases, there is no alternative drug to treat a patient's condition instead of the drug imputed in the HSR.[61] Thus, drug desensitization is indicated as an effective approach to the management of IgE- and non-IgE-mediated HSR.[62] Mainly for immediate HSR, rapid drug desensitization is the process of induction of a state of unresponsiveness to a drug responsible for an HSR in a short period of time, usually some hours.[61] Rapid drug desensitization is a therapeutic procedure indicated for patients with proven or highly suspected HSRs after an individual risk/benefit assessment showing that the benefits outweigh the risks. In case of DIA induced by antibiotics, chemotherapeutic agents, and monoclonal antibodies, it was demonstrated that rapid drug desensitization is cost effective and safe to maintain hypersensitive patients on first-line therapy.[63] Rapid drug desensitization should be performed by allergists with experience in those procedures, in a hospital basis, and sometimes in intensive care settings because of the intrinsic risk of inducing a severe anaphylaxis when re-exposing patients to the causative agent.[61,63]

SUMMARY

DIA can be life-threatening, and re-exposure to the agent involved in the initial reaction is common. However, many patients are labeled as "allergic" after unclear reactions not compatible with anaphylaxis, and avoid drugs that could be cost effective and safe. One should encourage patients and clinicians to undergo an allergist evaluation after an anaphylactic reaction, to complete investigation and to receive a conclusive medical report that helps in future drug management.

REFERENCES

1. Johansson SGO, Bieber T, Dahl R, et al. Revised nomenclature for allergy for global use: report of the Nomenclature Review Committee of the World Allergy Organization. J Allergy Clin Immunol 2004;113(5):832–6.
2. Demoly P, Adkinson NF, Brockow K, et al. International consensus on drug allergy. Allergy 2014;69(4):420–37.
3. Simons FE, Ardusso LR, Bilò MB, et al. International consensus on (ICON) anaphylaxis. World Allergy Organ J 2014;7(1):9.
4. Faria E, Rodrigues-Cernadas J, Gaspar A, et al. Drug-induced anaphylaxis survey in Portuguese Allergy Departments. J Investig Allergol Clin Immunol 2014; 24(1):40–8.
5. Gonzalez-Estrada A, Silvers SK, Klein A, et al. Epidemiology of anaphylaxis at a tertiary care center: a report of 730 cases. Ann Allergy Asthma Immunol 2017; 118(1):80–5.
6. Simons FE, Ebisawa M, Sanchez-Borges M, et al. 2015 update of the evidence base: World Allergy Organization anaphylaxis guidelines. World Allergy Organ J 2015;8(1):32.
7. Sampson HA, Muñoz-Furlong A, Campbell RL, et al. Second symposium on the definition and management of anaphylaxis: summary report–Second National Institute of Allergy and Infectious Disease/Food Allergy and Anaphylaxis Network symposium. J Allergy Clin Immunol 2006;117(2):391–7.
8. Simons FE, Ardusso LR, Bilò MB, et al. WAO Position Paper. World allergy organization guidelines for the assessment and management of anaphylaxis. World Allergy Organ J 2011;4(2):13–37.
9. Castells MC, Hornick JL, Akin C. Anaphylaxis after hymenoptera sting: is it venom allergy, a clonal disorder, or both? J Allergy Clin Immunol Pract 2015;3(3):350–5.
10. Bonadonna P, Lombardo C. Drug allergy in mastocytosis. Immunol Allergy Clin North Am 2014;34(2):397–405.
11. Techapornroong M, Akrawinthawong K, Cheungpasitporn W, et al. Anaphylaxis: a ten years inpatient retrospective study. Asian Pac J Allergy Immunol 2010;28(4): 262–9.
12. Tang ML, Osborne N, Allen K. Epidemiology of anaphylaxis. Curr Opin Allergy Clin Immunol 2009;9(4):351–6.
13. Yang MS, Kim JY, Kim BK, et al. True rise in anaphylaxis incidence: epidemiologic study based on a national health insurance database. Medicine (Baltimore) 2017; 96(5):e5750.
14. Liew WK, Williamson E, Tang MLK. Anaphylaxis fatalities and admissions in Australia. J Allergy Clin Immunol 2009;123(2):434–42.
15. Jerschow E, Lin RY, Scaperotti MM, et al. Fatal anaphylaxis in the United States, 1999-2010: temporal patterns and demographic associations. J Allergy Clin Immunol 2014;134(6):1318–28.
16. van der Klauw MM, Wilson JH, Stricker BH. Drug-associated anaphylaxis: 20 years of reporting in The Netherlands (1974-1994) and review of the literature. Clin Exp Allergy 1996;26(12):1355–63.
17. Wang DY, Forslund C, Persson U, et al. Drug-attributed anaphylaxis. Pharmacoepidemiol Drug Saf 1998;7(4):269–74.
18. Leone R, Conforti A, Venegoni M, et al. Drug-induced anaphylaxis: case/non-case study based on an Italian pharmacovigilance database. Drug Saf 2005; 28(6):547–56.

19. Aun MV, Blanca M, Garro LS, et al. Nonsteroidal anti-inflammatory drugs are major causes of drug-induced anaphylaxis. J Allergy Clin Immunol Pract 2014;2(4): 414–20.

20. Renaudin JM, Beaudouin E, Ponvert C, et al. Severe drug-induced anaphylaxis: analysis of 333 cases recorded by the Allergy Vigilance Network from 2002 to 2010. Allergy 2013;68(7):929–37.

21. Ribeiro-Vaz I, Marques J, Demoly P, et al. Drug-induced anaphylaxis: a decade review of reporting to the Portuguese Pharmacovigilance Authority. Eur J Clin Pharmacol 2013;69(3):673–81.

22. Ensina LF, de Lacerda AE, de Andrade DM, et al. Drug-induced anaphylaxis in children: nonsteroidal anti-inflammatory drugs and drug provocation test. J Allergy Clin Immunol Pract 2014;2(4):825.

23. Aun MV, Blanca M, Garro LS, et al. Reply: to PMID 25017529. J Allergy Clin Immunol Pract 2014;2(4):826.

24. Jares EJ, Baena-Cagnani CE, Sánchez-Borges M, et al. Drug-induced anaphylaxis in Latin American countries. J Allergy Clin Immunol Pract 2015;3(5):780–8.

25. Lee YS, Sun WZ. Epidemiology of anaphylaxis: a retrospective cohort study in Taiwan. Acta Anaesthesiol Taiwan 2017. [Epub ahead of print].

26. Park HK, Kang MG, Yang MS, et al. Epidemiology of drug-induced anaphylaxis in a tertiary hospital in Korea. Allergol Int 2017. [Epub ahead of print].

27. Tanno LK, Bierrenbach AL, Calderon MA, et al. Decreasing the undernotification of anaphylaxis deaths in Brazil through the International Classification of Diseases (ICD)-11 revision. Allergy 2017;72(1):120–5.

28. Kowalski ML, Makowska JS, Blanca M, et al. Hypersensitivity to nonsteroidal anti-inflammatory drugs (NSAIDs): classification, diagnosis and management: review of the EAACI/ENDA and GA2LEN/HANNA. Allergy 2011;66(7):818–29.

29. Kuruvilla M, Khan DA. Anaphylaxis to drugs. Immunol Allergy Clin North Am 2015;35(2):303–19.

30. Lieberman P. Definition and criteria for the diagnoses of anaphylaxis. In: Castells MC, editor. Anaphylaxis and hypersensitivity reactions. New York: Springer; 2011. p. 1–12.

31. Kemp SF, Lockey RF. Pathophysiology and organ damage in anaphylaxis. In: Castells MC, editor. Anaphylaxis and hypersensitivity reactions. New York: Springer; 2011. p. 33–46.

32. Muñoz-Cano R, Picado C, Valero A, et al. Mechanisms of anaphylaxis beyond IgE. J Investig Allergol Clin Immunol 2016;26(2):73–82.

33. Kishimoto TK, Viswanathan K, Ganguly T, et al. Contaminated heparin associated with adverse clinical events and activation of the contact system. N Engl J Med 2008;358(23):2457–67.

34. Karakaya G, Celebioglu E, Kalyoncu AF. Non-steroidal anti-inflammatory drug hypersensitivity in adults and the factors associated with asthma. Respir Med 2013; 107(7):967–74.

35. Giavina-Bianchi P, Aun MV, Jares EJ, et al. Angioedema associated with nonsteroidal anti-inflammatory drugs. Curr Opin Allergy Clin Immunol 2016;16(4): 323–32.

36. Simon RA. NSAIDs (including aspirin): allergic and pseudoallergic reactions. Up to Date; 2017. Available at: https://www.uptodate.com/contents/nsaids-including-aspirin-allergic-and-pseudoallergic-reactions?source=search_result&search=hipersensibilidade%20aine&selectedTitle=1~150.

37. McNeil BD, Pundir P, Meeker S, et al. Identification of a mast-cell-specific receptor crucial for pseudo-allergic drug reactions. Nature 2015;519(7542):237–41.

38. Subramanian H, Gupta K, Ali H. Roles of Mas-related G protein-coupled receptor X2 on mast cell-mediated host defense, pseudoallergic drug reactions, and chronic inflammatory diseases. J Allergy Clin Immunol 2016;138(3):700–10.
39. Decuyper II, Mangodt EA, Van Gasse AL, et al. In vitro diagnosis of immediate drug hypersensitivity Anno 2017: potentials and limitations. Drugs R D 2017;17:265.
40. Aranda A, Mayorga C, Ariza A, et al. In vitro evaluation of IgE-mediated hypersensitivity reactions to quinolones. Allergy 2011;66(2):247–54.
41. Ayso P, Blanca-López N, Doña I, et al. Advanced phenotyping in hypersensitivity drug reactions to NSAIDs. Clin Exp Allergy 2013;43(10):1097–109.
42. Giavina-Bianchi P, Galvão VR, Picard M, et al. Basophil activation test is a relevant biomarker of the outcome of rapid desensitization in platinum compounds-allergy. J Allergy Clin Immunol Pract 2017;5(3):728–36.
43. Caiado J, Castells M. Presentation and diagnosis of hypersensitivity to platinum drugs. Curr Allergy Asthma Rep 2015;15(4):15.
44. Giavina-Bianchi P, Patil SU, Banerji A. Immediate hypersensitivity reaction to chemotherapeutic agents. J Allergy Clin Immunol Pract 2017;5(3):593–9.
45. Picard M, Pur L, Caiado J, et al. Risk stratification and skin testing to guide re-exposure in taxane-induced hypersensitivity reactions. J Allergy Clin Immunol 2016;137(4):1154–64.
46. Prieto Garcia A, Pineda de la Losa F. Immunoglobulin E-mediated severe anaphylaxis to paclitaxel. J Investig Allergol Clin Immunol 2010;20(2):170–1.
47. Galvão VR, Castells MC. Hypersensitivity to biological agents-updated diagnosis, management, and treatment. J Allergy Clin Immunol Pract 2015;3(2):175–85.
48. Brennan PJ, Rodriguez Bouza T, Hsu FI, et al. Hypersensitivity reactions to mAbs: 105 desensitizations in 23 patients, from evaluation to treatment. J Allergy Clin Immunol 2009;124(6):1259–66.
49. Picard M, Galvão VR. Current knowledge and management of hypersensitivity reactions to monoclonal antibodies. J Allergy Clin Immunol Pract 2017;5(3):600–9.
50. Gaspar A, Faria E. Latex allergy. Rev Port Imunoalergologia 2012;20(3):173–92.
51. Galvão VR, Giavina-Bianchi P, Castells M. Perioperative anaphylaxis. Curr Allergy Asthma Rep 2014;14(8):452.
52. Mertes PM, Malinovsky JM, Jouffroy L, et al. Reducing the risk of anaphylaxis during anesthesia: 2011 updated guidelines for clinical practice. J Investig Allergol Clin Immunol 2011;21(6):442–53.
53. Kim YJ, Lim KH, Kim MY, et al. Cross-reactivity to acetaminophen and celecoxib according to the type of nonsteroidal anti-inflammatory drug hypersensitivity. Allergy Asthma Immunol Res 2014;6(2):156–62.
54. Krishna MT, York M, Chin T, et al. Multi-centre retrospective analysis of anaphylaxis during general anaesthesia in the United Kingdom: aetiology and diagnostic performance of acute serum tryptase. Clin Exp Immunol 2014;178(2):399–404.
55. Brockow K, Garvey LH, Aberer W, et al. ENDA/EAACI Drug Allergy Interest Group. Skin test concentrations for systemically administered drugs - an ENDA/EAACI Drug Allergy Interest Group position paper. Allergy 2013;68(6):702–12.
56. Aberer W, Bircher A, Romano A, et al. Drug provocation testing in the diagnosis of drug hypersensitivity reactions: general considerations. Allergy 2003;58(9):854–63.
57. Aun MV, Bisaccioni C, Garro LS, et al. Outcomes and safety of drug provocation tests. Allergy Asthma Proc 2011;32(4):301–6.

58. Pumphrey RSH. An epidemiological approach to reducing the risk of fatal anaphylaxis. In: Castells MC, editor. Anaphylaxis and hypersensitivity reactions. New York: Springer; 2011. p. 13–31.

59. Campbell RL, Bellolio MF, Knutson BD, et al. Epinephrine in anaphylaxis: higher risk of cardiovascular complications and overdose after administration of intravenous bolus epinephrine compared with intramuscular epinephrine. J Allergy Clin Immunol Pract 2015;3(1):76–80.

60. Hsu Blatman KS, Hepner DL. Current knowledge and management of hypersensitivity to perioperative drugs and radiocontrast media. J Allergy Clin Immunol Pract 2017;5(3):587–92.

61. Giavina-Bianchi P, Aun MV, Galvão VR, et al. Rapid desensitization in immediate hypersensitivity reaction to drugs. Curr Treat Options Allergy 2015;2:268–85.

62. Bonamichi-Santos R, Castells M. Desensitization for drug hypersensitivity to chemotherapy and monoclonal antibodies. Curr Pharm Des 2016;22(45): 6870–80.

63. Sloane D, Govindarajulu U, Harrow-Mortelliti J, et al. Safety, costs, and efficacy of rapid drug desensitizations to chemotherapy and monoclonal antibodies. J Allergy Clin Immunol Pract 2016;4(3):497–504.

Penicillin and Beta-Lactam Hypersensitivity

Daniel Har, MD[a,1], Roland Solensky, MD[b,c,]*

KEYWORDS

- Penicillin • Beta-lactam • Allergy • Hypersensitivity

KEY POINTS

- More than 90% of individuals with history of penicillin allergy tolerate penicillins, and skin testing is the optimal method for evaluation.
- "Penicillin allergy" is associated with antimicrobial resistance, prolonged hospitalizations, readmissions, and increased costs.
- There is minimal allergic cross-reactivity between penicillins and cephalosporins, except selective allergy to aminopenicillin R-group side chains, which greatly increase the risk of reactions to cephalosporins with identical R1 group side chains.
- There is minimal allergic cross-reactivity between penicillins and carbapenems.
- Allergy to cephalosporins is usually side-chain specific and may warrant graded challenge with cephalosporins containing dissimilar R1 or R2 group side chains.

PENICILLIN ALLERGY
Background

Drug allergy is defined as an unpredictable reaction, or type B reaction, which is mediated by immune mechanisms.[1] Penicillin allergy is the most commonly reported medication allergy.[2] Immunoglobulin (Ig)E-mediated (or type I) reactions are one type of drug allergy, and they are the focus of this review. For further information on delayed reactions, please refer Caitlin M.G. McNulty and Miguel A. Park's article, "Delayed Cutaneous Hypersensitivity Reactions to Antibiotics, Management with Desensitization," in this issue. IgE-related reactions are typically immediate, with symptoms occurring within minutes to 6 hours of last administered dose, although onset is classically within

Disclosure Statement: None.
[a] Division of Allergy and Immunology, UT Southwestern Medical Center, 5323 Harry Hines Blvd, Dallas, TX 75390, USA; [b] Division of Allergy and Immunology, The Corvallis Clinic, 3680 NW Samaritan Dr, Corvallis, OR 97330, USA; [c] Oregon State University/Oregon Health & Science University College of Pharmacy, 1601 SW Jefferson Way, Corvallis, OR 97331, USA
[1] Present address: 1955 Market Center Boulevard, Apartment 2201, Dallas, TX 75207.
* Corresponding author. 3680 Northwest Samaritan Drive, Corvallis, OR.
E-mail address: roland.solensky@corvallisclinic.com

1 hour. IgE-related symptoms may include pruritus, flushing, urticaria, angioedema, bronchospasm, laryngeal edema, nausea, emesis, and hypotension.

Epidemiology

Penicillin allergy is self-reported by approximately 10% of patients.[3] However, following thorough evaluation, 90% or more of individuals with a history of penicillin allergy tolerate penicillins.[4–7] As a result, a history of penicillin allergy is unreliable in predicting reactions with subsequent administration of the medication. There are various reasons for this incongruity. Often, reaction histories are poorly characterized and very remote. Symptoms may simply have been a consequence of an underlying illness, such as a viral infection, or from an interaction between a penicillin antibiotic and an infectious agent. A well-characterized example of the latter is when actively infected patients with Epstein-Barr virus are treated with ampicillin and develop a morbilliform rash.[8] Another important contributor to the discrepancy is loss of penicillin sensitivity over time. Approximately 50% of penicillin-allergic patients lose their sensitivity over 5 years, and approximately 80% over 10 years.[9,10]

Based on the rate of positive penicillin skin tests, the prevalence of immediate reactions to penicillin antibiotics is decreasing over the past 2 decades.[11,12] Penicillin-induced anaphylaxis is relatively rare, with several studies suggesting a rate of approximately 0.01% to 0.04% of treated patients.[13,14] In the United States, it has been estimated that 500 to 1000 deaths per year are secondary to penicillin-induced anaphylaxis.[15]

Detriment of "Penicillin Allergy" Label

Physicians frequently choose alternative antibiotics for those labeled with "penicillin allergy."[16–22] Unfortunately, this is associated with increased antimicrobial resistance, increased *Clostridium difficile* infections, prolonged length of hospital stays, increased intensive care admissions, increased hospital readmissions, and increased mortality.[19,23–26] Beyond compromising one's health, there are significantly higher costs associated with the "penicillin allergy" label.[18–21,27] Recently, King and colleagues[27] calculated that an average of $297 per patient would be saved if patients switched from a non–beta-lactam antibiotic to a beta-lactam antibiotic. Macy and Contreras[19] reported "penicillin-allergic" patients stayed an extra 0.59 days longer than control patients, resulting in an estimated $64.6 million cost. Cost-analysis studies thus far focus on one patient encounter, but extrapolating these data to the lifetime of a patient with potential future intensive care admissions, hospital readmissions, and expensive second-line antibiotic prescriptions could result in an overwhelming financial burden for patients.

Immunochemistry

Penicillin, like most drugs, is generally too small to be immunogenic; therefore, the immune response is directed against complexes of penicillin degradation products covalently bound to self-proteins.[28–30] The allergic components of penicillin are derived from either the beta-lactam core ring structure or from a specific side chain R group (**Fig. 1**). The core beta-lactam ring structure is shared among all penicillin antibiotics, whereas the R-group side chains differentiate penicillin antibiotics from each other.

After penicillin administration, the beta-lactam ring opens spontaneously to form several breakdown products. The most prevalent of these is penicilloyl polylysine, or major allergenic determinant, which comprises 95% of the breakdown products.

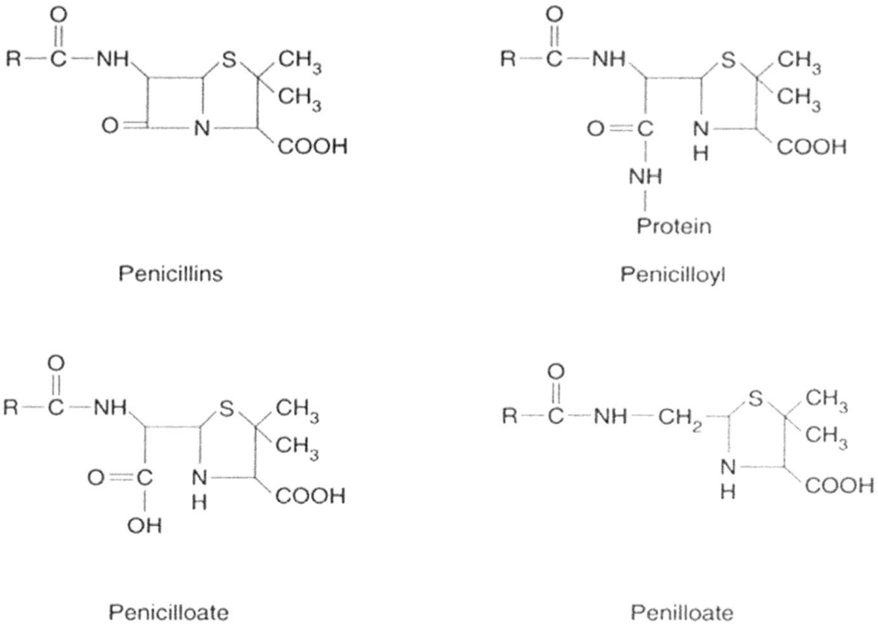

Penicillins

Penicilloyl

Penicilloate

Penilloate

Fig. 1. Structures of penicillin breakdown products. The 4-membered square-shaped ring is the beta-lactam ring, which opens up to form covalent bonds with self-proteins. The "R" represents the side chains which differentiate various penicillins. (*From* Solensky R. Drug hypersensitivity. Med Clin N Am 2006;90(1):238; with permission.)

Of the remaining minor allergenic determinants, penicilloate and penilloate are the most important. Some patients do not react to the core ring, but instead to the R-group side chain. For example, an individual may tolerate penicillin, but develop an allergic response to amoxicillin or ampicillin (eg, the aminopenicillins).[31–33] The prevalence of aminopenicillin-specific allergy is much lower in the United States (fewer than 5% of skin test–positive patients), compared with Southern Europe (25%–50% of skin test–positive patients).[34–37] Additionally, some patients react only to clavulanic acid, and not to other penicillin determinants. In other words, they tolerate amoxicillin but react to amoxicillin-clavulanate. The frequency of clavulanate-selective allergy is unclear due to limited data (all from Southern Europe).[38,39]

Penicillin Skin Test Reagents

Penicillin skin test reagents are based on the immunogenicity and include major and minor determinants. Penicilloyl polylysine (PPL) is the synthetically made major determinant, whereas penilloate, penicilloate, penicillin G, amoxicillin and ampicillin are grouped as minor determinants (**Table 1**). Sometimes the minor determinants are combined into a "minor determinant mixture" (MDM), and this consists of either penilloate and penicilloate, or penilloate, penicilloate, and penicillin G. PPL has been commercially available in the United States as Pre-Pen, but minor determinants have never been approved by the Food and Drug Administration. Some laboratories synthesize penicilloate and penilloate, whereas diluted penicillin G and ampicillin are used off-label for skin testing.

Table 1	
Penicillin skin test reagents	
Reagent	Concentration Used for Skin Testing
Penicilloyl-polylysine (Pre-Pen)	6×10^{-5} M
Penicillin G	10,000 units/mL
Penicilloate	0.01 M
Penilloate	0.01 M
Ampicillin/amoxicillin	3–25 mg/mL

Skin Testing Predictive Value

PPL is necessary for skin testing, as up to 84% of penicillin skin test–positive patients are positive to PPL, and up to 75% react to PPL only.[5,34,40–43] The positive predictive value (PPV) of PPL is unclear, given obvious patient safety and ethical concerns with challenging skin test–positive patients. However, limited retrospective data demonstrate that the PPV of penicillin skin testing is approximately 50% (with a range of 33%–100%).[32,40,42,44] The negative predictive value (NPV) of PPL ranges from 84% (in European studies) to 99%, with the theory that the variability is due to a higher prevalence of selectively allergic amoxicillin/ampicillin patients in Europe.[5,6,34,42,45–47]

With respect to minor determinants, approximately 10% of penicillin skin test–positive patients are positive to only penicilloate and/or penilloate.[11,34,35,48,49] Similar to PPL, there is a scarcity of literature regarding the PPV of penicilloate and/or penilloate.[29,50,51] As it is rare to skin test without PPL, the overall NPV of PPL and MDM (with all 3 reagents) is greater than 95%, which parallels that of PPL and penicillin G.[5,40,42,46,52–54] However, there is controversy regarding the accuracy of these NPVs, as selection bias and lack of standardized challenges may have effected results.[40,46,55] Regardless, many experts still favor penicilloate and penilloate as relevant skin testing reagents, and the Academy of Allergy, Asthma and Immunology supports the expedited approval by the Food and Drug Administration of a penicillin skin test kit that includes PPL, penicillin G, penilloate, penicilloate, and amoxicillin (Pre-Pen Plus).[56]

In Vitro Testing

In vitro tests using enzyme-linked immunosorbent assays to PPL, penicillin G, penicillin V, amoxicillin, and ampicillin are commercially available but are of limited value. Sensitivity of in vitro IgE antibodies is as low as 45% and studies with positive in vitro tests report a high number of false-positive results.[57,58] The basophil activation test, which uses flow cytometry, is another in vitro test that has been shown to be inferior to skin testing.[59,60]

Clinical Management

Role of history taking

As discussed earlier, most patients who claim they are allergic to penicillin can tolerate penicillin. Nevertheless, taking a detailed history is still critical for evaluation and management. Discounting reactions because they are vague may miss some truly allergic patients, because one-third of penicillin skin test–positive individuals have a vague reaction history.[61] When taking a history, the following questions are important to help guide management:

Are the symptoms consistent with a possible IgE-related mechanism? Did symptoms consist of pruritus, flushing, urticaria, angioedema, bronchospasm, laryngeal edema, nausea, emesis, or hypotension? If the answer is yes, the patient is a candidate for evaluation with an allergist for penicillin skin testing. The timing of the reaction (ie, soon after the last dose) is also suggestive of an IgE-mediated mechanism, but is often difficult to determine.

Are the symptoms consistent with a severe non–IgE-mediated mechanism? It is important to determine if the historical reaction had features of possible severe cutaneous adverse drug reaction, because strict avoidance of the culprit drug is required, and there is no role for skin testing or desensitization. These reactions include acute generalized exanthematous pustulosis, serum sickness–like reaction, Stevens-Johnson syndrome, toxic epidermal necrolysis, and drug rash with eosinophilia and systemic symptoms. Similarly, avoidance is the only option for other severe non–IgE-mediated reactions, such as immune cytopenias, drug fever, interstitial nephritis, and fixed drug eruption.

Is the reaction history unclear or not compatible with a possible allergy? Many times, patients are unable to provide useful details regarding their previous penicillin reactions, or, if they have experienced reactions due to more than 1 antibiotic, they may be unsure which antibiotic caused which type of reaction. Typically, in these cases, it is reasonable to pursue skin testing and challenge. If the reaction is incompatible with an allergy, such as isolated gastrointestinal symptoms or headache, then skin testing is not necessary and the patient may receive treatment with penicillins again.

When to evaluate

Penicillin allergy is ideally evaluated when the patient is well and not in need of antibiotic treatment. Because of the detrimental consequences resulting from a mislabeled penicillin allergy, all patients with a history of possible IgE-mediated penicillin allergy should be candidates for skin testing. Skin testing as a routine screen in the absence of clinical history is not recommended. Recent literature has shown via fine mapping genome-wise association studies and targeted genotyping that variants in HLA-DRA, HLA-DRB5, and interleukin-4 may be potential genetic predictors of penicillin allergy.[62,63] Regardless, patients who have never taken penicillin before but have a family history of penicillin allergy do not need evaluation and can safely take penicillins. Recently, the American Academy of Allergy Asthma & Immunology and others have urged more widespread use of drug allergy testing.[64,65]

Skin Testing

Penicillin skin testing is the most optimal method to evaluate for IgE-mediated penicillin allergy. When skin testing is executed properly, it is very safe; it has been studied in young children, pregnant women, emergency department patients, preoperative patients, and hospitalized critically ill patients. However, there is a rare risk of systemic reactions.[66,67] Therefore, skin testing should be performed only by trained personnel and in an environment capable of treating potential anaphylaxis.

Regarding the procedure itself, the first portion involves applying the skin test reagents along with positive (histamine) and negative (saline) controls via the prick technique. Measurements should be taken 15 minutes after placement. If the skin prick results are negative, intradermal testing should be performed with the same reagents and controls. Measurements should likewise be obtained 15 minutes after intradermal placement. If intradermal results are negative, the "penicillin allergy" label should be removed and patients should be educated about their tolerance to penicillins.

Challenge

In general, drug challenges should be performed when there is a low likelihood of a drug allergy, as the purpose is to confirm that a patient is not allergic and can tolerate the drug. Despite having a very high NPV, a survey by Warrington and colleagues[68] revealed that 52% of patients with negative penicillin skin tests still prefer to avoid penicillin, with some patients reporting that their family physicians thought it was safer to use an alternative antibiotic. For this reason, to unequivocally exclude the diagnosis of penicillin allergy, it has become standard of care to routinely perform a challenge immediately after a negative skin test.[7,53,69] Typically, the challenge is either a single dose or a 2-step graded challenge (one-tenth of full dose, followed 30–60 minutes later by the full dose). Amoxicillin is the preferable penicillin, because it has both the immunologically significant core beta-lactam ring and the potentially immunologically significant R-group side chain. If patients report reactions to amoxicillin-clavulanate, they should be challenged with that antibiotic, rather than amoxicillin.

Given the very low rate of positive penicillin skin tests, another recently studied approach is direct amoxicillin challenge without prior skin testing. Mill and colleagues[70] demonstrated that in 818 children with histories of cutaneous reactions to amoxicillin, a graded amoxicillin challenge was tolerated in 94%, with the remaining developing mild hives or a maculopapular rash. Of note, none of their patients had a history of anaphylaxis and most patients reported reactions during their first course of amoxicillin. Pending further research, this approach should be considered only in children with history of mild cutaneous reactions. Patients who fail challenges should either continue avoiding penicillin antibiotics or, if necessary, undergo desensitization.

Desensitization

Desensitization should be reserved for either those who have positive skin test results or are strongly suspected to have an IgE-mediated penicillin allergy, and for whom there are no alternative antibiotics available. Details will be further addressed in Sevim Bavbek and Min Jung Lee's article, "Subcutaneous Injectable Drugs Hypersensitivity and Desensitization: Insulin and Monoclonal Antibodies," in this issue.

Benefit of evaluation

There are significant benefits to an allergist's evaluation of penicillin allergy, namely the ability to remove a patient's "penicillin allergy" label. Most research up to this point has been pilot projects in hospital settings, where it is easier to track outcomes (such as transition to beta-lactam antibiotics and cost).[69,71–77] The most extensive penicillin skin-testing program is at the Mayo Clinic (Rochester, MN), where preoperative patients with a history of penicillin allergy routinely undergo penicillin skin testing. Because approximately 95% of the patients are skin test–negative, it allows surgeons to choose first-generation cephalosporins rather than vancomycin. In an effort to remove the "penicillin allergy" label on a more wide-scale level, some researchers have used clinical pharmacists along with allergists, both in inpatient and outpatient settings.[69,75] Despite recommendations to expand utilization of penicillin skin testing,[64,65] it is clear that there is a need for increased education.[78]

Remarkably, up to 49% of patients who are penicillin skin test–negative and 82% of those tolerant to penicillins may continue to be labeled as "penicillin-allergic."[78] Others are relabeled as allergic after having the label removed, with significant risk factors, including age older than 65 years ($P = .011$), acutely altered mentation ($P < .0001$), and dementia ($P < .0001$).[76] Interventions, such as detailed follow-up letters to primary care physicians succinctly listing antibiotic allergies, have decreased those not following recommendations from 26% to 15%.[79]

Resensitization

Resensitization is the redevelopment of penicillin allergy after initial resolution. Numerous studies have demonstrated that the rate of resensitization following treatment with oral penicillins is comparable to the rate of sensitization.[6,80,81] Therefore, the article by Solensky and colleagues,[82] Drug Allergy: An Updated Practice Parameter, does not recommend routine repeat penicillin skin testing in patients with a history of penicillin allergy who have tolerated 1 course or more of oral penicillins. Data on resensitization following parental penicillin are more limited; therefore, repeat penicillin skin testing may be considered in patients with a history of penicillin allergy who have tolerated parental penicillins.[82]

ALLERGIC CROSS-REACTIVITY BETWEEN PENICILLINS AND OTHER BETA-LACTAM ANTIBIOTICS
Penicillin/Cephalosporins

Penicillins and cephalosporins share a common beta-lactam ring and hence the potential for allergic cross-reactivity (**Fig. 2**). Additionally, some penicillins and cephalosporins share identical R-group side chains, and these are another source of potential allergic cross-reactivity (**Table 2**). There are 3 potential methods to evaluate cross-reactivity: (1) in vitro analysis, such as specific IgG, IgM, and IgE antibodies directed against penicillins and cephalosporins, (2) penicillin and cephalosporin skin testing,

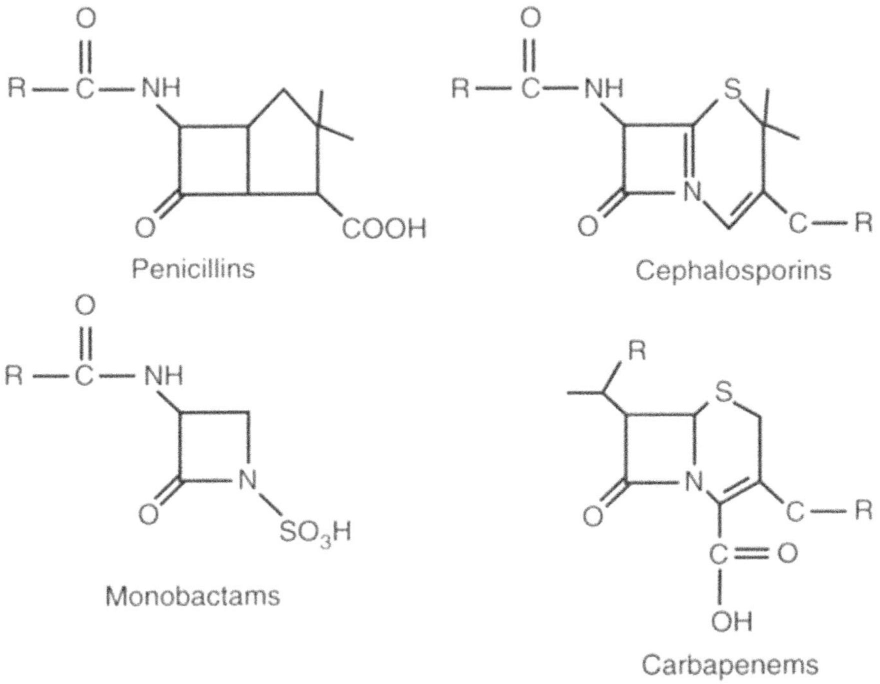

Fig. 2. Structures of beta-lactam antibiotics, which share a common beta-lactam ring (the 4-membered square-shaped ring). The "R" represents side chains; cephalosporins and carbapenems have 2, whereas monobactams have 1. (*From* Solensky R. Drug hypersensitivity. Med Clin N Am 2006;90(1):242; with permission.)

Table 2	
Aminopenicillins and cephalosporins with identical R/R1 group side chains	
Amoxicillin	**Ampicillin**
Cefadroxil	Cefaclor
Cefprozil	Cephalexin
Cefatrizine	Cephradine
	Cephaloglycin
	Loracarbef (a carbacephem)

and (3) cephalosporin challenges in patients with history of penicillin allergy (either with or without prior penicillin skin testing). Early studies using IgG and IgM antibodies and skin testing showed as much as 50% cross-reactivity between penicillin and first-generation cephalosporins,[83,84] but clinically, it became evident that cross-reactivity was much lower.

Several studies have evaluated patients with a history of penicillin allergy treated with cephalosporins (without preceding penicillin skin testing). As shown in **Table 3**, in the 1970s there appeared to be a fourfold to eightfold increased risk of cephalosporin reactions in patients with a history of penicillin allergy, compared with those without such a history.[85,86] However, very little detail was presented on the types of cephalosporin reactions observed. Also, before 1980, cephalosporins were contaminated with penicillin, meaning that exceptionally penicillin-allergic patients may have reacted to the penicillin within the cephalosporins rather than to the cephalosporin. Another limitation is that 90% or more of the subjects were probably not allergic to penicillins at time of cephalosporin treatment. Because these studies were retrospective in "real-world" settings, there was likely a selection bias in deciding which patients received cephalosporins versus other classes of antibiotics, meaning patients with more severe or recent penicillin reactions may have been less likely to be treated with cephalosporins. For example, in Daulat and colleagues,[87] inpatient pharmacists regularly denied cephalosporin prescription due to the severity of patients' penicillin allergy history (such as anaphylaxis). Furthermore, cephalosporin challenges were not blinded or placebo-controlled. Additionally, there was no attempt to include active controls, such as patients with a history of allergy to non–beta-lactam antibiotic treated with cephalosporins, or reaction rate of patients with history of penicillin allergy to non–beta-lactams. This is important because it is known that patients with a history of allergy to drugs are more likely to react to structurally unrelated drugs,[88,89] referred to as "multiple drug allergy syndrome."

Studies in which patients with a history of penicillin allergy were proven to be penicillin skin test–positive before cephalosporin challenge are most informative. Overall, as shown in **Table 4**, only approximately 3% of penicillin skin test–positive patients reacted to cephalosporins. Some investigators performed cephalosporin skin testing (using nonirritating concentrations) before challenging with cephalosporins, and that approach decreased the reaction rate to 0%. Some of the limitations discussed previously still apply, such as contamination of cephalosporins with penicillin (before 1980), lack of blinding, lack of inclusion of placebo or other controls, and "multiple drug allergy syndrome."

Patients who are selectively allergic to aminopenicillins (tolerant of penicillin VK) appear to have a higher risk of reacting to cephalosporins with identical R1 group side chains, but this conclusion is based on limited data.[90–92] Audicana and colleagues[90] challenged 10 patients selectively allergic to ampicillin with cephalexin (which has an identical R1 group side chain) and 1 (10%) reacted. Similarly, Sastre

Table 3
Cephalosporin challenges in patients with history of penicillin allergy (without prior penicillin skin testing)

Study	Cephalosporin Reaction Rate		Cephalosporins Administered	Type of Reaction
	History of Penicillin Allergy	No History of Penicillin Allergy		
Dash,[85] 1975	25/324 (7.7%)	140/17,216 (0.8%)	Cephalexin and cephaloridine	No details
Petz,[86] 1978	57/701 (8.1%)	285/15,007 (1.9%)	Cephalexin, cephaloridine, cephalothin, cefazolin,	No details
Goodman et al,[112] 2001	1/300 (0.3%)	1/2431 (0.04%)	Cefazolin (all but 1 patient)	Reaction questionable
Daulat et al,[87] 2004	1/606 (0.17%)	15/22,664 (0.07%)	1st generation (42%) 2nd generation (21%) 3rd generation (37%)	Eczema (cefazolin)
Fonacier et al,[113] 2006	7/83 (8.4%)	Not applicable	1st generation (59%) 2nd generation (8.4%) 3rd generation (25%) 4th generation (7%)	Reactions convincing: cephalexin-1, cefaclor-2, cefuroxime-2, cefixime-1, ceftriaxone-1
MacPherson et al,[114] 2006	0/84	Not applicable	Cefazolin, cefotetan, ceftriaxone	
Crotty et al,[115] 2015	7/186 (3.8%)	Not applicable	Cephalexin, cefoxitin, ceftriaxone, cefepime	6/7 cefepime; 3/7 immediate
Beltran et al,[116] 2015	1/153 (0.7%)	Not applicable	Cefazolin (84%) cefoxitin (17%)	Urticaria (cefazolin)

Table 4
Cephalosporin challenges in patients with history of penicillin allergy and positive penicillin skin testing

Study	No. of Patients	No. of Reactions (%)	Cephalosporin Skin Testing	Reaction(s) to
Girard,[117] 1968	23	2 (8.7)	No	Cephaloridine
Assem and Vickers,[84] 1974	3	3 (100)	No	Cephaloridine
Warrington et al,[118] 1978	3	0	Yes	
Solley et al,[32] 1982	27	0	No	
Saxon et al,[119] 1987	62	1 (1.6)	No	Not noted
Blanca et al,[120] 1989	16	2 (12.5)	No	Cefamandole
Shepherd and Burton,[121] 1993	9	0	No	
Audicana et al,[90] 1994	12		Yes	
Pichichero and Pichichero,[122] 1998	39	2 (5.1)	No	Cefaclor (other cephalosporin not indicated)
Novalbos et al,[123] 2001	23	0	Yes	
Macy and Burchette,[48] 2002	42	1 (2.4)	No	Cefixime
Romano et al,[124] 2004	75	0	Yes	
Greenberger and Klemens,[125] 2005	6	0	No	
Park et al,[3] 2010	85	2 (2.4)	No	Cefazolin and cephalexin
Ahmed et al,[126] 2012	21	0	No	
TOTAL	446	13 (2.9)		

and colleagues[92] and Miranda and colleagues[91] collectively challenged 37 patients selectively allergic to amoxicillin with cefadroxil and 10 (27%) reacted.

Based a comprehensive review of the published literature and consensus opinion, The American Academy of Allergy, Asthma and Immunology Cephalosporin Administration to Patients with a History of Penicillin Allergy Workgroup Report made the following recommendations.[93] The use of penicillin skin testing was encouraged, because by virtue of ruling out penicillin allergy in the vast majority of patients, it greatly simplifies the approach to treatment of cephalosporins. Namely, penicillin skin test–negative patients may receive any beta-lactams safely without increased risk of allergic reactions. If penicillin skin testing is positive, then cephalosporins should be given via graded challenge or desensitization, but given that the risk of reaction is only approximately 3%, graded challenge is preferred. If penicillin skin testing is unavailable and patients with history of "severe" penicillin allergy are excluded, then cephalosporins may be given via full dose or graded challenge, depending on the reaction history, stability of the patient, and route of administration. There is no uniform definition for what constitutes a "severe" penicillin allergy, but exclusion of these patients was a common theme in **Table 3** studies, and hence the basis for the Workgroup Report recommendation. For patients believed to be selectively allergic to aminopenicillins, cephalosporins with identical R1 group side chains should be avoided (cefadroxil, cefprozil, and cefatrizine for amoxicillin; cephalexin, cefaclor, cephradine, and cephaloglycin for ampicillin). However, these patients may receive other cephalosporins via full dose or graded challenge, as outlined previously. Last, cephalosporin skin test may be considered to further reduce the risk of reaction, but this is not standardized and only possible with intravenous (IV) cephalosporins, not oral ones. The article by Solensky and colleagues,[82] Drug Allergy: An Updated Practice Parameter, made similar recommendations regarding cephalosporin administration to patients with a history of penicillin allergy.

A novel approach to decrease overuse of broad-spectrum antibiotics in hospitalized patients with a history of penicillin allergy, targeting nonallergist inpatient providers, has been implemented in several hospitals in Boston.[94,95] After educational intervention, a drug allergy history–based clinical guideline was developed specifically for use by general inpatient providers. Depending on type of penicillin reaction history, the treatment algorithm allowed cephalosporin treatment either via graded challenge or full dose. This novel strategy does not require specialty consultation services or training to perform penicillin skin testing. Studies of this approach have shown that it results in increased use of beta-lactams instead of broad-spectrum antibiotics such as vancomycin and quinolones.[94,95]

Penicillins/Carbapenems

The data on allergic cross-reactivity between penicillins and carbapenems mirrors the discussion on penicillin/cephalosporin cross-reactivity. **Table 5** summarizes published studies in which patients with a history of penicillin allergy were challenged with carbapenems (without preceding penicillin skin testing), and they showed an increased rate of reactions. The studies are subject to several confounding factors including lack of confirmation of penicillin allergy, lack of placebo and other controls, probable selection bias in avoiding carbapenems in patients with more severe or recent penicillin allergy histories, and "multiple drug allergy syndrome." Studies in which patients were proven to be penicillin-allergic before being challenged with carbapenems are superior in design. **Table 6** summarizes studies in which penicillin skin test–positive patients were challenged with carbapenems, and remarkably the reaction rate was 0%. Moreover, all the patients underwent carbapenem skin testing, but only 1% were positive (and therefore were not challenged with carbapenems). The PPV of carbapenem skin testing is uncertain, meaning that at least 99% of penicillin-allergic patients tolerate carbapenems. Solensky and colleagues[82] recommend that penicillin skin test–positive patients and patients with a history of penicillin allergy who do not undergo skin testing receive carbapenems via graded challenge.

Penicillins/Monobactams

Aztreonam is the only monobactam and the only beta-lactam antibiotic that contains a monocyclic ring structure, in contrast to the bicyclic core of other beta-lactams.

Table 5
Carbapenem in patients with history of penicillin allergy (without prior penicillin skin testing)

	Carbapenem Reaction Rate		
Study	History of Penicillin Allergy	No History of Penicillin Allergy	P
McConnell SA,[127] 2000	4/63 (6.3%)	N/A	N/A
Prescott et al,[128] 2004	11/100 (11%)	3/111 (2.7%)	.024
Sodhi et al,[129] 2004	15/163 (9.2%)	4/103 (0.04%)	.164
Cunha et al,[130] 2008	0/110	N/A	N/A
Crotty et al,[115] 2015	3/56 (5%)	N/A	N/A

Abbreviation: N/A, not indicated.

Table 6
Carbapenem challenges in patients with history of penicillin allergy and positive penicillin skin testing

Study	No. of Patients	No. of Reactions (%)	Carbapenem Given	Comments
Romano et al,[131] 2006	110	0	Imipenem	1 patient imipenem skin test–positive
Romano et al,[132] 2007	103	0	Meropenem	1 patient meropenem skin test–positive
Atanaskovic et al,[133] 2008	107	0	Meropenem	1 patient meropenem skin test–positive
Atanaskovic et al,[134] 2009	123	0	Imipenem	1 patient imipenem skin test–positive
Gaeta et al,[135] 2015	211	0	Imipenem Meropenem Ertapenem	No patients carbapenem skin test–positive Patients challenged with all 3 carbapenems
TOTAL	654	0		

All patients also underwent skin testing with carbapenems and only those who were skin test–negative were challenged.

In vitro studies demonstrated virtually no immunologic cross-reactivity between penicillins and aztreonam.[96–99] Likewise, skin testing and challenge studies revealed no evidence of allergic cross-reactivity between penicillins and aztreonam, including no positive aztreonam challenges in penicillin skin test–positive patients.[96,98,100,101] Therefore, patients with history of penicillin allergy may receive aztreonam in usual fashion, without special precautions. The only beta-lactam that shows cross-reactivity with aztreonam is ceftazidime, and these 2 antibiotics share an identical R-group side chain.

ALLERGY TO CEPHALOSPORINS

Allergic reactions to cephalosporins are not as common as those to penicillins. The incidence of beta-lactam–related cutaneous reactions (mostly maculopapular eruptions and urticaria) in a large inpatient prospective trial was 5.1% of exposed patients (amoxicillin), 4.5% (ampicillin), 1.6% (penicillin G), and 1.5% (cephalosporins).[102,103] It is not known how many were due to drug-specific IgE antibodies. Limited data suggest that the incidence of anaphylaxis due to cephalosporins is approximately 1 order of magnitude lower than penicillins.[104]

The lack of standardized validated skin testing makes evaluation of possible cephalosporin-induced IgE-mediated allergy more difficult than penicillin allergy. Skin testing (prick/puncture followed by intradermal, analogous to penicillin skin testing) with nonirritating concentrations of native cephalosporins can be of some value, but its predictive value is unknown. A positive skin test using a nonirritating concentration is suggestive of IgE-mediated allergy, but a negative result does not necessarily rule out sensitivity. Also, intradermal skin testing is usually limited to IV cephalosporins, not with cephalosporins available only in oral forms. Several studies have investigated nonirritating skin test concentrations of cephalosporins in healthy nonallergic control subjects. Empedrad and colleagues[105] found cefuroxime, cefotaxime, ceftriaxone, and ceftazidime to be nonirritating at 10 mg/mL, whereas cefazolin was nonirritating at 33 mg/mL. Similarly, Testi and colleagues[106] reported the same 5 cephalosporins to be nonirritating at 20 mg/mL, whereas cefepime was irritating at 20 mg/mL. Romano and colleagues[107] showed cephalexin, cefaclor, cefadroxil, cefazolin, and ceftibuten to be nonirritating at 20 mg/mL, whereas other cephalosporins (cefamandole, cefuroxime, ceftazidime, ceftriaxone, cefotaxime, cefepime, cefoperazone, cefodizime) were nonirritating at 2 mg/mL.

When evaluating allergies to cephalosporins, a common dilemma is whether patients who have reacted to one cephalosporin are able to tolerate other cephalosporins. The immune response in IgE-mediated allergy to cephalosporins is likely directed mostly at the R1 or R2 group side chains, implying that patients allergic to some cephalosporins can tolerate cephalosporins with dissimilar side chains. However, the evidence for this is limited to largely single-patient case reports and small case series,[108–111] and one recently published larger case series.[107] In the largest case series, Romano and colleagues[107] studied 102 patients with recent convincing immediate-type allergic reactions to cephalosporins. A total of 83% of the patients reported anaphylaxis (including hypotension in two-thirds and loss of consciousness in three-eighths) and 9% urticaria. All the patients underwent skin testing with at least 11 different cephalosporins (including the culprit cephalosporins), and based on the skin test responses, were categorized into 4 groups. Group A comprised 73 patients and included patients who had historical reactions to and were skin test–positive to ceftriaxone or other cephalosporins with identical/similar R1 group side chains (cefotaxime, cefuroxime, cefepime, ceftazidime, and cefodizime). Thirteen patients in group B reported historical reactions and were skin test–positive to so called amino-cephalosporins (cephalosporins that contain R1 group side chains identical to amoxicillin or ampicillin: cephalexin, cefaclor, and cefadroxil). Group C contained 7 patients and the following cephalosporins with similar R1 group side chains: cefazolin, cefamandole, cefoperazone, and ceftibutin. Group D (9 patients) showed skin test positivity to cephalosporins from more than 1 group, which suggests the immune response was directed at cross-reacting core determinants, rather than side chains. Graded challenges were performed with selected (not all) cephalosporins to which skin tests were negative, and none of the patients reacted. Notably, patients were not challenged with cephalosporins with similar R-group side chains as the culprit cephalosporin, even if skin testing to those cephalosporins was negative. To summarize, approximately 90% of patients were found to have IgE-mediated allergies to cephalosporins directed at R-group side chains, whereas 10% showed positivity to various cephalosporins with dissimilar side chains.

Based on the available evidence, the approach to patients with history of cephalosporin reactions that could be IgE-mediated, and who require treatment with other cephalosporins, is 2-step to 3-step graded challenge with a cephalosporin with dissimilar side chains. If possible, a negative skin test using a nonirritating concentration of the cephalosporin to be administered may provide additional evidence of lack of allergy. A positive skin test should be assumed to indicate IgE-mediated allergy and the patient should avoid that cephalosporin (and similar ones), or receive it via rapid desensitization if there are no alternate treatment options.

REFERENCES

1. Rawlins MD, Thompson W. Mechanisms of adverse drug reactions. In: Davies DM, editor. Textbook of adverse drug reactions. New York: Oxford University Press; 1991. p. 18–45.

2. Macy E, Poon K. Self-reported antibiotic allergy incidence and prevalence: age and sex effects. Am J Med 2009;122:778.e1-7.

3. Park MA, Markus PJ, Matesic D, et al. Safety and effectiveness of a preoperative allergy clinic in decreasing vancomycin use in patients with a history of penicillin allergy. Ann Allergy Asthma Immunol 2006;97:681–7.

4. Abrams EM, Wakeman A, Gerstner TV, et al. Prevalence of beta-lactam allergy: a retrospective chart review of drug allergy assessment in a predominantly pediatric population. Allergy Asthma Clin Immunol 2016;12:59.

5. Gadde J, Spence M, Wheeler B, et al. Clinical experience with penicillin skin testing in a large inner-city STD clinic. JAMA 1993;270:2456–63.

6. Mendelson LM, Ressler C, Rosen JP, et al. Routine elective penicillin allergy skin testing in children and adolescents: study of sensitization. J Allergy Clin Immunol 1984;73:76–81.

7. Meng J, Thursfield D, Lukawska JJ. Allergy test outcomes in patients self-reported as having penicillin allergy: two-year experience. Ann Allergy Asthma Immunol 2016;117(3):273–9.

8. Patel BM. Skin rash with infectious mononucleosis and ampicillin. Pediatrics 1967;40:910–1.

9. Blanca M, Torres MJ, Garcia JJ, et al. Natural evolution of skin test sensitivity in patients allergic to beta-lactam antibiotics. J Allergy Clin Immunol 1999;103: 918–24.

10. Sullivan TJ, Wedner HJ, Shatz GS, et al. Skin testing to detect penicillin allergy. J Allergy Clin Immunol 1981;68:171–80.

11. Jost BC, Wedner HJ, Bloomberg GR. Elective penicillin skin testing in a pediatric outpatient setting. Ann Allergy Asthma Immunol 2006;97:807–12.

12. Macy E, Schatz M, Lin CK, et al. The falling rate of positive penicillin skin tests from 1995 to 2007. Perm J 2009;13:12–8.

13. Idsoe O, Guthe T, Willcox RR, et al. Nature and extent of penicillin side-reactions, with particular reference to fatalities from anaphylactic shock. Bull World Health Organ 1968;38:159–88.

14. Napoli DC, Neeno TA. Anaphylaxis to benzathine penicillin G. Pediatr Asthma Allergy Immunol 2000;14:329–32.

15. Neugut AI, Ghatak AT, Miller RL. Anaphylaxis in the United States. An investigation into its epidemiology. Arch Intern Med 2001;161:15–21.

16. Kwan T, Lin F, Ngai B, et al. Vancomycin use in 2 Ontario tertiary care hospitals: a survey. Clin Invest Med 1999;22:256–64.

17. Lee CE, Zembower TR, Fotis MA, et al. The incidence of antimicrobial allergies in hospitalized patients: implications regarding prescribing patterns and emerging bacterial resistance. Arch Intern Med 2000;160:2819–22.

18. MacLaughlin EJ, Saseen JJ, Malone DC. Costs of beta-lactam allergies: selection and costs of antibiotics for patients with a reported beta-lactam allergy. Arch Fam Med 2000;9:722–6.

19. Macy E, Contreras R. Healthcare utilization and serious infection prevalence associated with penicillin "allergy" in hospitalized patients: a cohort study. J Allergy Clin Immunol 2014;133:790–6.

20. Picard M, Begin P, Bouchard H, et al. Treatment of patients with a history of penicillin allergy in a large tertiary-care academic hospital. J Allergy Clin Immunol Pract 2013;1(3):252–7.

21. Sade K, Holtzer I, Levo Y, et al. The economic burden of antibiotic treatment of penicillin-allergic patients in internal medicine wards of a general tertiary care hospital. Clin Exp Allergy 2003;33:501–6.

22. Solensky R, Earl HS, Gruchalla RS. Clinical approach to penicillin allergic patients: a survey. Ann Allergy Asthma Immunol 2000;84:329–33.

23. Charneski L, Deshpande G, Smith SW. Impact of an antimicrobial allergy label in the medical record on clinical outcomes in hospitalized patients. Pharmacotherapy 2011;31(8):742–7.

24. MacFadden DR, LaDelfa A, Leen J, et al. Impact of reported beta-lactam allergy on inpatient outcomes: a multicenter prospective cohort study. Clin Infect Dis 2016;63(7):904–10.

25. Martinez JA, Ruthazer R, Hansjosten K, et al. Role of environmental contamination as a risk factor for acquisition of vancomycin-resistant enterococci in patients treated in a medical intensive care unit. Arch Intern Med 2003;163: 1905–12.

26. Weiss K. *Clostridium difficile* and fluoroquinolones: is there a link. Int J Antimicrob Agents 2009;33(Suppl 1):S29–32.

27. King EA, Challa S, Curtin P, et al. Penicillin skin testing in hospitalized patients with beta-lactam allergies: effect on antibiotic selection and cost. Ann Allergy Asthma Immunol 2016;117(1):67–71.

28. Levine BB, Ovary Z. Studies on the mechanism of the formation of the penicillin antigen. III. The N-(D-alpha-benzyl-penicilloyl) group as an antigenic determinant responsible for hypersensitivity to penicillin G. J Exp Med 1961;114: 875–904.

29. Levine BB, Redmond AP. Minor haptenic determinant-specific reagins of penicillin hypersensitivity in man. Int Arch Allergy Appl Immunol 1969;35:445–55.

30. Parker CW, Shapiro J, Kern M, et al. Hypersensitivity to penicillenic acid derivatives in human beings with penicillin allergy. J Exp Med 1962;115:821–38.

31. Blanca M, Perez E, Garcia J, et al. Anaphylaxis to amoxycillin but good tolerance for benzyl penicillin. In vivo and in vitro studies of specific IgE antibodies. Allergy 1988;43:508–10.

32. Solley GO, Gleich GJ, Dellen RGV. Penicillin allergy: clinical experience with a battery of skin-test reagents. J Allergy Clin Immunol 1982;69:238–44.

33. Vega JM, Blanca M, Garcia JJ, et al. Immediate allergic reactions to amoxicillin. Allergy 1994;49:317–22.

34. Bousquet PJ, Co-Minh HB, Arnoux B, et al. Importance of mixture of minor determinants and benzylpenicilloyl poly-L-lysine skin testing in the diagnosis of beta-lactam allergy. J Allergy Clin Immunol 2005;115:1314–6.

35. Matheu V, Perez E, Gonzalez R, et al. Assessment of a new brand of determinants for skin testing in a large group of patients with suspected beta-lactam allergy. J Investig Allergol Clin Immunol 2007;17:257–60.

36. Romano A, Bousquet-Rouanet L, Viola M, et al. Benzylpenicillin skin testing is still important in diagnosing immediate hypersensitivity reactions to penicillins. Allergy 2009;64:249–53.

37. Torres MJ, Romano A, Mayorga C, et al. Diagnostic evaluation of a large group of patients with immediate allergy to penicillins: the role of skin testing. Allergy 2001;56:850–6.

38. Fernandez-Rivas M, Perez Carral C, Cuevas M, et al. Selective allergic reactions to clavulanic acid. J Allergy Clin Immunol 1995;95(3):748–50.

39. Torres MJ, Ariza A, Mayorga C, et al. Clavulanic acid can be the component in amoxicillin-clavulanic acid responsible for immediate hypersensitivity reactions. J Allergy Clin Immunol 2010;125(2):502–5.e502.

40. Green GR, Rosenblum AH, Sweet LC. Evaluation of penicillin hypersensitivity: value of clinical history and skin testing with penicilloyl-polylysine and penicillin G. J Allergy Clin Immunol 1977;60:339–45.

41. Macy E, Richter PK, Falkoff R, et al. Skin testing with penicilloate and penilloate prepared by an improved method: amoxicillin oral challenge in patients with negative skin test responses to penicillin reagents. J Allergy Clin Immunol 1997;100:586–91.

42. Sogn DD, Evans R, Shepherd GM, et al. Results of the National Institute of Allergy and Infectious Diseases collaborative clinical trial to test the predictive value of skin testing with major and minor penicillin derivatives in hospitalized adults. Arch Intern Med 1992;152:1025–32.

43. Van Dellen RG, Walsh WE, Peters GA, et al. Differing patterns of wheal and flare skin reactivity in patients allergic to the penicillins. J Allergy 1971;47(4):230–6.

44. Adkinson NF, Thompson WL, Maddrey WC, et al. Routine use of penicillin skin testing on an inpatient service. N Engl J Med 1971;46:457–60.

45. Bousquet PJ, Pipet A, Bousquet-Rouanet L, et al. Oral challenges are needed in the diagnosis of beta-lactam hypersensitivity. Clin Exp Allergy 2008;38:185–90.

46. del Real GA, Rose ME, Ramirez-Atamoros MT, et al. Penicillin skin testing in patients with a history of beta-lactam allergy. Ann Allergy Asthma Immunol 2007; 98:355–9.

47. Matheu V, Perez-Rodriguez E, Sanchez-Machin I, et al. Major and minor determinants are high-performance skin tests in beta-lactam allergy diagnosis. J Allergy Clin Immunol 2005;116:1167–8.

48. Macy E, Burchette R. Oral antibiotic adverse reactions after penicillin skin testing: multi-year follow-up. Allergy 2002;57:1151–8.

49. Park M, Matesic D, Markus PJ, et al. Female sex as a risk factor for penicillin allergy. Ann Allergy Asthma Immunol 2007;99:54–8.

50. Levine BB, Zolov DM. Prediction of penicillin allergy by immunological tests. J Allergy 1969;43:231–44.

51. Macy E, Ho N. Adverse reactions associated with therapeutic antibiotic use after penicillin skin testing. Perm J 2011;15:31–7.

52. Fox S, Park M. Penicillin allergy testing is a safe and effective tool for evaluating penicillin allergy in the pediatric population. J Allergy Clin Immunol Pract 2014; 2:439–44.

53. Macy E, Mangat R, Burchette RJ. Penicillin skin testing in advance of need: multiyear follow-up in 568 test result-negative subjects exposed to oral penicillins. J Allergy Clin Immunol 2003;111:1111–5.

54. Macy E, Ngor EW. Safely diagnosing clinically significant penicillin allergy using only penicilloyl-polylysine, penicillin, and oral amoxicillin. J Allergy Clin Immunol Pract 2013;1:258–63.

55. Solensky R, Macy E. Minor determinants are essential for optimal penicillin allergy testing: a pro/con debate. J Allergy Clin Immunol Pract 2015;3:883–7.

56. Park MA, Solensky R, Khan DA, et al. Patients with positive skin test results to penicillin should not undergo penicillin or amoxicillin challenge. J Allergy Clin Immunol 2015;135:816–7.

57. Johansson SG, Adedoyin J, van Hage M, et al. False-positive penicillin immunoassay: an unnoticed common problem. J Allergy Clin Immunol 2013;132(1): 235–7.

58. Macy E, Goldberg B, Poon K. Use of commercial anti–penicillin IgE fluorometric enzyme immunoassays to diagnose penicillin allergy. Ann Allergy Asthma Immunol 2010;105:136–41.

59. Sanz ML, Gamboa PM, Antepara I, et al. Flow cytometric basophil activation test by detection of CD63 expression in patients with immediate-type reactions to betalactam antibiotics. Clin Exp Allergy 2002;32:277–86.
60. Torres MJ, Padial A, Mayorga C, et al. The diagnostic interpretation of basophil activation test in immediate allergic reactions to betalactams. Clin Exp Allergy 2004;34:1768–75.
61. Solensky R, Earl HS, Gruchalla RS. Penicillin allergy: prevalence of vague history in skin test-positive patients. Ann Allergy Asthma Immunol 2000;85:195–9.
62. Apter AJ, Schelleman H, Walker A, et al. Clinical and genetic risk factors of self-reported penicillin allergy. J Allergy Clin Immunol 2008;122:152–8.
63. Guéant JL, Romano A, Cornejo-Garcia JA, et al. HLA-DRA variants predict penicillin allergy in genome-wide fine-mapping genotyping. J Allergy Clin Immunol 2015;135:253–9.
64. Barlam TF, Cosgrove SE, Abbo LM, et al. Implementing an antibiotic stewardship program: guidelines by the Iinfectious Diseases Society of America and the Society for Healthcare Epidemiology of America. Clin Infect Dis 2016; 62(10):e51–77.
65. ChoosingWisely. Available at: http://www.choosingwisely.org/clinician-lists/american-academy-allergy-asthma-immunlogy-non-beta-lactam-antibiotics-penicillin-allergy/. Accessed April 1, 2017.
66. Co Minh HB, Bousquet PJ, Fontaine C, et al. Systemic reactions during skin tests with beta-lactams: a risk factor analysis. J Allergy Clin Immunol 2006; 117(2):466–8.
67. Valyasevi MA, VanDellen RG. Frequency of systematic reactions to penicillin skin tests. Ann Allergy Asthma Immunol 2000;85:363–5.
68. Warrington RJ, Burton R, Tsai E. The value of routine penicillin allergy skin testing in an outpatient population. Allergy Asthma Proc 2003;24:199–202.
69. Chen J, Tarver S, Alvarez K, et al. A proactive approach to penicillin allergy testing in hospitalized patients. J Allergy Clin Immunol Pract 2017;5(3):686–93.
70. Mill C, Primeau MN, Medoff E, et al. Assessing the diagnostic properties of a graded oral provocation challenge for the diagnosis of immediate and nonimmediate reactions to amoxicillin in children. JAMA Pediatr 2016;170(6):e160033.
71. Arroliga ME, Radojicic C, Gordon SM, et al. A prospective observational study of the effect of penicillin skin testing on antibiotic use in the intensive care unit. Infect Control Hosp Epidemiol 2003;24:347–50.
72. Frigas E, Park MA, Narr BJ, et al. Preoperative evaluation of patients with history of allergy to penicillin: comparison of 2 models of practice. Mayo Clin Proc 2008; 83(6):651–62.
73. Li JT, Markus PJ, Osmon DR, et al. Reduction of vancomycin use in orthopedic patients with a history of antibiotic allergy. Mayo Clin Proc 2000;75:902–6.
74. Nadarajah K, Green GR, Naglak M. Clinical outcomes of penicillin skin testing. Ann Allergy Asthma Immunol 2005;95:541–5.
75. Park MA, McClimon BJ, Ferguson B, et al. Collaboration between allergists and pharmacists increases beta-lactam antibiotic prescriptions in patients with a history of penicillin allergy. Int Arch Allergy Immunol 2011;15:57–62.
76. Rimawi RH, Shah KB, Cook PP. Risk of redocumenting penicillin allergy in a cohort of patients with negative penicillin skin tests. J Hosp Med 2013;8(11): 615–8.
77. Warrington RJ, Lee KR, McPhillips S. The value of skin testing for penicillin allergy in an inpatient population: analysis of the subsequent patient management. Allergy Asthma Proc 2000;21:297–9.

78. Blumenthal KG, Shenoy ES, Hurwitz S, et al. Effect of a drug allergy educational program and antibiotic prescribing guideline on inpatient clinical providers' antibiotic prescribing knowledge. J Allergy Clin Immunol Pract 2014;2(4):407–13.

79. Bourke J, Pavlos R, James I, et al. Improving the effectiveness of penicillin allergy de-labeling. J Allergy Clin Immunol Pract 2015;3(3):365–74.e1.

80. Hershkovich J, Broides A, Kirjner L, et al. Beta lactam allergy and resensitization in children with suspected beta lactam allergy. Clin Exp Allergy 2009;39:726–30.

81. Solensky R, Earl HS, Gruchalla RS. Lack of penicillin resensitization in patients with a history of penicillin allergy after receiving repeated penicillin courses. Arch Intern Med 2002;162:822–6.

82. Solensky R, Khan DA, Bernstein IL, et al. Drug allergy: an updated practice parameter. Ann Allergy Asthma Immunol 2010;105:259–73.e278.

83. Abraham GN, Petz LD, Fudenberg HH. Immunohaematological cross-allergenicity between penicillin and cephalothin in humans. Clin Exp Immunol 1968;3:343–57.

84. Assem ESK, Vickers MR. Tests for penicillin allergy in man II. The immunological cross-reaction between penicillins and cephalosporins. Immunology 1974;27: 255–69.

85. Dash CH. Penicillin allergy and the cephalosporins. J Antimicrob Chemother 1975;1(Suppl):107–18.

86. Petz LD. Immunologic cross-reactivity between penicillins and cephalosporins: a review. J Infect Dis 1978;137(Suppl):S74–9.

87. Daulat SB, Solensky R, Earl HS, et al. Safety of cephalosporin administration to patients with histories of penicillin allergy. J Allergy Clin Immunol 2004;113: 1220–2.

88. Apter AJ, Kinman JL, Bilker WB, et al. Is there cross-reactivity between penicillins and cephalosporins? Am J Med 2006;119:354.e11-20.

89. Strom BL, Schinnar R, Apter AJ, et al. Absence of cross-reactivity between sulfonamide antibiotics and sulfonamide nonantibiotics. N Engl J Med 2003;349: 1628–35.

90. Audicana M, Bernaola G, Urrutia I, et al. Allergic reactions to betalactams: studies in a group of patients allergic to penicillin and evaluation of cross-reactivity with cephalosporin. Allergy 1994;49:108–13.

91. Miranda A, Blanca M, Vega JM, et al. Cross-reactivity between a penicillin and a cephalosporin with the same side chain. J Allergy Clin Immunol 1996;98:671–7.

92. Sastre J, Quijano LD, Novalbos A, et al. Clinical cross-reactivity between amoxicillin and cephadroxil in patients allergic to amoxicillin and with good tolerance of penicillin. Allergy 1996;51:383–6.

93. AAAAI Workgroup Report. Available at: http://www.aaaai.org/Aaaai/media/Media Library/PDF%20Documents/Practice%20and%20Parameters/Cephalosporin-administration-2009.pdf. Accessed April 1, 2017.

94. Blumenthal K, Shenoy E, Varughese C, et al. Impact of a clinical guideline for prescribing antibiotics to inpatients reporting penicillin or cephalosporin allergy. Ann Allergy Asthma Immunol 2015;115:294–300.

95. Blumenthal KG, Shenoy ES, Wolfson AR, et al. Addressing inpatient beta-lactam allergies: a multihospital implementation. J Allergy Clin Immunol Pract 2017;5: 616–25.

96. Adkinson NF. Immunogenicity and cross-allergenicity of aztreonam. Am J Med 1990;88(Suppl 3C):S3–14.

97. Adkinson NF, Swabb EA, Sugerman AA. Immunology of the monobactam aztreonam. Antimicrob Agents Chemother 1984;25:93–7.

98. Saxon A, Hassner A, Swabb EA, et al. Lack of cross-reactivity between aztreonam, a monobactam antibiotic, and penicillin in penicillin-allergic subjects. J Infect Dis 1984;149:16–22.

99. Saxon A, Swabb EA, Adkinson NF. Investigation into the immunologic cross-reactivity of aztreonam with other beta-lactam antibiotics. Am J Med 1985; 78(Suppl 2A):19–26.

100. Graninger W, Pirich K, Schindler I, et al. Aztreonam efficacy in difficult-to-treat infections and tolerance in patients with betalactam hypersensitivity. Chemioterapia 1985;4(Suppl 1):64–6.

101. Vega JM, Blanca M, Garcia JJ, et al. Tolerance to aztreonam in patients allergic to betalactam antibiotics. Allergy 1991;46:196–202.

102. Arndt KA, Jick H. Rates of cutaneous reactions to drugs: a report from the Boston Collaborative Drug Surveillance Program. JAMA 1976;235:918–22.

103. Bigby M, Jick S, Jick H, et al. Drug-induced cutaneous reactions. A report from the Boston Collaborative Drug Surveillance Program on 15,438 consecutive inpatients, 1975 to 1982. JAMA 1986;256:3358–63.

104. Lin RY. A perspective on penicillin allergy. Arch Intern Med 1992;152:930–7.

105. Empedrad R, Darter AL, Earl HS, et al. Nonirritating intradermal skin test concentrations for commonly prescribed antibiotics. J Allergy Clin Immunol 2003; 112:629–30.

106. Testi S, Severino M, Iorno M, et al. Nonirritating concentration for skin testing with cephalosporins. J Investig Allergol Clin Immunol 2010;20:170–6.

107. Romano A, Gaeta F, Valluzzi R, et al. IgE-mediated hypersensitivity to cephalosporins: cross-reactivity and tolerability of alternative cephalosporins. J Allergy Clin Immunol 2015;136:685–91.e683.

108. Igea JM, Fraj J, Davila I, et al. Allergy to cefazolin: study of in vivo cross reactivity with other betalactams. Ann Allergy 1992;68:515–9.

109. Marcos Bravo C, Luna Ortiz I, Vazquez Gonzalez R. Hypersensitivity to cefuroxime with good tolerance to other beta-lactams. Allergy 1995;50:359–61.

110. Romano A, Quaratino D, Venuti A, et al. Selective type-1 hypersensitivity to cefuroxime. J Allergy Clin Immunol 1998;101:564–5.

111. Romano A, Quaratino D, Venemalm L, et al. A case of IgE-mediated hypersensitivity to ceftriaxone. J Allergy Clin Immunol 1999;104:1113–4.

112. Goodman EJ, Morgan MJ, Johnson PA, et al. Cephalosporins can be given to penicillin-allergic patients who do not exhibit an anaphylactic response. J Clin Anesth 2001;13:561–4.

113. Fonacier L, Hirschberg R, Gerson S. Adverse drug reactions to a cephalosporins in hospitalized patients with a history of penicillin allergy. Allergy Asthma Proc 2005;26:135–41.

114. MacPherson RD, Willcox C, Chow C, et al. Anaesthetist's responses to patients' self-reported drug allergies. Br J Anaesth 2006;97:634–9.

115. Crotty DJ, Chen XJ, Scipione MR, et al. Allergic reactions in hospitalized patients with a self-reported penicillin allergy who receive a cephalosporin or meropenem. J Pharm Pract 2017;30:42–8.

116. Beltran RJ, Kako H, Chovanec T, et al. Penicillin allergy and surgical prophylaxis: cephalosporin cross-reactivity risk in a pediatric tertiary care center. J Pediatr Surg 2015;50:856–9.

117. Girard JP. Common antigenic determinants of penicillin G, ampicillin and the cephalosporins demonstrated in men. Int Arch Allergy Appl Immunol 1968;33: 428–38.

118. Warrington RJ, Simons FER, Ho HW, et al. Diagnosis of penicillin allergy by skin testing: the Manitoba experience. Can Med Assoc J 1978;118:787–91.
119. Saxon A, Beall GN, Rohr AS, et al. Immediate hypersensitivity reactions to beta-lactam antibiotics. Ann Intern Med 1987;107:204–15.
120. Blanca M, Fernandez J, Miranda A, et al. Cross-reactivity between penicillins and cephalosporins: clinical and immunologic studies. J Allergy Clin Immunol 1989;83:381–5.
121. Shepherd GM, Burton DA. Administration of cephalosporin antibiotics to patients with a history of penicillin allergy (abstract). J Allergy Clin Immunol 1993;91:262
122. Pichichero ME, Pichichero DM. Diagnosis of penicillin, amoxicillin, and cephalosporin allergy: reliability of examination assessed by skin testing and oral challenge. J Pediatr 1998;132:137–43.
123. Novalbos A, Sastre J, Cuesta J, et al. Lack of allergic cross-reactivity to cephalosporins among patients allergic to penicillins. Clin Exp Allergy 2001;31:438–43.
124. Romano A, Gueant-Rodriguez RM, Viola M, et al. Cross-reactivity and tolerability of cephalosporins in patients with immediate hypersensitivity to penicillins. Ann Intern Med 2004;141:16–22.
125. Greenberger PA, Klemens JC. Utility of penicillin major and minor determinants for identification of allergic reactions to cephalosporins (abstract). J Allergy Clin Immunol 2005;115:S182
126. Ahmed KA, Fox SJ, Frigas E, et al. Clinical outcome in the use of cephalosporins in pediatric patients with a history of penicillin allergy. Int Arch Allergy Immunol 2012;158:405–10.
127. McConnell SA, Penzak SR, Warmack TS, et al. Incidence of imipenem hypersensitivity reactions in febrile neutropenic bone marrow transplant patients with a history of penicillin allergy. Clin Infect Dis 2000;31:1512–4.
128. Prescott WA, DeDepestel DD, Ellis JJ, et al. Incidence of carbapenem-associated allergic-type reactions among patients with versus patients without a reported penicillin allergy. Clin Infect Dis 2004;38:1102–7.
129. Sodhi M, Axtell SS, Callahan J, et al. Is it safe to use carbapenems in patients with a history of allergy to penicillin? J Antimicrob Chemother 2004;54:1155–7.
130. Cunha BA, Hamid NS, Krol V, et al. Safety of meropenem in patients reporting penicillin allergy: lack of allergic cross reactions. J Chemother 2008;20:233–7.
131. Romano A, Viola M, Gueant-Rodriquez RA, et al. Imipenem in patients with immediate hypersensitivity to penicillins. N Engl J Med 2006;354:2835–7.
132. Romano A, Viola M, Gueant-Rodriguez RM, et al. Brief communication: tolerability of meropenem in patients with IgE-mediated hypersensitivity to penicillins. Ann Intern Med 2007;146:266–9.
133. Atanaskovic-Markovic M, Gaeta F, Medjo B, et al. Tolerability of meropenem in children with IgE-mediated hypersensitivity to penicillins. Allergy 2008;63:237–40.
134. Atanaskovic-Markovic M, Gaeta F, Gavrovic-Jankulovic M, et al. Tolerability of imipenem in children with IgE-mediated hypersensitivity to penicillins. J Allergy Clin Immunol 2009;124:167–9.
135. Gaeta F, Valluzzi RL, Alonzi C, et al. Tolerability of aztreonam and carbapenems in patients with IgE-mediated hypersensitivity to penicillins. J Allergy Clin Immunol 2015;135:972–6.

Platinum Chemotherapy Hypersensitivity

Prevalence and Management

Iris M. Otani, MD[a],*, Johnson Wong, MD[b], Aleena Banerji, MD[b]

KEYWORDS

- Platinum agent • Carboplatin • Cisplatin • Oxaliplatin • Chemotherapy allergy
- Chemotherapy hypersensitivity • Chemotherapy desensitization

KEY POINTS

- Hypersensitivity reactions to platinum agents are common. For carboplatin and cisplatin, the incidence of the first hypersensitivity reaction is typically clustered around the second and third reexposure during the second line of therapy (eighth and ninth courses overall). For oxaliplatin, the first hypersensitivity reactions occurred throughout the treatment course.
- Skin testing is helpful for risk stratification to choose desensitization protocols and assess risk for breakthrough hypersensitivity reactions during the desensitization.
- A risk-stratification protocol using 3 serial skin tests has been shown to be safe and effective in managing patients with a history of hypersensitivity reactions to platinum-based chemotherapeutic agents.
- The most widely accepted desensitization protocols for platinum agents are the 8-step and 12-step (or modified 13-step) protocols.
- With appropriate clinical history and evaluation, patients can receive first-line chemotherapy treatment safely despite a history of hypersensitivity reactions to platinum-based chemotherapeutic agents.

INTRODUCTION

Cancer is a leading cause of death worldwide and although the incidence continues to rise, cancer mortality has declined over the past decade in large part due to more efficacious chemotherapeutic regimens.[1] The ability to use first-line chemotherapeutic

Disclosure Statement: Nothing to disclose.
[a] Department of Medicine, Division of Pulmonary, Critical Care, Allergy, and Sleep Medicine, UCSF Medical Center, 400 Parnassus Avenue, Fifth Floor, San Francisco, CA 94143, USA;
[b] Department of Medicine, Division of Rheumatology, Allergy, and Immunology, Massachusetts General Hospital, 55 Fruit Street, Boston, MA 02114, USA
* Corresponding author.
E-mail address: iris.otani@ucsf.edu

Immunol Allergy Clin N Am 37 (2017) 663–677
http://dx.doi.org/10.1016/j.iac.2017.06.003
0889-8561/17/© 2017 Elsevier Inc. All rights reserved.

immunology.theclinics.com

agents in the treatment of patients with cancer is critical to good patient outcomes. However, hypersensitivity reactions (HSRs) have emerged as a significant complication to therapy and an increasing incidence of HSRs to first-line chemotherapeutic agents are limiting their use.

As an example, it is well-described that ovarian cancer is the most fatal gynecologic malignancy.[2] The standard treatment approach for newly diagnosed ovarian cancer involves multidisciplinary treatment, including surgical cytoreduction followed by a platinum-based therapy.[3,4] Despite achieving initial complete clinical remission, the vast majority will go on to develop recurrent ovarian cancer.[5] For women with recurrent ovarian cancer, repeat treatment with carboplatin is the treatment of choice. However, carboplatin retreatment in these patients is associated with a high rate of HSRs ranging from 21% to 47%.[6-8] Unfortunately, patients with recurrent ovarian cancer presenting with drug HSRs are frequently and irreversibly labeled as allergic, preventing the use of first-line therapies. The lack of understanding the standard approach to management after an initial HSR leads to suboptimal outcomes, including needless avoidance of first-line chemotherapeutic agents in patients who could tolerate rechallenge without desensitization or intentional rechallenge with a drug that may cause a recurrent and severe HSR. However, there is significant research and experience showing that an accurate clinical history and proper management can improve patient outcomes despite a reported HSR.

This review focuses on HSRs induced by platinum-based chemotherapeutic agents. We review the epidemiology, clinical presentation, and management of HSRs to platinum-based chemotherapeutic agents.

BACKGROUND AND EPIDEMIOLOGY

Carboplatin and cisplatin are platinum-based chemotherapeutic agents commonly used for ovarian, lung, and head and neck cancers. Carboplatin and cisplatin are classified as DNA alkylating agents. Carboplatin was introduced in the late 1980s and has since gained popularity in clinical treatment due to its vastly reduced side effects compared with its parent compound cisplatin. HSRs are rarely reported during the initial treatment and the frequency of HSRs appears directly related to the number of exposures. HSRs are typically noted after multiple cycles have been administered and occur most frequently with the second line of treatment.

With carboplatin, the incidence increases from 1% in individuals who have received 6 or fewer carboplatin infusions to 27% in those who received 7 or more, and up to 46% in patients who have received more than 15 infusions.[6,9] The peak incidence of HSRs occurs with the eighth or ninth exposure, which generally corresponds to the second or third cycle of retreatment after recurrence of malignancy.[9] It is important to note that women with inherited mutations in BRCA 1 or 2 appear to have a higher risk for carboplatin infusion reactions and reactions occur at a lower cumulative exposure.[10,11] Patients with a BRCA 1 or 2 mutation are also at higher risk for reacting during desensitization.[11]

Cisplatin was the first of the platinum drugs to be used but is often limited by side effects, including neurotoxicity, nephrotoxicity, and ototoxicity. These side effects are less common with equal efficacy, making carboplatin a better treatment option for most patients with cancer requiring platinum-based therapy. The incidence of cisplatin hypersensitivity exhibits similar characteristics to those observed with carboplatin. One of the first publications on cisplatin as a treatment for lung cancer described that, among patients receiving 6 or more cycles of combination chemotherapy, 5 of 21 patients experienced "anaphylaxis."[12] In general, the frequency of cisplatin HSRs ranges from 5% to 20% and increases with concomitant radiation therapy.[13]

Oxaliplatin is another platinum-based chemotherapy drug in the same family as carboplatin and cisplatin and is similarly a DNA alkylating agent. It is typically administered in combination with other agents for the treatment of colorectal cancer. Colorectal cancer is the third-leading cause of cancer death in the United States. Initial reports of HSRs to oxaliplatin were low, but more recent data suggest the incidence of HSRs to oxaliplatin is similar to that of the earlier-generation platinum agents. This rising incidence of HSRs to oxaliplatin is likely the result of increasing clinical use. The reported incidence of HSRs associated with oxaliplatin in patients with colorectal cancer is approximately 12%, with 1% to 2% of patients developing moderate to severe reactions.[14]

MECHANISMS AND CLINICAL PRESENTATION

HSRs to platinum agents are likely primarily mast cell mediated, although the exact mechanism remains unclear. HSRs to platinum agents are thought to be primarily immunoglobulin (Ig)E-mediated, because a period of sensitization and/or re-sensitization is required, skin tests are often positive, skin test reactivity correlates with the risk of reaction during desensitization, and skin test conversion from negative to positive is seen following reexposure and after developing a reaction.[15–19] A different mechanism may be responsible for a subgroup that remains skin test negative despite repeat testing, although mechanistic studies are needed to investigate this hypothesis.

IgE-mediated mechanisms were first observed in workers who were repeatedly exposed to platinum salts. Workers sensitized to platinum agents developed sinopulmonary symptoms (rhinitis, conjunctivitis, bronchospasm) when challenged with platinum-containing solutions.[20] IgE-mediated mechanisms were also supported by the fact that skin reactivity can be passively transferred via serum of sensitized workers.[21] Specific IgE has been identified in patients who experienced HSRs to platinum agents (this is discussed further in the section on diagnostic testing).[22–24]

It has been observed that approximately half of HSRs due to carboplatin present with moderately severe symptoms, including diffuse erythroderma, wheezing, facial swelling, nausea and/or vomiting, diarrhea, dyspnea, and hypotension.[9,19] The distribution of clinical characteristics of HSRs to carboplatin and oxaliplatin observed in our original studies are summarized in **Table 1**.[16,18]

Delayed HSRs that are likely due to T-cell–mediated mechanisms may also occur after platinum agent administration.[25,26] These HSRs range from mild to severe cutaneous manifestations, with mild reactions being more common, and severe cutaneous reactions including desquamation.[26]

DIAGNOSTIC TESTING
Carboplatin Skin Testing

Carboplatin skin testing was first developed in the 1990s. Initial studies used 0.05 to 0.1 mg/mL of carboplatin for epicutaneous and intradermal skin testing.[27–29] Subsequent studies investigating carboplatin skin testing have established a standard concentration of 10 mg/mL for the epicutaneous step followed by increasing stepwise concentrations from 0.2 to 30.0 µg (0.02–0.04-mL injection of 0.01–1 mg/mL carboplatin) to 20.0 to 300.0 µg (0.02–0.04-mL injection of 1–10 mg/mL carboplatin) for the intradermal steps.[15,16,19,25,30–32] At our institution, we perform skin testing at the nonirritating concentrations listed in **Table 2**.

Table 1
Clinical characteristics of hypersensitivity reactions

Clinical Characteristics	Carboplatin (n = 38) No. of Patients (%)[15]	Oxaliplatin (n = 48) No. of Patients (%)[17]

Oropharynx
  Throat tightness
  Tongue swelling
  Hoarseness
	6 (16)	9 (19)

Cardiovascular
  Tachycardia/bradycardia
  Hypertension/hypotension
  Chest pain
  Dizziness
  Light-headed
	11 (29)	16 (33)

Pulmonary
  Chest tightness
  Shortness of breath
  Cough
  Nasal symptoms
	11 (29)	17 (35)

Gastrointestinal
  Nausea/vomiting/diarrhea
  Abdominal pain
	14 (37)	14 (29)

Genitourinary Urethral burning	2 (5)	0 (0)

Musculoskeletal
  Arthralgia
  Spasm
  Pain
	0 (0)	3 (6)

Cutaneous
  Erythema/flushing pruritus
  Urticarial
  Palmar erythema
	30 (79)	38 (78)

Delayed cutaneous
  Rash
  Erythema/flushing
  Pruritus
	3 (8)	1 (2)

Neurologic
  Tingling
  Dizziness
  Tunnel vision
  Jittery
  Seizure
  Difficulty focusing[a]
	0 (0)	6 (13)

Systemic
  Fever
  Chills/rigors
  Somnolence
	0 (0)	9 (19)

Drug-induced immune-mediated
  Thrombocytopenia (DITP)
  Hemolytic anemia (DIHA)
	0 (0)	1 (6)[b]

[a] One patient had tunnel vision, jitters, seizure, difficulty focusing, and tingling.
[b] One additional patient developed DITP and DIHA after undergoing additional desensitization among the original 48 patients with oxaliplatin HSRs.

Table 2
Nonirritating concentrations for platinum agent skin testing

Platinum Agent	Skin Prick Test Dilutions, mg/mL	Intradermal Test Dilutions, mg/mL
Carboplatin	10	0.1
		1
		5[a]
Oxaliplatin	5	0.05
		0.5
		5
Cisplatin	1	0.01
		0.1
		1

Abbreviation: ID, intradermal.
[a] Higher 10 mg/mL ID concentration has been reported to cause local skin necrosis, and is therefore not used.

Epicutaneous and intradermal steps are both important for carboplatin skin testing. Performing the epicutaneous step can decrease the risk of inducing HSRs with skin testing, whereas the intradermal step is needed to achieve adequate sensitivity, as 86.4% of positive skin testing is elicited during the intradermal step.[33] The final concentration for intradermal skin testing also affects skin-testing results. Among patients who had a history of HSR, using a final step of 0.02 to 0.03 mL of a 10-mg/mL dilution resulted in positive skin testing for 81% to 88% of patients,[19,31] whereas using 0.02 mL of 1 to 5 mg/mL dilutions resulted in positive skin testing for 41% to 75% of patients (83% among patients who experienced recent HSRs within the past 3 months).[15,16,22,25] However, skin necrosis has been reported with the higher concentration of 10 mg/mL.[16] The rate of positive skin testing also may depend on the severity of the HSR. A cohort of 23 patients with moderate to severe carboplatin-induced HSRs had a 100% positive skin-testing rate.[32]

The length of time between last exposure to carboplatin (typically when the carboplatin-induced HSR occurred) and initial skin testing must be taken into consideration when interpreting carboplatin skin testing.

Data from hymenoptera venom skin testing suggest that the risk for false-negative skin testing is higher due to "anergy" during the first 4 to 6 weeks following a systemic reaction.[34] We have similarly seen a small number of patients who experienced HSRs less than 6 weeks before the initial skin test, who initially had negative skin testing that later converted to positive when the skin testing was repeated outside the 6-week window (unpublished observation). Therefore, if skin testing performed during the first 4 to 6 weeks following carboplatin-induced HSR is negative, it is typically repeated outside of the 4-week to 6-week window.

We have found that a longer interval of time (ie, >6 months) between carboplatin-induced HSRs and skin testing is associated with a higher frequency of an initial false-negative skin test. The frequency of positive skin testing has been shown to be significantly lower among patients who experienced recent HSRs within the past 3 months (83%, 20/24) compared with patients who experienced a remote HSR more than 9 months before (36%, 5/14).[16] Most of the latter group, 71% (5/7) converted to positive skin testing on retesting after 1 reexposure to carboplatin via desensitization.[16] Two other studies have also shown that patients who converted from negative to positive skin testing after reexposure to carboplatin via desensitization were more likely to have a time interval of at least 6 months between the carboplatin-induced HSR and initial skin testing compared with patients with persistently negative skin testing.[15,17] In our experience, 3 repeat skin tests before each desensitization was adequate for risk stratification for patients who undergo initial skin testing more than 6 months after the initial carboplatin-induced HSR.[15–18,33]

Predictive values of carboplatin skin testing are discussed further in the "Risk Stratification and Desensitization" section.

Cisplatin Skin Testing

Nonirritating concentrations have been reported for both epicutaneous (highest 10 mg/mL) and intradermal skin-testing steps (highest 1 mg/mL).[19,25,35]

Predictive values for skin testing have been the least studied for cisplatin out of the 3 platinum agents. In 1 report, 2 patients with cisplatin-induced HSR had positive skin testing and subsequently received cisplatin via desensitization.[19] In another report, of 2 patients with cisplatin-induced HSRs, 1 patient had positive skin testing and subsequently did not receive any platinum agent, and 1 patient had negative skin testing and subsequently tolerated carboplatin without reaction.[25]

Oxaliplatin Skin Testing

Skin testing has been performed at 0.01 to 5 mg/mL for the epicutaneous step, 0.001 to 0.05 mg/mL for the initial intradermal step, and 0.5 to 5 mg/mL for the final intradermal step.[18,24,25,36,37] At our institution, we perform skin testing at the nonirritating concentrations listed in **Table 2**.

Skin testing following oxaliplatin-induced HSR has a reported 26% to 100% positive rate.[18,24,25,36,37] Skin testing in patients who tolerated infusions of oxaliplatin and in oxaliplatin-naïve patients has a reported 100% negative rate. Pagani and colleagues[37] reported that oxaliplatin skin testing was negative for 100% (15/15) of patients never exposed to platinum agents and 100% (18/18) of patients who had received oxaliplatin therapy without reactions.

The negative predictive value of oxaliplatin skin testing remains unclear. Although a prospective study of 101 patients reported a 5% false-negative rate,[38] another study reported 70% (7/10) of patients with negative skin testing who subsequently received oxaliplatin via graded challenge had a positive reaction.[24]

Therefore, as with carboplatin skin testing, the main utility of oxaliplatin skin testing appears to be risk stratification of patients who have experienced oxaliplatin-induced HSRs (see section on risk stratification).

Specific IgE

Specific IgE to platinum agents has been investigated as a diagnostic tool.

In a report of only 3 patients with carboplatin-induced HSR, 100% (3/3) had specific IgE to carboplatin (Carbo-sIgE) $\geq$ 0.35 kU/L and 33% (1/3) had specific IgE to cisplatin (Cis-sIgE) $\geq$ 0.35 kU/L. Interestingly, the 2 patients with undetectable Cis-sIgE had breakthrough HSRs during the initial carboplatin desensitizations that were mild enough to allow completion of the desensitization protocol, and tolerated carboplatin subsequent desensitizations without breakthrough HSRs. The 1 patient with Cis-sIgE elevated at 4.2 kU/L experienced a severe breakthrough HSR (anaphylaxis) during the initial carboplatin desensitization and subsequent administration of platinum agents was deferred.[22]

In a much larger study, Caiado and colleagues,[23] measured Carbo-sIgE and specific IgE to oxaliplatin (Oxali-sIgE) in 24 patients who had experienced HSRs due to platinum agents (carboplatin, 12; oxaliplatin 12). Cis-sIgE was measured in 21 of these patients. Of the 12 patients who had experienced HSRs due to carboplatin, 59% (7/12) had positive Carbo-sIgE, 17% (2/12) also had positive Cis-sIgE, and all had negative

Oxali-sIgE. Of the 12 patients with oxaliplatin-induced HSRs, 75% (9/12) had positive Oxali-sIgE, 67% (8/12) had positive Carbo-sIgE and Cis-sIgE. Carbo-sIgE and Oxali-sIgE were measured in 17 control patients who had been exposed to platinum agents and did not experience HSRs (carboplatin, 5; oxaliplatin, 12). All 5 carboplatin-exposed, nonreactive controls had negative Carbo-sIgE and Oxali-sIgE. Of the 12 oxaliplatin-exposed, nonreactive controls, 25% (3/12) had positive Carbo-sIgE and 2 had positive Oxali-sIgE. Based on these results, the investigators concluded that Carbo-sIgE likely had higher specificity and lower sensitivity compared with Oxali-sIgE, and that oxaliplatin was more immunogenic (given the positive Carbo-sIgE and Cis-sIgE observed in patients exposed only to oxaliplatin).

In a separate study, Oxali-sIgE was reported to have a sensitivity of 38% to 54% depending on the cutoff (0.10–0.35 kU/L).[24]

Basophil Activation Test

The basophil activation test, or BAT, has been evaluated as a diagnostic test for platinum-induced HSRs. Basophil CD63 and CD203c expression were compared between patients with history of carboplatin-induced HSRs (n = 12) and oxaliplatin-induced HSRs (n = 3), control patients who had previously tolerated carboplatin (n = 6), and control patients who had never been exposed to platinum agents (n = 6). BAT was positive for 67% (8/12) of patients with carboplatin-induced HSRs and 100% (3/3) of patients with oxaliplatin-induced HSRs. All 15 patients with history of platinum-induced HSRs had positive skin testing results. Patients from both control groups had negative BAT results. Based on these results, the Giavina-Bianchi and colleagues[39] calculated that BAT has a sensitivity of 73% and specificity of 100% for platinum-induced HSRs.

The same investigators also correlated BAT with breakthrough reactions during 27 desensitization procedures. Nine patients experienced 13 breakthrough reactions during desensitization, and BAT was positive in 92% (12/13) with increased CD203c expression in 92% (12/13) and increased CD63 expression in 69% (9/13). Although BAT was also positive in 50% (7/14) of desensitization procedures without breakthrough reactions, there was a statistically significant difference in BAT positivity between desensitization procedures with and without breakthrough reactions (P = .02). The 13 breakthrough reactions during desensitization ranged in severity from grade 1 (n = 10), grade 2 (n = 2), to grade 3 (n = 1). The grade 2 and 3 breakthrough reactions (n = 3) had positive BAT for both markers (100%), suggesting that positive BAT for both activation markers could possibly be a biomarker predictive of higher risk of grade 2 to 3 breakthrough reactions during desensitization.[39]

RISK STRATIFICATION AND DESENSITIZATION
Carboplatin

Predictive values before hypersensitivity reaction
Carboplatin skin testing has been investigated as a predictive tool for the development of HSRs in patients with recurrent platinum-sensitive gynecologic cancer who required retreatment with carboplatin before HSR.[30,40,41] The overall frequency of positive skin testing (31%–36%) is similar to the frequency of HSR observed in patients being retreated with carboplatin.[33] Carboplatin skin testing was shown to have a negative predictive value between 81% and 92% and a positive predictive value of 86%.[33] Further studies are needed to investigate the clinical utility of skin testing before retreatment.

Predictive values after hypersensitivity reaction: utilization for risk stratification with desensitization

The positive predictive value of skin testing after HSR without desensitization is unknown, as carboplatin rechallenge without desensitization in patients with positive skin testing has not been reported in the literature. The negative predictive value of skin testing after HSR is also unclear, although data from 4 patients suggest that the negative predictive value is low. These 4 patients had negative skin testing after carboplatin-induced HSR but developed mild HSRs when they received carboplatin without desensitization.[19]

Skin testing appears to have the most utility in risk stratification of patients who have experienced carboplatin-induced HSR. Positive skin testing indicates a risk for additional HSRs during reexposure even if desensitization is used (37% of patients and 17% of desensitizations).[16] This is true for both patients with initial positive skin testing and patients who convert from negative to positive skin testing after reexposure. The percentage of desensitizations complicated by HSRs are comparable between patients with initial positive skin testing and patients who convert from negative to positive skin testing after reexposure (58.5% vs 56.1%, $P = 5.87$).[15] Serial negative skin testing can help identify patients who can safely return to receiving carboplatin in the outpatient setting without desensitization. Patients with serial negative skin testing are significantly less likely to have desensitizations complicated by HSRs compared with patients who convert from negative to positive skin testing after reexposure (4.5% vs 56.1%, $P<.001$).[15]

A risk-stratification protocol using 3 serial skin tests has been shown to be safe and effective in managing patients with carboplatin-induced HSRs.[15,17] This protocol safely differentiates allergic from nonallergic patients and helps prevent unnecessary desensitizations.[17]

Cisplatin

Multiple studies have shown that desensitization is a safe and effective way to reintroduce cisplatin to patients who have experienced cisplatin-induced HSRs.[19,42] At our institution, we have been following the same risk-stratification protocol for cisplatin as carboplatin and oxaliplatin with success.

Oxaliplatin

Multiple studies have shown that desensitization is a safe and effective way to reintroduce oxaliplatin to patients who have experienced oxaliplatin-induced HSRs.[17–19,43]

As with carboplatin skin testing, oxaliplatin skin testing is useful for risk stratification of patients who have experienced oxaliplatin-induced HSRs. We have shown that patients with positive skin testing are more likely to experience HSRs during desensitization compared with patients with negative skin testing. Among the 25 patients who had positive initial skin test, 48% (12/25 patients) developed an HSR during at least 1 of their desensitizations, with 24% (34/144) of the desensitizations complicated by HSRs. In contrast, the respective incidences for patients who were initially skin test negative were 24% (5/21 patients) and 11% (6/54 desensitizations), respectively, despite using a more rapid desensitization protocol. When considering the results of repeat skin testing, a higher percentage of patients had breakthrough reactions if their initial skin testing was positive and remained positive (45%, 10/22) or if their skin testing converted from negative to positive (50%, 1/2), than if their skin testing remained negative (21%, 4/19).[18]

As with carboplatin, the timing of skin testing is important in determining the interpretation of the results for risk stratification and management.[17,18] The risk-stratification protocol used for carboplatin has been investigated and found to be safe and effective for oxaliplatin as well, and is described in the following section.[17]

It has also been found that HSRs are less common when oxaliplatin is administered using a slowed, stepwise infusion (one-fifth of the total dose over 1 hour followed by the remaining four-fifths of the total dose over 6 hours vs the total dose over 2 hours) (3.4% vs 13.6%, $P<.01$).[44]

Desensitization Protocols Based on Risk Stratification

The most widely accepted desensitization protocols for platinum agents are the 8-step and 12-step (or modified 13-step) protocols.[15–17,19,31,45] The 8-step and modified 13-step protocols are outlined in **Table 3**.

The choice of protocol for a particular desensitization is based on risk stratification from the skin-testing results. Based on our studies, patients with positive skin testing are considered allergic and are reintroduced to the platinum agent using a 13-step desensitization procedure.[15,17] The 13-step desensitization procedure is identical to a previously published 12-step procedure with the addition of a 60-mL/h step between steps 11 and 12 in the third bag.[45] Patients with initial negative skin testing are reintroduced to the platinum agent using an 8-step desensitization procedure,[16] followed by repeat skin testing before each subsequent desensitization. If repeat skin testing is negative, subsequent desensitizations are performed using the 8-step desensitization procedure. After 3 consecutive negative skin tests and 8-step desensitizations tolerated without breakthrough reactions, patients are considered not allergic to the platinum gent and receive subsequent treatments in the outpatient setting at a 50% infusion rate. If skin tests convert from negative to positive, or if an HSR is experienced during an 8-step desensitization, a 12-step desensitization is used for subsequent treatments and skin testing is not repeated.[17]

Taking into consideration data regarding skin-testing anergy during the first 4 to 6 weeks after an HSR and data suggesting that most false-negative initial skin testing occurs when the time interval between the initial HSR and the initial skin test is at least 6 months, we have updated the risk-stratification protocol at our institution to risk stratify patients with 1 skin test only if the time interval between the initial HSR and the initial skin test is at least 6 weeks but less than 6 months (**Fig. 1**).

Desensitization also has been shown to be effective from both a medical and health care cost perspective. Sloane and colleagues[46] investigated health care costs and outcomes in carboplatin-allergic patients (patients with a history of carboplatin-induced HSRs) compared with nonallergic control patients (patients who tolerated carboplatin via standard administration). The investigators found that average hospital costs were 31% higher for nonallergic control patients (n = 186) than carboplatin-allergic patients (n = 171). Desensitization costs were not included in this calculation. The investigators also found that there was a trend toward increased life expectancy in the carboplatin-allergic patients (n = 155) with recurrent ovarian cancer who received carboplatin via desensitization compared with nonallergic control patients (n = 81) with recurrent ovarian cancer who received carboplatin via standard administration.

Cross-Reactivity Between Platinum Agents

Studies have investigated the use of oxaliplatin and/or cisplatin as alternative agents following carboplatin-induced HSRs.

Studies investigating the use of cisplatin as an alternative agent following carboplatin-induced HSRs suggest that although many carboplatin-allergic patients tolerate cisplatin, there is some degree of potentially fatal cross-reactivity between carboplatin and cisplatin. In 1 study, 100% (19/19) of patients were able to tolerate

Table 3
Desensitization protocols for carboplatin (target dose 297.6 mg)

13-Step Protocol

Solution	Concentration, mg/mL	Amount Infused, mL
1	0.011904	9.375
2	0.11904	18.75
3	1.1810256	250

Step	Solution	Infusion Duration, min	Cumulative Time, min	Infusion Rate, mL/h	Volume Infused per Step, mL	Dose per Step, mg	Cumulative Dose, mg
1	1	15	15	2.5	0.625	0.00744	0.00744
2	1	15	30	5	1.25	0.01488	0.02232
3	1	15	45	10	2.5	0.02976	0.05208
4	1	15	60	20	5	0.05952	0.1116
5	2	15	75	5	1.25	0.1488	0.2604
6	2	15	90	10	2.5	0.2976	0.558
7	2	15	105	20	5	0.5952	1.1532
8	2	15	120	40	10	1.1904	2.3436
9	3	15	135	10	2.5	2.952564	5.296164
0	3	15	150	20	5	5.905128	11.201292
11	3	15	165	40	10	11.810256	23.011548
12	3	15	180	60	15	17.715384	40.726932
13	3	163	343	80	217.5	256.873068	297.6

8-Step Protocol

Solution	Concentration, mg/mL	Amount Infused, mL
1	0.011904	18.75
2	1.1895072	250

Step	Solution	Infusion Duration, min	Cumulative Time, min	Infusion Rate, mL/h	Volume Infused per Step, mL	Dose per Step, mg	Cumulative Dose, mg
1	1	15	15	5	1.25	0.01488	0.0435
2	1	15	30	10	2.5	0.02976	0.1305
3	1	15	45	20	5	0.05952	0.3045
4	1	15	60	40	10	0.11904	0.6525
5	2	15	75	10	2.5	2.973768	1.516
6	2	15	90	20	5	5.947536	3.2429
7	2	15	105	40	10	11.895072	6.6968
8	2	15	120	80	232.5	276.560424	87

cisplatin after carboplatin-induced HSRs.[47] In another case series of 6 patients who received cisplatin after developing a carboplatin-induced HSR, 5 patients were able to tolerate cisplatin with premedication, but 1 patient developed a cisplatin-induced HSR that precluded further treatment with cisplatin.[48] In a case series of 24 patients who received cisplatin without desensitization after experiencing carboplatin-induced HSRs, 6 (24%) developed cisplatin-induced HSRs at some point during cisplatin therapy.[49] Furthermore, there have been 2 cases reported of patients with

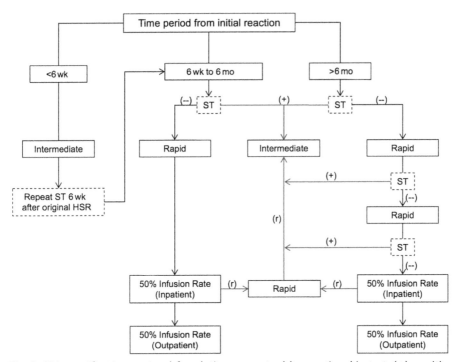

Fig. 1. Risk stratification protocol for platinum agents. (–), negative skin test; (+), positive skin test; Intermediate, 13-step protocol as outlined in **Table 3**; (r), reaction; Rapid, 8-step protocol as outlined in **Table 3**; ST, skin test.

carboplatin-induced HSRs who were switched to cisplatin and developed fatal HSRs.[48,50]

Studies investigating the use of oxaliplatin as an alternative agent following carboplatin-induced HSRs suggest that there is some degree of potentially fatal cross-reactivity between carboplatin and oxaliplatin. In one study, 27 patients received oxaliplatin after experiencing carboplatin-induced HSRs, and 7% (2/27) of patients experienced HSRs to oxaliplatin.[47] Another study reported that 2 of 11 patients who received oxaliplatin via desensitization after experiencing an HSR during carboplatin desensitization also developed an HSR during oxaliplatin desensitization.[51]

The results of specific IgE testing for carboplatin, oxaliplatin, and cisplatin among patients with and without a history of platin-induced HSRs suggest that the risk of patients sensitized to oxaliplatin also being sensitized to carboplatin and cisplatin is higher than the risk of patients sensitized to carboplatin also being sensitized to oxaliplatin. Patients who experienced carboplatin-induced HSRs had positive Carbo-sIgE (59%, 7/12) and negative Oxali-sIgE (100%, 12/12), but patients who experienced oxaliplatin-induced HSRs had not only positive Oxali-sIgE (75%, 9/12), but positive Carbo-sIgE and Cis-sIgE as well (67%, 8/12).[23]

Negative skin testing may be helpful in selecting an alternative platinum agent. Leguy-Seguin and colleagues[25] found that 100% (8/8) of patients who had negative skin testing to an alternative platinum agent were able to tolerate that alternative platinum agent (4/4 with carboplatin-induced HSRs tolerated cisplatin, 1/1 with a cisplatin-induced HSR tolerated carboplatin, 2/2 with oxaliplatin-induced HSRs tolerated cisplatin, and 1/1 with an oxaliplatin-induced HSR tolerated carboplatin). Elligers and colleagues,[52] reported 1 patient with an oxaliplatin-induced HSR and negative cisplatin skin testing subsequently tolerated cisplatin. Enrique and colleagues[53] reported 2 patients with carboplatin-induced HSRs who had negative cisplatin skin testing and subsequently tolerated cisplatin. Syrigou and colleagues[54] reported 3 patients with carboplatin-induced HSRs who had negative cisplatin skin testing and subsequently tolerated cisplatin. Taken together, 100% (14/14) of patients who had negative skin testing to an alternative platinum agent were able to tolerate that alternative platinum agent.

SUMMARY

HSRs to platinum agents are common. For carboplatin and cisplatin, the first HSR typically occurs around the second and third re-exposure during the second line of therapy (eighth and ninth courses overall). For oxaliplatin, the first HSR can occur throughout the treatment course. Skin testing helps risk stratify patients to appropriate desensitization protocols and assess risk for breakthrough HSRs during desensitization. Patients with platinum agent hypersensitivity may be managed with a risk-stratification protocol using 3 serial skin tests and desensitization protocols. Patients with a negative result on the initial skin test should be retested if their HSRs were less than 6 weeks or more than 6 months from the initial skin test, as they are at risk for converting to a positive result on subsequent skin testing. Those who convert to a positive skin test result should be treated with a slower desensitization protocol. Those who have 3 consecutive negative skin test results may progress to outpatient slowed infusion protocols. Specific IgE to platinum agents are promising as a diagnostic tool, but remain investigational. In summary, with appropriate clinical history and management, patients can receive first-line chemotherapy treatment safely despite a history of HSRs to platinum-based chemotherapeutic agents.

REFERENCES

1. Hunn J, Rodriguez GC. Ovarian cancer: etiology, risk factors, and epidemiology. Clin Obstet Gynecol 2012;55(1):3–23.
2. Siegel R, Naishadham D, Jemal A. Cancer statistics, 2012. CA Cancer J Clin 2012;62(1):10–29.
3. Markman M. Pharmaceutical management of ovarian cancer: current status. Drugs 2008;68(6):771–89. Available at: http://www.ncbi.nlm.nih.gov/pubmed/18416585. Accessed April 7, 2017.
4. Schorge JO, Eisenhauer EE, Chi DS. Current surgical management of ovarian cancer. Hematol Oncol Clin North Am 2012;26(1):93–109.
5. Thigpen T. A rational approach to the management of recurrent or persistent ovarian carcinoma. Clin Obstet Gynecol 2012;55(1):114–30.
6. Koshiba H, Hosokawa K, Kubo A, et al. Incidence of carboplatin-related hypersensitivity reactions in Japanese patients with gynecologic malignancies. Int J Gynecol Cancer 2009;19(3):460–5.
7. Schwartz JR, Bandera C, Bradley A, et al. Does the platinum-free interval predict the incidence or severity of hypersensitivity reactions to carboplatin? The experience from Women and Infants' Hospital. Gynecol Oncol 2007;105(1):81–3.
8. Zanotti KM, Rybicki LA, Kennedy AW, et al. Carboplatin skin testing: a skin-testing protocol for predicting hypersensitivity to carboplatin chemotherapy. J Clin Oncol 2001;19(12):3126–9.

9. Markman M, Kennedy A, Webster K, et al. Clinical features of hypersensitivity reactions to carboplatin. J Clin Oncol 1999;17(4):1141.

10. Moon DH, Lee J-M, Noonan AM, et al. Deleterious BRCA1/2 mutation is an independent risk factor for carboplatin hypersensitivity reactions. Br J Cancer 2013; 109(4):1072–8.

11. Galvao VR, Phillips E, Giavina-Bianchi P, et al. Carboplatin-allergic patients undergoing desensitization: prevalence and impact of the BRCA 1/2 mutation. J Allergy Clin Immunol Pract 2016;5(3):816–8.

12. Gralla RJ, Casper ES, Kelsen DP, et al. Cisplatin and vindesine combination chemotherapy for advanced carcinoma of the lung: a randomized trial investigating two dosage schedules. Ann Intern Med 1981;95(4):414–20. Available at: http://www.ncbi.nlm.nih.gov/pubmed/7025719. Accessed April 7, 2017.

13. Koren C, Yerushalmi R, Katz A, et al. Hypersensitivity reaction to cisplatin during chemoradiation therapy for gynecologic malignancy. Am J Clin Oncol 2002;25(6): 625–6. Available at: http://www.ncbi.nlm.nih.gov/pubmed/12478013. Accessed April 7, 2017.

14. Saif MW. Hypersensitivity reactions associated with oxaliplatin. Expert Opin Drug Saf 2006;5(5):687–94.

15. Patil SU, Long AA, Ling M, et al. A protocol for risk stratification of patients with carboplatin-induced hypersensitivity reactions. J Allergy Clin Immunol 2012; 129(2):443–7.

16. Hesterberg PE, Banerji A, Oren E, et al. Risk stratification for desensitization of patients with carboplatin hypersensitivity: clinical presentation and management. J Allergy Clin Immunol 2009;123(6):1262–7.e1.

17. Wang AL, Patil SU, Long AA, et al. Risk-stratification protocol for carboplatin and oxaliplatin hypersensitivity: repeat skin testing to identify drug allergy. Ann Allergy Asthma Immunol 2015;115(5):422–8.

18. Wong JT, Ling M, Patil S, et al. Oxaliplatin hypersensitivity: evaluation, implications of skin testing, and desensitization. J Allergy Clin Immunol Pract 2014; 2(1):40–5.

19. Castells MC, Tennant NM, Sloane DE, et al. Hypersensitivity reactions to chemotherapy: outcomes and safety of rapid desensitization in 413 cases. J Allergy Clin Immunol 2008;122(3):574–80.

20. Pickering CA. Inhalation tests with chemical allergens: complex salts of platinum. Proc R Soc Med 1972;65(3):272–4. Available at: http://www.ncbi.nlm.nih.gov/ pubmed/5083317. Accessed April 22, 2017.

21. Pepys J, Parish WE, Cromwell O, et al. Passive transfer in man and the monkey of Type I allergy due to heat labile and heat stable antibody to complex salts of platinum. Clin Allergy 1979;9(2):99–108. Available at: http://www.ncbi.nlm.nih.gov/ pubmed/87286. Accessed April 22, 2017.

22. Pagani M, Venemalm L, Bonnadona P, et al. An experimental biological test to diagnose hypersensitivity reactions to carboplatin: new horizons for an old problem. Jpn J Clin Oncol 2012;42(4):347–50.

23. Caiado J, Venemalm L, Pereira-Santos MC, et al. Carboplatin-, oxaliplatin-, and cisplatin-specific IgE: cross-reactivity and value in the diagnosis of carboplatin and oxaliplatin allergy. J Allergy Clin Immunol Pract 2013;1(5):494–500.

24. Madrigal-Burgaleta R, Berges-Gimeno MP, Angel-Pereira D, et al. Hypersensitivity and desensitization to antineoplastic agents: outcomes of 189 procedures with a new short protocol and novel diagnostic tools assessment. Allergy 2013;68(7): 853–61.

25. Leguy-Seguin V, Jolimoy G, Coudert B, et al. Diagnostic and predictive value of skin testing in platinum salt hypersensitivity. J Allergy Clin Immunol 2007;119(3): 726–30.

26. Robinson JB, Singh D, Bodurka-Bevers DC, et al. Hypersensitivity reactions and the utility of oral and intravenous desensitization in patients with gynecologic malignancies. Gynecol Oncol 2001;82(3):550–8.

27. Goldberg A, Confino-Cohen R, Fishman A, et al. A modified, prolonged desensitization protocol in carboplatin allergy. J Allergy Clin Immunol 1996;98(4):841–3.

28. Sood AK, Gelder MS, Huang S-W, et al. Anaphylaxis to carboplatin following multiple previous uncomplicated courses. Gynecol Oncol 1995;57(1):131–2.

29. Broome CB, Schiff RI, Friedman HS. Successful desensitization to carboplatin in patients with systemic hypersensitivity reactions. Med Pediatr Oncol 1996;26(2): 105–10.

30. Markman M, Zanotti K, Peterson G, et al. Expanded experience with an intradermal skin test to predict for the presence or absence of carboplatin hypersensitivity. J Clin Oncol 2003;21(24):4611–4.

31. Lee C-W, Matulonis UA, Castells MC, et al. Rapid inpatient/outpatient desensitization for chemotherapy hypersensitivity: standard protocol effective in 57 patients for 255 courses. Gynecol Oncol 2005;99(2):393–9.

32. Confino-Cohen R, Fishman A, Altaras M, et al. Successful carboplatin desensitization in patients with proven carboplatin allergy. Cancer 2005;104(3):640–3.

33. Lax T, Long A, Banerji A, et al. Skin testing in the evaluation and management of carboplatin-related hypersensitivity reactions. J Allergy Clin Immunol Pract 2015; 3(6):856–62.

34. Goldberg A, Confino-Cohen R, Georgitis J, et al. Timing of venom skin tests and IgE determinations after insect sting anaphylaxis. J Allergy Clin Immunol 1997; 100(2):182–4.

35. Brockow K, Garvey LH, Aberer W, et al. Skin test concentrations for systemically administered drugs—an ENDA/EAACI Drug Allergy Interest Group position paper. Allergy 2013;68(6):702–12.

36. Herrero T, Tornero P, Infante S, et al. Diagnosis and management of hypersensitivity reactions caused by oxaliplatin. J Investig Allergol Clin Immunol 2006;16(5): 327–30. Available at: http://www.ncbi.nlm.nih.gov/pubmed/17039675. Accessed March 18, 2017.

37. Pagani M, Bonadonna P, Senna GE, et al. Standardization of skin tests for diagnosis and prevention of hypersensitivity reactions to oxaliplatin. Int Arch Allergy Immunol 2007;145(1):54–7.

38. Pagani M, Bonadonna P. Skin test protocol for the prevention of hypersensitivity reactions to oxaliplatin. Anticancer Res 2014;34(1):537–40. Available at: http:// www.ncbi.nlm.nih.gov/pubmed/24403513. Accessed March 19, 2017.

39. Giavina-Bianchi P, Galvão VR, Picard M, et al. Basophil activation test is a relevant biomarker of the outcome of rapid desensitization in platinum compounds-allergy. J Allergy Clin Immunol Pract 2017;5(3):728–36.

40. McAlpine JN, Kelly MG, O'malley DM, et al. Atypical presentations of carboplatin hypersensitivity reactions: characterization and management in patients with gynecologic malignancies. Gynecol Oncol 2006;103(1):288–92.

41. Gomez R, Harter P, Lück H-J, et al. Carboplatin hypersensitivity. Int J Gynecol Cancer 2009;19(7):1284–7.

42. Li Q, Cohn D, Waller A, et al. Outpatient rapid 4-step desensitization for gynecologic oncology patients with mild to low-risk, moderate hypersensitivity reactions to carboplatin/cisplatin. Gynecol Oncol 2014;135(1):90–4.

43. Park H, Lee J, Kim S, et al. A new practical desensitization protocol for oxaliplatin-induced immediate hypersensitivity reactions: a necessary and useful approach. J Investig Allergol Clin Immunol 2016;26(3):168–76.
44. Zhang X, Zhao Y, Zheng Y, et al. The effects of prolonged infusion on reducing oxaliplatin hypersensitivity reactions. J Investig Allergol Clin Immunol 2017; 27(1):65–6.
45. Lee C-W, Matulonis UA, Castells MC. Carboplatin hypersensitivity: a 6-h 12-step protocol effective in 35 desensitizations in patients with gynecological malignancies and mast cell/IgE-mediated reactions. Gynecol Oncol 2004;95(2):370–6.
46. Sloane D, Govindarajulu U, Harrow-Mortelliti J, et al. Safety, costs, and efficacy of rapid drug desensitizations to chemotherapy and monoclonal antibodies. J Allergy Clin Immunol Pract 2016;4(3):497–504.
47. Kolomeyevskaya NV, Lele SB, Miller A, et al. Oxaliplatin is a safe alternative option for patients with recurrent gynecologic cancers after hypersensitivity reaction to carboplatin. Int J Gynecol Cancer 2015;25(1):42–8.
48. Dizon DS, Sabbatini PJ, Aghajanian C, et al. Analysis of patients with epithelial ovarian cancer or fallopian tube carcinoma retreated with cisplatin after the development of a carboplatin allergy. Gynecol Oncol 2002;84(3):378–82.
49. Callahan MB, Lachance JA, Stone RL, et al. Use of cisplatin without desensitization after carboplatin hypersensitivity reaction in epithelial ovarian and primary peritoneal cancer. Am J Obstet Gynecol 2007;197(2):199.e1-4.
50. Zweizig S, Roman LD, Muderspach LI. Death from anaphylaxis to cisplatin: a case report. Gynecol Oncol 1994;53(1):121–2.
51. Rose PG, Metz C, Link N. Desensitization with oxaliplatin in patients intolerant of carboplatin desensitization. Int J Gynecol Cancer 2014;24(9):1603–6.
52. Elligers KT, Davies M, Sanchis D, et al. Rechallenge with cisplatin in a patient with pancreatic cancer who developed a hypersensitivity reaction to oxaliplatin. Is skin test useful in this setting? JOP 2008;9(2):197–202. Available at: http://www.ncbi.nlm.nih.gov/pubmed/18326929. Accessed March 19, 2017.
53. Enrique E, Malek T, Castelló JV, et al. Usefulness of skin testing with platinum salts to demonstrate lack of cross-reactivity between carboplatin and cisplatin. Ann Allergy Asthma Immunol 2008;100(1):86.
54. Syrigou E, Makrilia N, Vassias A, et al. Administration of cisplatin in three patients with carboplatin hypersensitivity: is skin testing useful? Anticancer Drugs 2010; 21(3):333–8.

Management of Hypersensitivity Reactions to Taxanes

Matthieu Picard, MD, FRCPC

KEYWORDS

- Taxane • Paclitaxel • Docetaxel • Allergy • Hypersensitivity • Skin test
- Desensitization and challenge

KEY POINTS

- The incidence of immediate hypersensitivity reaction (HSR) to taxanes varies greatly between molecules from 10% with paclitaxel to less than 1% with cabazitaxel.
- Two mechanisms could account for immediate HSRs to taxanes: complement activation caused by the emulsifying agents (Cremophor EL and polysorbate 80) used in their formulation and an IgE-mediated reaction.
- Almost all patients who experienced an immediate HSR to taxanes can be safely retreated and many of those do not require desensitization.
- The decision to re-expose a patient to taxanes through desensitization or challenge should be based on the severity of the reaction and on the skin test result.
- Because the risk of recurrent reaction decreases with repeated exposures to taxanes, desensitization protocols can be progressively shortened in patients with good tolerance with the aim of eventually resuming regular infusions.

INTRODUCTION

Paclitaxel (taxol) is a taxane antineoplastic agent that is widely used in the treatment of various types of cancers, such as ovarian, breast, and lung cancer.[1] However, it causes immediate hypersensitivity reactions (HSRs) in around 10% of patients despite premedication with antihistamines and a corticosteroid.[2–4] Docetaxel (taxotere) is another taxane molecule and is used for treating a wide variety of cancers.[5] It must also be administered along with a corticosteroid premedication to reduce the incidence of immediate HSRs.[5–7] The newer taxanes, nanoparticle albumin-bound

Disclosures: No funding was received for this work. M. Picard has received consultancy fees from Algorithme Pharma, and has received lecture fees from Sanofi and Nestle.
Department of Medicine, Division of Allergy and Immunology, Hôpital Maisonneuve-Rosemont, Université de Montréal, 5415 boulevard de l'Assomption, Montréal, Québec H1T 2M4, Canada
E-mail address: matthieu.picard@umontreal.ca

(nab)-paclitaxel (abraxane) and cabazitaxel (jevtana) can also cause immediate HSRs, although more rarely than the older taxanes.[8-11] This article reviews the clinical presentation, diagnosis, and management of HSRs to taxanes and discusses the different options for their safe readministration.

TERMINOLOGY

The International Consensus on drug allergy defines HSRs as reactions that clinically resemble an allergic reaction even if an immunologic mechanism has not been demonstrated.[12] It also differentiates between immediate and nonimmediate HSRs depending on the onset of the reaction (immediate, ≤ 1 hour after drug administration; nonimmediate, >1 hour). Occasionally, immediate HSRs to taxanes can occur a few hours after the infusion. This terminology is used in this review.

EPIDEMIOLOGY

Table 1 gives a brief description of the different taxanes in clinical use and the incidence of immediate HSRs associated with each molecule.

Paclitaxel

Phase I studies of paclitaxel revealed that a high percentage of patients suffered from immediate HSRs, most commonly during the first administration of the drug.[13-15] Premedication with antihistamines and a corticosteroid was soon implemented to mitigate this important adverse event.[13] Currently, around 10% of patients treated with paclitaxel will develop an immediate HSR despite premedication.[2-4] Two premedication regimens can be used. Both regimens contain an H1 (diphenhydramine) and an H2 (ranitidine, cimetidine, or famotidine) antihistamine given 30 to 60 minutes before the infusion.[1,4] They differ in that the standard regimen consists of 2 doses of dexamethasone administered the night before and the morning of the infusion, whereas the simplified protocol consists of a single dose of dexamethasone given 30 to 60 minutes before the infusion.[4] Although the single-dose protocol could entail a slightly higher risk of reaction, both protocols are considered acceptable options for premedication.[4,16,17]

Docetaxel

Early clinical trials of docetaxel were also complicated by a high incidence of immediate HSRs and by an adverse event specific to this taxane: fluid retention caused by capillary protein leak.[18-21] Premedication with dexamethasone given for 3 days starting the day before docetaxel administration helped reduce the incidence of immediate HSRs to around 5% and that of fluid retention to between 3.5% and 16.5%.[6,7,22,23]

Nab-Paclitaxel

Nab-paclitaxel is a newer paclitaxel formulation that does not contain Cremophor EL, which is considered responsible for most immediate HSRs to paclitaxel.[8,24,25] Thus, it can be infused without premedication and at a faster rate than paclitaxel.[8] Although, immediate HSRs are much less frequent than with paclitaxel,[10,11] severe and even fatal reactions have been reported with nab-paclitaxel.[8] Given its ease of administration and safety profile, nab-paclitaxel is increasingly used in place of conventional paclitaxel despite its much higher cost.[26]

Table 1
Description of the different taxanes in clinical use

	Paclitaxel	Docetaxel	Nab-Paclitaxel	Cabazitaxel
Solubilizer	Cremophor-EL	Polysorbate 80	Human serum albumin	Polysorbate 80
FDA-approved indications	Ovarian cancer, breast cancer, non-small cell lung carcinoma, AIDS-related Kaposi sarcoma	Breast cancer, prostate cancer, non-small cell lung carcinoma, head and neck cancer, gastric adenocarcinoma	Breast cancer, non-small cell lung carcinoma, pancreatic adenocarcinoma	Prostate cancer
Administration	Over 3 h every 3 wk or over 1 h every week	Over 1 h every 3 wk	Over 30 min every 3 wk or weekly	Over 1 h every 3 wk
Premedication	Diphenhydramine Ranitidine Dexamethasone	Dexamethasone	None	Diphenhydramine Ranitidine Dexamethasone
Incidence of immediate HSR	10%	5%	4%	<1%[a]

Abbreviations: AIDS, acquired immune deficiency syndrome; FDA, US Food and Drug Administration.
[a] In patients on concomitant prednisone therapy as part of the treatment regimen for prostate cancer.

Cabazitaxel

Cabazitaxel was developed to treat castration-resistant prostate cancer in patients whose tumor had progressed after treatment with docetaxel.[9,27] It is administered with premedication consisting of antihistamines and a corticosteroid.[9] Phase III clinical trials in subjects with prostate cancer did not detect any HSR.[28,29] This is in contrast with a phase II clinical trial performed on subjects with breast cancer that found a 6% incidence of immediate HSRs.[30]

PATHOPHYSIOLOGY

Taxanes are poorly soluble molecules. Therefore, to allow intravenous administration, emulsifying agents were used in their formulation: Cremophor EL for paclitaxel and polysorbate 80 for docetaxel and cabazitaxel.[22,27,31] In contrast, nab-paclitaxel uses human serum albumin to create nanoparticles of paclitaxel molecules.[24] Cremophor EL and polysorbate 80 are capable of causing complement activation in vitro and it is hypothesized that through production of anaphylatoxins they could trigger immediate HSRs in vivo, thereby explaining why most patients experience immediate HSRs on first exposure to taxanes if no premedication is used.[32,33] More recently, the possibility of an immunoglobulin (Ig)E-mediated mechanism has been raised based on the finding that a positive skin test result to paclitaxel and/or docetaxel could be elicited in a subset of patients who had experienced an immediate HSR to these molecules.[34–37] Also, acute elevations in serum tryptase and 24-hour urine N-methylhistamine have been reported following severe immediate HSRs to taxanes, thus indicating mast cell activation.[34,38] An IgE-mediated mechanism may be more likely if the HSR was severe and involved flushing.[34] Interestingly, patients with a positive skin test result generally experienced the HSR on their first exposure to taxane, raising the possibility that sensitization had occurred beforehand.[34] Taxanes molecules can be isolated from yew tree pollen, as well as from hazelnut trees and its nuts, providing potential sources of environmental exposure.[39,40] Finally, atopy seems to be a risk factor for immediate HSR to taxanes and to increase the risk of a recurrent HSR on re-exposure.[34,38]

CLINICAL FEATURES
Immediate Hypersensitivity Reactions

Immediate HSRs to taxanes generally occur during the first cycle, within minutes of starting the infusion, and usually resolve promptly after the infusion is stopped.[3,34,41] Cutaneous symptoms (most commonly flushing) are present in most patients.[34,41] Chest, back, and abdominal pain are also frequently seen, as well as respiratory symptoms.[34,41] More severe reactions are characterized by oxygen desaturation and/or hypotension.[34,41] It is clinically useful to divide immediate HSRs as mild (grade 1), moderate (grade 2), and severe (grade 3) because this classification can guide the strategy used for re-exposure (**Table 2**).[34,41]

Nonimmediate Hypersensitivity Reactions

Nonimmediate HSRs to taxanes usually consist of a skin eruption, described as maculopapular and sometimes as flushing, with onset from several hours to 15 days after the drug infusion.[34] The mechanism of these reactions is unknown but a short course of corticosteroids for several days after the infusion is sometimes used to help prevent a recurrence.[34] Although in most patients these HSRs usually abide after several exposures, in some they can be the prelude to an immediate HSR.[34] Skin testing could be useful in detecting this particular subset of patients.[34] Cases of severe

Table 2		
Severity grading of immediate hypersensitivity reactions		
Grade	**Severity**	**Description**
1	Mild	Symptoms are limited to the skin (eg, flushing) or involve a single organ or system and are mild (eg, mild back pain)
2	Moderate	Symptoms involve at least 2 organs or systems (eg, flushing and dyspnea) but there is no significant drop in blood pressure or in oxygen saturation.
3	Severe	Symptoms typically involve at least 2 organs or systems and there is a significant drop in blood pressure (systolic≤90 mm Hg and/or syncope) and/or oxygen saturation (≤92%).

Adapted from Picard M, Pur L, Caiado J, et al. Risk stratification and skin testing to guide re-exposure in taxane-induced hypersensitivity reactions. J Allergy Clin Immunol 2016;137(4):1156; with permission.

nonimmediate HSRs (Stevens-Johnson syndrome, toxic epidermal necrolysis, acute interstitial pneumonitis, and subacute cutaneous lupus erythematosus) have been reported in association with paclitaxel, docetaxel, and nab-paclitaxel.[8,42–50] Re-exposure to taxanes should not be reattempted in those patients.

DIAGNOSTIC TESTS

Although the diagnosis of an immediate HSR to taxane is usually straightforward, several diagnostic tests can be useful to guide the re-treatment strategy and to sometimes rule out an alternative diagnosis.

Tryptase

It could be useful to measure the serum tryptase level within 4 hours of a severe immediate HSR.[34] The result should be compared with a baseline tryptase value, which is usually obtained several days or weeks after the reaction. An increase in the tryptase level by a factor of 1.2 times plus 2 ng/ml compared with baseline would indicate mast cell activation even if the absolute value is equal to or less than11.4 ng/ml.[51] In addition, if the baseline level is greater than the upper limit of normal, it should prompt an investigation for an underlying mast cell disease.[52] This information should be taken into account when re-exposing the patient to taxanes by using a more prudent approach in patients with documented elevations in mast cell mediators.[34]

Skin Testing

Skin testing could be useful to identify a subset of patients in whom an IgE-mediated mechanism is present and who would, therefore, benefit from re-exposure through desensitization.[34–37] The proportion of patients with an IgE-mediated allergy among all patients with immediate HSRs to taxanes varies greatly between populations from less than 10% to around 70%.[34,35,53] Therefore, the necessity for a skin test may vary according to the likelihood of eliciting a positive result. As previously mentioned, patients with more severe reactions and those whose reaction involved flushing may be more likely to have a positive skin test result.[34] Re-exposure to taxane should never be delayed only to allow skin testing, which should ideally be performed at least 2 weeks after the reaction to avoid false-negative results.[34] Skin testing concentrations for paclitaxel are 1 mg/ml for a skin prick test (SPT) and up to 0.01 mg/ml for an intradermal test (IDT).[34] For docetaxel, SPT and IDT should be performed at

0.4 mg/ml.[34] One group has reported that higher concentrations were nonirritating but they encountered false-positive results with paclitaxel at 6 mg/ml IDT.[36] Skin testing with nab-paclitaxel and cabazitaxel has not been studied.

DIFFERENTIAL DIAGNOSIS

Several other medications that are often administered shortly before or after taxanes can elicit immediate HSRs. Ondansetron, an antiemetic drug; ranitidine, an H2 antihistamine; and dexamethasone, a corticosteroid, are often given shortly before the start of the taxane infusion. IgE-mediated reactions have been reported with these drugs, albeit rarely.[54–56] The possibility that these medications are the cause of the HSR rather than the taxane should be entertained if atypical features are present. For example, if the reaction occurred after several well-tolerated cycles of taxane or if the reaction recurred despite desensitization and very early in its course (eg, during step 1), one should evaluate the possibility that a drug given as premedication is responsible for the reaction through skin testing. Carboplatin is often given right after the end of the taxane infusion and is associated with an increasing incidence of immediate HSRs from the sixth cycle onwards.[57,58] Therefore, immediate HSRs that occur during or shortly after the end of the carboplatin infusion are more likely to be caused by this medication, especially if prior taxane cycles were well tolerated.[34] Finally, dexamethasone can cause facial flushing with onset, usually several hours after intake, which lasts for several days.[59] However, this condition is usually benign and does not require any treatment.

RE-EXPOSURE TO TAXANES AFTER A HYPERSENSITIVITY REACTION

Almost all patients, regardless of the severity of the immediate HSR, can be safely re-exposed to taxanes either through desensitization or a regular infusion.[3,34,41] Also, the risk of having a recurrent reaction steadily decreases with repeated exposures regardless of the method used for re-exposure.[3,13,34,41] After an immediate HSR, many patients will tolerate the next infusion through a regular infusion without the need for desensitization.[3,13,36,41] However, depending on the population studied, a significant proportion of patients will have a recurrent HSR with this approach that is sometimes more severe than the initial reaction.[34,36,41] Also, it may be difficult to convince a patient with a recent HSR to receive the same medication without any additional precaution.[36] In contrast, desensitization using the 3-bag, 12-step desensitization protocol developed at Brigham and Women's Hospital and Dana-Farber Cancer Institute (BWH-DFCI) has been shown to be safe and has a very high success rate, allowing patients with HSR of any severity to be retreated with taxanes.[34,38,60,61] A suggested approach to taxane reintroduction is depicted in **Fig. 1**. It is generally agreed that the severity of the initial HSR should guide the method chosen for re-exposure: desensitization versus challenge.[3,34,36,41] In addition, skin testing could also be useful because a positive skin test result may indicate an IgE-mediated mechanism and thus a higher risk of reaction on re-exposure.[34,35] Therefore, patients with a positive skin test result should be retreated as if they had a severe HSR (see **Fig. 1**). Patients with mild reactions are often rechallenged by their treating oncologist and referred to an allergy specialist only in the event of a recurrent HSR.[3,41] Almost all patients with mild HSRs tolerates a rechallenge and can safely continue treatment with regular infusions.[3,41] In contrast, even if some patients with a severe HSR can tolerate a rechallenge without reaction, it is generally advisable to re-expose those patients through desensitization.[34,41] A 3-bag, 12-step protocol or, in very severe cases, a 4-bag, 16-step protocol can be used (**Table 3**).[34] If no HSR occurs with desensitization,

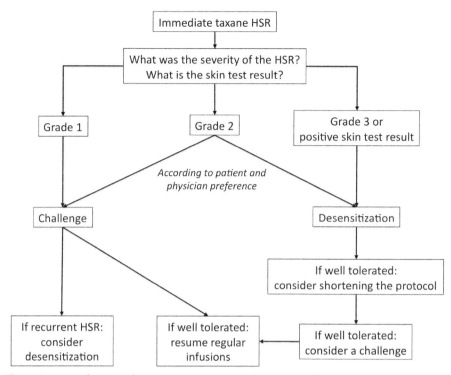

Fig. 1. Suggested approach to taxane re-exposure in patients who experienced an immediate HSR.

the protocol could then be progressively shortened by cutting 1 bag at a time and/or by increasing the final infusion rate to 160 mL/h.[34] If a 1-bag desensitization protocol is well-tolerated, a challenge procedure can be attempted and, if well-tolerated, the patient could then resume regular infusions (**Table 4**).[34] For patients with a moderate HSR, the decision between desensitization and challenge is often made on a case-by-case basis. For example, if the patient is reluctant to undergo retreatment with taxanes because of the fear of a recurrent HSR, despite adequate reassurance, or if the physician, based on personal experience, considers that there is a significant risk of recurrent reaction, a desensitization protocol should be chosen.[34]

DESENSITIZATION PROTOCOLS AND PREMEDICATION

Various desensitization protocols for taxanes have been studied with variable safety outcomes.[3,7,36,37,62–64] The BWH-DFCI 3-bag, 12-step protocol has been the most studied and has an excellent safety record (see **Table 3**).[34,38,60,61] Patients are premedicated, as for regular infusions, before these procedures, which should be performed with a 1-to-1 nursing ratio and under the supervision of an allergist with expertise in drug desensitization.[34] When second-generation antihistamines are available, it is customary to replace diphenhydramine with cetirizine.[34] In patients with a severe HSR or with a recurrent HSR despite desensitization, it may be useful to add a single dose of montelukast (10 mg) and/or aspirin (325 mg) 30 to 60 minutes before the infusion to the premedication regimen.[34,65] To alleviate the anxiety associated with these procedures, a benzodiazepine such as lorazepam can be used.[34] Approximately

Table 3
Desensitization protocols for taxanes

Example with paclitaxel 250 mg

Volume per bag: 250 ml

Bag A: contains total dose minus cumulative dose administered with previous bags (eg, 250 mg minus (varies depending on the protocol from 1.875 to 1.973 mg)/250 mL)

Bag B: contains 1/10th of the total dose to be administered (eg, 25 mg/250 mL)

Bag C: contains 1/100th of the total dose to be administered (eg, 2.5 mg/250 mL)

Bag D: contains 1/1000th of the total dose to be administered (eg, 0.25 mg/250 mL)

Only Bag A is completely infused. A fraction of the total volume of Bags B, C and D is infused to the patient. What remains is discarded.

Protocols					4-bag	3-bag	2-bag	1-bag
Bag	Step	Infusion rate (mL/h)	Time (minutes)		Cumulative Dose (mg)	Cumulative Dose (mg)	Cumulative dose (mg)	Cumulative dose (mg)
D	1	2.5	15		0.0006	NA	NA	NA
D	2	5	15		0.001	NA	NA	NA
D	3	10	15		0.002	NA	NA	NA
D	4	20	15		0.005	NA	NA	NA
C	5	2.5	15		0.011	0.005	NA	NA
C	6	5	15		0.023	0.018	NA	NA
C	7	10	15		0.048	0.043	NA	NA
C	8	20	15		0.098	0.093	NA	NA

B	9	5	15	0.223	0.218	0.125	NA
B	10	10	15	0.473	0.468	0.375	NA
B	11	20	15	0.973	0.968	0.875	NA
B	12	40	15	1.973	1.968	1.875	NA
A	13	10	15	4.454	4.448	4.356	2.5
A	14	20	15	9.414	9.409	9.319	7.5
A	15	40	15	19.335	19.330	19.244	17.5
A	16	80	174	250	250	250	250

The final infusion rate can be increased to 120 mL/h and then to 160 mL/h if well tolerated, waiting 15 min between steps.

Duration of the protocols (hours) compared with a regular infusion (3 h)

4-bag: 6.7
3-bag: 5.7
2-bag: 4.7
1-bag: 3.7

Increasing the final infusion rate to 160 mL/h reduces the duration of the protocol by approximately 1 hour.

Abbreviation: NA, not applicable.
Data from Picard M, Pur L, Caiado J, et al. Risk stratification and skin testing to guide re-exposure in taxane-induced hypersensitivity reactions. J Allergy Clin Immunol 2016;137(4):1154–64.e1–12.

Table 4
Challenge protocols for taxanes

Paclitaxel (135–175 mg/m²) Infused Every 3 wk Over 3 h (Example = 294 mg)

Bag	Volume (mL) per Bag	Concentration (mg/mL) per Bag	Amount (mL) of Bag Infused	Dose Infused (mg) per Bag	Dose Infused (mg) per Step	Cumulative dose (mg)
Solution 1	250	1.176	250	294		
Step	Rate (mL/h)	Time (min)	Volume Infused (mL)			
1	2	15	0.5		0.588	0.588
2	8	15	2		2.352	2.940
3	80	185.625	247.5		291.06	294.0

Total time (hours) = 3.59

Paclitaxel (50–80 mg/m²) Infused Weekly Over 1 h (Example = 134 mg)

Bag	Volume (mL) per Bag	Concentration (mg/mL) per Bag	Amount (mL) of Bag Infused	Dose Infused (mg) per Bag	Dose Infused (mg) per Step	Cumulative Dose (mg)
Solution 1	250	0.536	250	134		
Step	Rate (mL/h)	Time (min)	Volume Infused (mL)			
1	2.5	15	0.625		0.335	0.335
2	25	15	6.25		3.35	3.685
3	250	58.35	243.125		290.315	294.0

Total time (hours) = 1.47

Data from Picard M, Pur L, Caiado J, et al. Risk stratification and skin testing to guide re-exposure in taxane-induced hypersensitivity reactions. J Allergy Clin Immunol 2016;137(4):1154–64.e1–12.

20% of patients who undergo desensitization to taxanes will experience an immediate HSR, most commonly during the last step of the protocol.[34] However, these reactions are usually mild and almost never severe.[34] With repeated exposures, the risk of recurrent reactions steadily decreases to around 2%.[34]

CHALLENGE PROCEDURE

The goal of the challenge procedure is to insure that the patient will thereafter tolerate a regular infusion of the drug while minimizing the risks associated with such a reaction (see **Table 4**). One bag of the medication is prepared as if it was to be administered through a regular infusion protocol.[34] However, the infusion is started at a 10-fold to 100-fold slower rate than the regular infusion for 15 minutes, then increased to the regular infusion rate by 10-fold increments.[34] Premedication should be administered as for a regular infusion.[34]

CURRENT CONTROVERSIES

Taxane skin testing remains controversial because most immediate HSRs to these molecules are considered non–IgE-mediated.[41] It is also unclear if the risk of recurrent reaction on re-exposure is increased in patients with a positive skin test result because those patients are usually treated more conservatively than those with a negative result.[34] Another caveat is that the proportion of patients with a positive skin test result varies greatly depending on the population studied.[34–36] Therefore, in a population in which a positive result on taxane skin testing is rare, it may not be necessary to routinely skin test all patients with a taxane HSR. Finally, skin testing may not be feasible in patients who receive weekly treatments of paclitaxel.[34] Skin testing is most useful when it affects the retreatment strategy used in a particular patient.[34] For example, a patient who experiences a recurrent HSR on re-exposure, either through challenge or desensitization, could benefit from skin testing. If skin testing is positive, it likely indicates an IgE-mediated phenomenon and it argues for pursuing desensitization procedures. In contrast, if skin testing is negative, it remains possible that the patient will eventually tolerate regular infusions and a challenge procedure could be reattempted. Likewise, a patient with a severe HSR would benefit from skin testing because, if it were negative, a challenge procedure could be attempted once tolerance to desensitization is established, whereas, if it were positive, a challenge would be discouraged even if the patient tolerates desensitization.[34]

Because many patients with an immediate taxane HSR tolerate re-exposure through a regular infusion, it remains to be defined which patients truly benefit from desensitization.[3,36,41] Some investigators consider desensitization only in patients with a recurrent reaction on rechallenge or who suffered a severe HSR.[3,36] Recently, Banerji and colleagues[41] reviewed all cases of patients with immediate HSRs to paclitaxel at Massachusetts General Hospital over a 5-year period. They concluded that patients with mild reactions (flushing and/or back pain) could be safely rechallenged, albeit at half the normal infusion rate, and that patients with moderate to severe reactions should be re-exposed through desensitization.[41] It should be kept in mind that severe HSRs, some fatal, have been described during rechallenge procedures to paclitaxel despite a slower infusion rate and added premedication.[13,36,41,66] In contrast, the safety of desensitization to taxanes using the BWH-DFCI protocol has been clearly established.[34,38,60,61]

SUMMARY

Although immediate HSRs to taxanes are common, they should not lead to drug discontinuation because almost all patients can be safely retreated with these molecules either through desensitization or rechallenge. The severity of the HSR and the taxane skin test result can help the clinician decide between these 2 options. Future studies on the subject will certainly allow a better understanding of these HSRs and will help refine the approach to retreatment.

REFERENCES

1. Taxol Prescribing Information. 2014. Available at: http://packageinserts.bms.com/pi/pi_taxol.pdf. Accessed January 13, 2014.
2. Ratanajarusiri T, Sriuranpong V, Sitthideatphaiboon P, et al. A difference in the incidences of hypersensitivity reactions to original and generic taxanes. Chemotherapy 2017;62(2):134–9.
3. Markman M, Kennedy A, Webster K, et al. Paclitaxel-associated hypersensitivity reactions: experience of the gynecologic oncology program of the Cleveland Clinic Cancer Center. J Clin Oncol 2000;18(1):102–5.
4. Kwon JS, Elit L, Finn M, et al. A comparison of two prophylactic regimens for hypersensitivity reactions to paclitaxel. Gynecol Oncol 2002;84(3):420–5.
5. Taxotere Prescribing Information. 2013. Available at: http://products.sanofi.us/Taxotere/taxotere.html. Accessed December 24, 2013.
6. Vasey PA, Jayson GC, Gordon A, et al. Phase III randomized trial of docetaxel-carboplatin versus paclitaxel-carboplatin as first-line chemotherapy for ovarian carcinoma. J Natl Cancer Inst 2004;96(22):1682–91.
7. Syrigou E, Dannos I, Kotteas E, et al. Hypersensitivity reactions to docetaxel: retrospective evaluation and development of a desensitization protocol. Int Arch Allergy Immunol 2011;156(3):320–4.
8. Abraxane Prescribing Information. 2014. Available at: http://abraxane.com/downloads/Abraxane_PrescribingInformation.pdf. Accessed January 3, 2014.
9. Cabazitaxel Prescribing Information. 2014. Available at: http://products.sanofi.us/jevtana/jevtana.html. Accessed January 12, 2014.
10. Gradishar WJ, Tjulandin S, Davidson N, et al. Phase III trial of nanoparticle albumin-bound paclitaxel compared with polyethylated castor oil-based paclitaxel in women with breast cancer. J Clin Oncol 2005;23(31):7794–803.
11. Yamamoto Y, Kawano I, Iwase H. Nab-paclitaxel for the treatment of breast cancer: efficacy, safety, and approval. Onco Targets Ther 2011;4:123–36.
12. Demoly P, Adkinson NF, Brockow K, et al. International Consensus on drug allergy. Allergy 2014;69(4):420–37.
13. Weiss RB, Donehower RC, Wiernik PH, et al. Hypersensitivity reactions from taxol. J Clin Oncol 1990;8(7):1263–8.
14. Wiernik PH, Schwartz EL, Strauman JJ, et al. Phase I clinical and pharmacokinetic study of taxol. Cancer Res 1987;47(9):2486–93.
15. Kris MG, O'Connell JP, Gralla RJ, et al. Phase I trial of taxol given as a 3-hour infusion every 21 days. Cancer Treat Rep 1986;70(5):605–7.
16. Markman M, Kennedy A, Webster K, et al. Simplified regimen for the prevention of paclitaxel-associated hypersensitivity reactions. J Clin Oncol 1997;15(12):3517.
17. Chen FC, Wang LH, Zheng XY, et al. Meta-analysis of the effects of oral and intravenous dexamethasone premedication in the prevention of paclitaxel-induced allergic reactions. Oncotarget 2016;8:19236–43.

18. Mertens WC, Eisenhauer EA, Jolivet J, et al. Docetaxel in advanced renal carcinoma. A phase II trial of the National Cancer Institute of Canada Clinical Trials Group. Ann Oncol 1994;5(2):185–7.

19. Pazdur R, Lassere Y, Soh LT, et al. Phase II trial of docetaxel (Taxotere) in metastatic colorectal carcinoma. Ann Oncol 1994;5(5):468–70.

20. Francis PA, Rigas JR, Kris MG, et al. Phase II trial of docetaxel in patients with stage III and IV non-small-cell lung cancer. J Clin Oncol 1994;12(6):1232–7.

21. Semb KA, Aamdal S, Oian P. Capillary protein leak syndrome appears to explain fluid retention in cancer patients who receive docetaxel treatment. J Clin Oncol 1998;16(10):3426–32.

22. Cortes JE, Pazdur R. Docetaxel. J Clin Oncol 1995;13(10):2643–55.

23. Piccart MJ, Klijn J, Paridaens R, et al. Corticosteroids significantly delay the onset of docetaxel-induced fluid retention: final results of a randomized study of the European Organization for Research and Treatment of Cancer Investigational Drug Branch for Breast Cancer. J Clin Oncol 1997;15(9):3149–55.

24. Stinchcombe TE. Nanoparticle albumin-bound paclitaxel: a novel Cremphor-EL-free formulation of paclitaxel. Nanomedicine (Lond) 2007;2(4):415–23.

25. Cucinotto I, Fiorillo L, Gualtieri S, et al. Nanoparticle albumin bound Paclitaxel in the treatment of human cancer: nanodelivery reaches prime-time? J Drug Deliv 2013;2013:905091.

26. Sofias AM, Dunne M, Storm G, et al. The battle of "nano" paclitaxel. Adv Drug Deliv Rev 2017. [Epub ahead of print].

27. Galsky MD, Dritselis A, Kirkpatrick P, et al. Cabazitaxel. Nat Rev Drug Discov 2010;9(9):677–8.

28. de Bono JS, Oudard S, Ozguroglu M, et al. Prednisone plus cabazitaxel or mitoxantrone for metastatic castration-resistant prostate cancer progressing after docetaxel treatment: a randomised open-label trial. Lancet 2010;376(9747): 1147–54.

29. Bracarda S, Gernone A, Gasparro D, et al. Real-world cabazitaxel safety: the Italian early-access program in metastatic castration-resistant prostate cancer. Future Oncol 2013;10:975–83.

30. Pivot X, Koralewski P, Hidalgo JL, et al. A multicenter phase II study of XRP6258 administered as a 1-h i.v. infusion every 3 weeks in taxane-resistant metastatic breast cancer patients. Ann Oncol 2008;19(9):1547–52.

31. Exposito O, Bonfill M, Moyano E, et al. Biotechnological production of taxol and related taxoids: current state and prospects. Anticancer Agents Med Chem 2009; 9(1):109–21.

32. Szebeni J, Muggia FM, Alving CR. Complement activation by Cremophor EL as a possible contributor to hypersensitivity to paclitaxel: an in vitro study. J Natl Cancer Inst 1998;90(4):300–6.

33. Weiszhar Z, Czucz J, Revesz C, et al. Complement activation by polyethoxylated pharmaceutical surfactants: Cremophor-EL, Tween-80 and Tween-20. Eur J Pharm Sci 2012;45(4):492–8.

34. Picard M, Pur L, Caiado J, et al. Risk stratification and skin testing to guide reexposure in taxane-induced hypersensitivity reactions. J Allergy Clin Immunol 2016;137(4):1154–64.e1112.

35. Prieto Garcia A, Pineda de la Losa F. Immunoglobulin E-mediated severe anaphylaxis to paclitaxel. J Investig Allergol Clin Immunol 2010;20(2):170–1.

36. Alvarez-Cuesta E, Madrigal-Burgaleta R, Angel-Pereira D, et al. Delving into cornerstones of hypersensitivity to antineoplastic and biological agents: value of diagnostic tools prior to desensitization. Allergy 2015;70(7):784–94.

37. Madrigal-Burgaleta R, Berges-Gimeno MP, Angel-Pereira D, et al. Hypersensitivity and desensitization to antineoplastic agents: outcomes of 189 procedures with a new short protocol and novel diagnostic tools assessment. Allergy 2013;68: 853–61.

38. Feldweg AM, Lee CW, Matulonis UA, et al. Rapid desensitization for hypersensitivity reactions to paclitaxel and docetaxel: a new standard protocol used in 77 successful treatments. Gynecol Oncol 2005;96(3):824–9.

39. Vanhaelen M, Duchateau J, Vanhaelen-Fastre R, et al. Taxanes in *Taxus baccata* pollen: cardiotoxicity and/or allergenicity? Planta Med 2002;68(1):36–40.

40. Bukacel DG, Bander R, Ibrahim RB. Cross-reactivity between paclitaxel and hazelnut: a case report. J Oncol Pharm Pract 2007;13(1):53–5.

41. Banerji A, Lax T, Guyer A, et al. Management of hypersensitivity reactions to Carboplatin and Paclitaxel in an outpatient oncology infusion center: a 5-year review. J Allergy Clin Immunol Pract 2014;2(4):428–33.

42. Hiraki A, Aoe K, Murakami T, et al. Stevens-Johnson syndrome induced by paclitaxel in a patient with squamous cell carcinoma of the lung: a case report. Anticancer Res 2004;24(2C):1135–7.

43. Sawada Y, Sugita K, Kabashima R, et al. Docetaxel-induced Stevens-Johnson syndrome with regenerating epidermis composed of atypical keratinocytes. J Eur Acad Dermatol Venereol 2009;23(11):1333–5.

44. Taj A. Docetaxel-induced hypersensitivity pneumonitis mimicking lymphangitic carcinomatosis in a patient with metastatic adenocarcinoma of the lung. Hematol Oncol Stem Cell Ther 2013;6(3–4):117–9.

45. Nagata S, Ueda N, Yoshida Y, et al. Severe interstitial pneumonitis associated with the administration of taxanes. J Infect Chemother 2010;16(5):340–4.

46. Read WL, Mortimer JE, Picus J. Severe interstitial pneumonitis associated with docetaxel administration. Cancer 2002;94(3):847–53.

47. Von Hoff DD, Ervin T, Arena FP, et al. Increased survival in pancreatic cancer with nab-paclitaxel plus gemcitabine. N Engl J Med 2013;369(18):1691–703.

48. Chen M, Crowson AN, Woofter M, et al. Docetaxel (taxotere) induced subacute cutaneous lupus erythematosus: report of 4 cases. J Rheumatol 2004;31(4): 818–20.

49. Marchetti MA, Noland MM, Dillon PM, et al. Taxane associated subacute cutaneous lupus erythematosus. Dermatol Online J 2013;19(8):19259.

50. Lamond NW, Younis T, Purdy K, et al. Drug-induced subacute cutaneous lupus erythematosus associated with nab-paclitaxel therapy. Curr Oncol 2013;20(5): e484–7.

51. Valent P, Akin C, Arock M, et al. Definitions, criteria and global classification of mast cell disorders with special reference to mast cell activation syndromes: a consensus proposal. Int Arch Allergy Immunol 2012;157(3):215–25.

52. Picard M, Giavina-Bianchi P, Mezzano V, et al. Expanding spectrum of mast cell activation disorders: monoclonal and idiopathic mast cell activation syndromes. Clin Ther 2013;35(5):548–62.

53. Giavina-Bianchi P, Caiado J, Picard M, et al. Rapid desensitization to chemotherapy and monoclonal antibodies is effective and safe. Allergy 2013;68(11): 1482–4.

54. Leung J, Guyer A, Banerji A. IgE-mediated hypersensitivity to ondansetron and safe use of palonosetron. J Allergy Clin Immunol Pract 2013;1(5):526–7.

55. Park KH, Pai J, Song DG, et al. Ranitidine-induced anaphylaxis: clinical features, cross-reactivity, and skin testing. Clin Exp Allergy 2016;46(4):631–9.

56. Rachid R, Leslie D, Schneider L, et al. Hypersensitivity to systemic corticosteroids: an infrequent but potentially life-threatening condition. J Allergy Clin Immunol 2011;127(2):524–8.
57. Zanotti KM, Rybicki LA, Kennedy AW, et al. Carboplatin skin testing: a skin-testing protocol for predicting hypersensitivity to carboplatin chemotherapy. J Clin Oncol 2001;19(12):3126–9.
58. Schwartz JR, Bandera C, Bradley A, et al. Does the platinum-free interval predict the incidence or severity of hypersensitivity reactions to carboplatin? The experience from Women and Infants' Hospital. Gynecol Oncol 2007;105(1):81–3.
59. Decadron. Available at: https://www.accessdata.fda.gov/drugsatfda_docs/label/2004/11664slr062_decadron_lbl.pdf. Accessed March 31, 2017.
60. Lee CW, Matulonis UA, Castells MC. Rapid inpatient/outpatient desensitization for chemotherapy hypersensitivity: standard protocol effective in 57 patients for 255 courses. Gynecol Oncol 2005;99(2):393–9.
61. Castells MC, Tennant NM, Sloane DE, et al. Hypersensitivity reactions to chemotherapy: outcomes and safety of rapid desensitization in 413 cases. J Allergy Clin Immunol 2008;122(3):574–80.
62. Essayan DM, Kagey-Sobotka A, Colarusso PJ, et al. Successful parenteral desensitization to paclitaxel. J Allergy Clin Immunol 1996;97(1 Pt 1):42–6.
63. Robinson JB, Singh D, Bodurka-Bevers DC, et al. Hypersensitivity reactions and the utility of oral and intravenous desensitization in patients with gynecologic malignancies. Gynecol Oncol 2001;82(3):550–8.
64. Gastaminza G, de la Borbolla JM, Goikoetxea MJ, et al. A new rapid desensitization protocol for chemotherapy agents. J Investig Allergol Clin Immunol 2011;21(2):108–12.
65. Breslow RG, Caiado J, Castells MC. Acetylsalicylic acid and montelukast block mast cell mediator-related symptoms during rapid desensitization. Ann Allergy Asthma Immunol 2009;102(2):155–60.
66. A fatal anaphylactic reaction to paclitaxel is described, which was preceded by a possible delayed reaction to the initial infusion. Allergy Asthma Proc 2011;32(1):79.

Monoclonal Antibodies Hypersensitivity
Prevalence and Management

Rafael Bonamichi Santos, MD, Violeta Régnier Galvão, MD, PhD*

KEYWORDS

- Monoclonal antibodies • Biological agents • Rapid drug desensitization
- Drug allergy • Skin test • Immunoglobulin E • Tryptase

KEY POINTS

- Monoclonal antibodies (mAbs) are effective in the treatment of autoimmune, neoplastic, and inflammatory diseases.
- Hypersensitivity reactions (HSR) secondary to mAbs are being more reported.
- Some of the main mAbs in clinical use and their associated HSR are reviewed.
- The authors propose algorithms for the treatment of mAb-related HSR and for desensitization indications.

INTRODUCTION

The first monoclonal antibodies (mAbs) were created in the mid 1970s to target specific mutations and defects in protein structures expressed in several diseases and conditions. They are now part of mainstream treatments for neoplastic, autoimmune, and chronic inflammatory diseases, which led to an increase in the reports of hypersensitivity reactions (HSR) secondary to this drug class.

First-generation mAbs are monospecific/bifunctional antibodies, with one binding site to a specific antigen and an intact Fc-part binding to an Fc receptor on accessory cells. In 2009, catumaxomab, a bispecific/trifunctional mAb, was approved for the treatment of malignant ascites in patients with cancer.[1]

There are 3 types of bispecific mAbs, as follows:

- Trifunctional antibody: presents binding sites for 2 different antigens. In addition, its intact Fc-part can bind to an Fc receptor, on monocytes/macrophages,

Disclosure Statement: The authors have nothing to disclose.
Division of Clinical Immunology and Allergy, University of São Paulo, School of Medicine, Av. Dr. Arnaldo, 455-Cerqueira César, São Paulo, São Paulo 01246-903, Brazil
* Corresponding author.
E-mail address: violeta_galvao@yahoo.com.br

natural killers, dendritic cells, or other Fc receptor–expressing cells to the tumor cells, leading to their destruction.[2]

- Chemically linked Fab: consists only of Fab regions. It is considered non–mmunoglobulin G (IgG)-like.
- Bispecific T-cell engager: fusion proteins consisting of 2 single-chain variable fragments. The protein sources are different antibodies, or amino acid sequences from 4 different genes, on a single peptide chain.

Some of mAbs' mechanisms of action include the following:

- Neutralization of targeted molecule's functions (infliximab: anti–tumor necrosis factor-α [TNF-α]).
- Modulating signaling pathways by blocking targeted cell receptors, also known as checkpoint therapy (ipilimumab: anti–CTLA-4).
- Cell apoptosis mechanisms:
  - Antibody-dependent cell-mediated cytotoxicity
  - Complement-mediated cell lysis
  - Toxic effect of a conjugate drug molecule linked to the mAb Fc region (tositumomab: radioactively conjugated and brentuximab vedotin: cytotoxic-conjugated).

PHENOTYPES AND ENDOTYPES
Type I Hypersensitivity

Type I hypersensitivity typically occurs within 30 to 120 minutes of the infusion. This type of reaction usually requires a previous exposure to the drug for sensitization to occur,[3] but a notable exception to this rule is a cetuximab-induced HSR.[4] IgE-mediated reactions to this drug might occur because of a previous tick bite (lone star tick, *Amblyomma americanum*) and the consequent development of an anti-α-1,3-galactose antibody.[4]

Various systems can be involved (cutaneous, respiratory, gastrointestinal, cardiovascular, and neurologic), and the severity can range from mild cutaneous symptoms to life-threatening reactions.[5]

Applied subcutaneously, mAbs may cause an IgE-mediated injection-site reaction (ISR), characterized by local redness, warmth, burning, stinging, itching, urticaria. These symptoms usually appear within the first hour of the injection.

Immunoglobulin G–Mediated Reactions

IgG-mediated HSRs are still being studied. On animal models, it was demonstrated that mAbs can stimulate anti-mAb IgGs bound to Fc-gamma-receptors, found on macrophages, basophils, and neutrophils, leading to the release of platelet-activating factor.[6]

Another mechanism could be the activation of the complement system by large immune complexes, generating anaphylatoxins.[6,7] In this case, the clinical presentation would be like that of an IgE-mediated HSR.

Type III Hypersensitivity Reactions

Type III HSRs are secondary to immune complex deposition (mAb + anti-mAb IgG) in small blood vessels located in the skin, kidney, and other organs. This deposition typically occurs 5 to 7 days after the drug exposure.[8,9] Symptoms can include fever, malaise, myalgia, arthralgia/arthritis, jaw pain or tightness, rash, pruritus, erythematous (sometimes urticarial) skin eruption, edema, purpura, and conjunctival hyperemia.[10,11]

Type IV Hypersensitivity Reactions

Delayed, cell-mediated HSRs can be seen at some subcutaneous injection sites, typically following the fourth injection.[12] Such reactions can start in the first hour of the injection and tend to resolve in the subsequent days.[6] Recall reactions, local reactions at the site of the previous injections, are known to occur simultaneously.[12] Severe delayed HSRs to biologicals have been reported, with reports of Stevens-Johnson syndrome and toxic epidermal necrolysis.[13–16]

Cytokine Storm Reactions

Cytokine storm reactions are due to the release of proinflammatory cytokines (TNF-α, interleukin-1 [IL-1] and IL-6) from activated macrophages and other immune cells with FcγR receptors.[17] Patients may experience chills, fever, nausea, malaise, myalgia, and flushing. This type of reaction does not tend to be severe, but it is important to mention the TGN1412 trial, in which 6 volunteers developed multiorgan failure because of a severe cytokine storm caused by an anti-CD28 mAb.[18]

Desensitization may be considered in selected cases. If treatment is well tolerated, a progressive shortening of the rapid drug desensitization (RDD) protocol may be considered.[19,20]

Mixed Reactions

Mixed reactions are characterized by features of a cytokine storm reaction associated with type I HSR features. Increased levels of tryptase, IL-1, IL-6, and TNF-α can all be found; positive skin testing and/or detection of specific IgE antibodies can also occur.

MONOCLONAL ANTIBODIES

Table 1 presents frequently used mAbs, their molecular targets, HSR incidence, and immunologic mechanisms. The nomenclature of mAbs can be found in **Table 2**.[21]

Anti–Tumor Necrosis Factor-α

Infliximab (Remicade)
Infliximab is a chimeric mAb against TNF-α.[22] First-exposure HSRs may occur, but the occurrences peak around the seventh infusion.[19,23]

Patients with anti-infliximab IgGs tend to present a higher risk of immediate HSRs.[24] A subset of infliximab-immediate HSRs has been found to be IgE-mediated reactions. Positive immediate skin tests to infliximab and anti-infliximab IgE were seen on average in 28% and 21% of reactive patients, versus 3% and 10% in tolerant patients, respectively.[25]

Delayed HRS to infliximab may occur 1 to 14 days after infusion[8] and mimic type III HSR, with myalgia, rash, fever, polyarthralgia, pruritus, edema, and malaise.

Etanercept (Enbrel)
Etanercept is a TNF receptor–IgG fusion protein. ISR can occur in up to 37% patients. IgE-mediated HSRs have been described,[26] and desensitization to the drug has been successfully performed.

Adalimumab (Humira)
Adalimumab is a fully human mAb anti-TNF-α. ISRs occur in 20% of patients.[27] Immediate and prolonged ISRs have been reported as well as immediate HSR with a positive intradermal test.[28–30]

Table 1
Monoclonal antibodies hypersensitivity reactions and mechanisms

Target	Drug and Route of Administration	HSR	HSR Mechanisms Based on Clinical Manifestations and/or Laboratory Analysis
TNF-α	Infliximab (Remicade) IV	1%[a,22]	Type I and III[8,24,25,73,77,78]
	Etanercept (Enbrel) SC	<2%[a,79]	Type I and IV[12,26,74]
	Adalimumab (Humira) SC	1%[80]	Type I and III[26,73]
	Golimumab (Simponi) SC	[b]	—
	Certolizumab (Cimzia) SC	[b]	—
CD20	Rituximab (Rituxan) IV	5%–10%[81]	Type I III and cytokine storm[3,9,37]
	Ofatumumab (Arzerra) IV	2%[82]	Type I and cytokine storm[38,39,83]
	Obinutuzumab (Gazyva) IV	Up to 20%[a,42,84]	Cytokine storm[42]
HER-2	Trastuzumab (Herceptin) IV	0.6%–5%[43]	Type I and cytokine storm[19,20,36,44]
	Pertuzumab (Perjeta) IV	11.3[a,46,47]	Type I[47]
IgE	Omalizumab (Xolair) SC	0.09%–0.2%[48,85]	Type III[5]
CD30	Brentuximab (Adcetris) IV	(61–63)[a]	Type I[53–55,86]
EGFR	Cetuximab (Erbitux) IV	1.1–5%[87–90] 14%–27% (Southern USA)[91–93]	Type I[4,94]
VEGF-A	Bevacizumab (Avastin) IV	3 patients[20,62]	Type I and IV[20,62]
IL-6	Tocilizumab (Actemra) IV	0.1%–7%[a,64,95]	Type I and IV[10,64,96]
CCR4	Mogamulizumab (Poteligeo) IV	1 patient[16]	Type IV[16]
EpCAM/CD3	Catumaxomab (Removab) IP	0.8%–5.1%[65]	Cytokine storm[65]

Abbreviations: IP, intraperitoneal; IV, intravenous; SC, subcutaneous.
[a] Case reports of anaphylaxis.
[b] No report to date.

Golimumab (Simponi)

Golimumab is a human IgG1k mAb against TNF-α.[31] It has been shown to induce ISR in 4.4% to 20% of patients and rash in 3.1% to 10.9% of patients.[32,33]

Certolizumab pegol (Cimzia)

Certolizumab is a humanized antigen-binding fragment of an mAb against TNF-α.[34] The incidence of ISR ranged from 0.8% to 2.3% in a study with patients with Rheumatoid arthritis. There were no reports of anaphylactic reactions.[35]

Anti-CD20

Rituximab (Rituxan)

Rituximab is a chimeric mAb against CD20. Reactions consistent with IgE-mediated HSR are estimated to account for 5% to 10% of infusion reactions.[5] Rituximab can cause immediate HSR upon first exposure, as seen in approximately half of patients with a B-cell malignancy, even after premedication.[36] Reactions due to cytokine release have been reported[37] as well as serum sickness–like reactions.[9]

Table 2
Monoclonal antibodies nomenclature

Disease or Target (Substem A)		Immunoglobulin Source (Substem B)
-b(a)- bacterial	Tumors	-xi- chimeric
-c(i)- cardiovascular	-co(l)- colon	-zu- humanized
-f(u)- fungal	-go(t)- testis	-xizu- chimeric-humanized
-k(i)- interleukin	-go(v)- ovary	-u- human
-l(i)- immunomodulating	-ma(r)- mammary	-o- mouse
-s(o)- bone	-me(l)- melanoma	-a- rat
tox(a)- toxin	-pr(o)- prostate	-e- hamster
-v(i)- viral	-tu(m)- miscellaneous	-i- primate
EX: omaLizumab	EX: riTuximab	EX: cetuXimab
bevaCizumab	trasTuzumab	tociliZumab
		adalimUmab

Adapted from International Nonproprietary Names (INN) for biological and biotechnological substances. World Health Organization. 2013. Available at: http://www.who.int/medicines/services/inn/BioRev2013.pdf. Accessed March 12, 2017; with permission.

Ofatumumab (Arzerra)

Ofatumumab is a fully human anti-CD20 mAb. Half of patients tend to present immediate infusion reactions, which are thought to be caused by cytokine release.[38,39] Infusion reactions are less common after the first 2 infusions.[40]

Obinutuzumab (Gazyva)

Obinutuzumab is an anti-CD20 cytolytic mAb.[41] Infusion-related reactions elicited by the drug are common, occurring in 38% to 65% of patients on their first exposure.[41] The most common infusion-related symptoms include nausea, fatigue, dizziness, vomiting, diarrhea, hypertension, flushing, headache, pyrexia, and chills.[41]

Severe infusion reactions were described in 20% of patients on their first infusion, but not on subsequent infusions.[42]

Classic immediate HSR signs and symptoms have been reported, such as hypotension, tachycardia, dyspnea, bronchospasm, and wheezing.

Anti–Human Epidermal Growth Factor Receptor-2

Trastuzumab (Herceptin)

Trastuzumab is a humanized mAb against the human epidermal growth factor receptor 2 (HER2). Up to 40% of patients can present first-time infusion reactions with chills and/or fever, but serious infusion reactions are rare.[43,44]

IgE-mediated HSR with positive skin testing may occur, and desensitization is an effective method of reexposure.[19,20]

Papulopustular acneiform skin eruptions have also been reported.[45]

Pertuzumab (Perjeta)

Pertuzumab is a humanized mAb targeting HER-2 and is approved for use in specific HER2-positive breast cancer cases, in combination with trastuzumab and docetaxel.[46]

Infusion-related reactions can present with fever, chills, fatigue, headache, asthenia, and vomiting.

An IgE-mediated HSR, with a positive basophil activation test (BAT) and increased tryptase levels, was reported in a 38-year-old woman with breast cancer on her second infusion.[47] She was safely reexposed to the drug through RDD.

Anti–Immunoglobulin E

Omalizumab (Xolair)

Omalizumab is a humanized mAb that targets the high-affinity receptor binding site on the human IgE. Anaphylaxis can occur in up to 0.2% of patients, but its mechanism remains to be clarified,[48] because tryptase levels are unaltered and specific IgE/IgG have not been detected.[49,50] Delayed-onset anaphylaxis has also been reported, with reports after 1 day of the administration.[51]

Possible reactions to the excipient polysorbate have been reported but remain to be confirmed by other groups.[49]

Serum sickness–like symptoms can occur after 1 to 5 days of the administration of omalizumab.[5] ISR are reported in 45% of patients, usually within 1 hour and subsiding in 8 days.[48]

Desensitizations to the drug have been reported, followed by weekly or biweekly administration to preserve the desensitized state.[52]

Anti-CD30

Brentuximab vedotin (Adcetris)

Brentuximab vedotin is a chimeric mAb anti-CD30. Infusion reactions occur in approximately 12% patients, with chills, nausea, dyspnea, pruritus, pyrexia, and cough. Successful RDDs due to anaphylaxis have been performed.[53–55]

Anti–Epidermal Growth Factor Receptor

Cetuximab (Erbitux)

Cetuximab is an IgG1 chimeric mAb that binds to the extracellular domain of the human epidermal growth factor receptor (EGFR). Most patients presenting with severe immediate HSR on their first exposure to cetuximab have preexisting IgE antibodies against α-1,3-galactose.[4] This antibody is also associated with delayed allergic reactions to red meat[56] and may be induced by a tick bite (A americanum, lone star tick, with a characteristic geographic distribution[57]). Severe anaphylaxis cases with elevated tryptase levels and positive pretreatment anti-cetuximab IgE levels have been reported,[58] suggesting that screening with anti-cetuximab IgE might be useful to identify high-risk patients.

Anti–Vascular Endothelial Growth Factor-A

Bevacizumab (Avastin)

Bevacizumab is a humanized IgG1 mAb.[59] Its administration can elicit skin manifestations, such as a nonspecific rash and exfoliative dermatitis.[59–61] Intravitreal injections of the drug have been performed, and there are case reports of delayed skin reactions following this application.[62] Immediate HSR symptoms secondary to intravenous infusions have also been reported,[63] such as itching, urticaria, erythematous rash, and facial swelling. Successful desensitization procedures to the drug have been reported.[20]

Anti–Interleukin-6

Tocilizumab (Actemra)

Tocilizumab is a humanized mAb that binds to IL-6 receptors. The role of intradermal testing to tocilizumab in anaphylaxis cases has been shown,[64] and desensitizations have been reported. Delayed HSR, characterized by skin lesions with CD4 T-cell and eosinophil infiltrates, has been described.[10]

Anti–CC Chemokine Receptor 4

Mogamulizumab (Poteligeo)

Mogamulizumab is a humanized monoclonal IgG1 antibody against C-C chemokine receptor 4. A case of Stevens-Johnson syndrome has been reported in a 71-year-old woman with T-cell leukemia/lymphoma after her eighth infusion.[16]

Anti Epithelial Cell Adhesion Molecule/CD3

Catumaxomab (Removab)

Catumaxomab is a rat-mouse hybrid IgG2 mAb. Cytokine release–related symptoms have been observed, such as fever, chills, nausea, and vomiting.[65]

BIOMARKERS

Following the identification of the suspected mechanism, some procedures can help pinpoint the immunologic mechanism involved.

Type I HSR can be investigated with tryptase levels, immediate response to skin testing (prick test/intradermal test), and BAT.

A blood sample for tryptase measurement should be obtained 30 to 120 minutes after the onset of reaction, and if levels are elevated, the test should be repeated at least 2 days after the HSR. Mast cell activation is suspected when acute serum tryptase levels are greater than normal range or increased by 20% plus 2 ng/mL beyond baseline level.[66]

It is worth mentioning that some immediate HSR might present with normal tryptase levels, which can be attributed to anaphylaxis secondary to basophil mediators.

When an IgE-mediated reaction is suspected, skin testing to the culprit mAb can be done 2 to 4 weeks following the reaction. Positive skin testing has been shown to wane over time, so it should be done as soon as possible.[25] Nonirritating concentrations for skin testing are described in **Table 3**.

BAT has been shown to be a useful tool in the investigation of mAb-related immediate HSR. Piva and colleagues[67] showed an increased CD63 expression in patients presenting HSR reactions to rituximab, and a report of pertuzumab anaphylaxis with increased serum tryptase levels and positive BAT was published.[47]

Cytokine storm reactions can be investigated by measuring serum levels of IL-1, IL-6, and TNF-α, when available. Type IV reactions might induce positive delayed-reading intradermal tests.

MANAGEMENT
Acute Care

The priority in the management of acute mAb-related HSR is the prompt stabilization of the patient, which requires the immediate interruption of the infusion and a rapid assessment of vital signs. **Fig. 1** illustrates the management of immediate HSR to mAbs.

In the event of an anaphylactic reaction secondary to mAb administration, an intramuscular dose of epinephrine should be administered.[5] Additional doses may be required and should not be delayed, because of an increase in mortality when postponed.[68] The patient should be placed on their back with elevated lower extremities (if no respiratory distress or vomiting), and volume expansion with isotonic crystalloid solutions can be instituted if hypotension or shock occurs.[69] Lack of response to epinephrine could be secondary to intravascular volume depletion or use of beta-blockers.[70,71] The administration of large amounts of IV fluids and glucagon can be helpful, respectively.

Table 3
Proposed skin testing concentrations

Medication	Prick (mg/mL)	Intradermal (mg/mL)
Rituximab	10	0.1, 1, and 10
Infliximab	10	0.1, 1, and 10
Tocilizumab	20	0.2, 2, and 20
Cetuximab	20	0.2, 2, and 20
Trastuzumab	21	0.21, 2.1, and 21
Bevacizumab	25	0.25, 2.5, and 25
Adalimumab	40	0.4
Etanercept	50	0.025, 0.05, and 0.5
Omalizumab	125	0.00125
Pertuzumab	1.6	0.16
Brentuximab vedotin	0.0018	0.0018, 0.018, 0.18

Oxygen should be supplemented for patients with any respiratory distress.[72]

Corticosteroids and antihistamines (H1 and H2) should not substitute the prompt administration of epinephrine, but they can be helpful as adjuvant medications in the management of immediate HSR. Acetylsalicylic acid (ASA) can be used in the

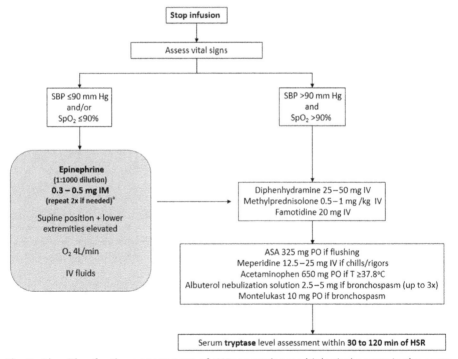

Fig. 1. Algorithm for the management of HSRs secondary to biological agents in the acute care setting. C, Celsius; IM, intramuscular; O₂, oxygen; PO, per os; SBP, systolic blood pressure; SpO₂, peripheral oxygen saturation; T, axillary temperature. [a] If the patient is on β-blockers: consider glucagon.

case of flushing, meperidine for chills and/or rigors, acetaminophen for hyperthermia, and albuterol nebulization and montelukast for bronchospasm.

A blood sample for tryptase measurement should be obtained within 30 to 120 minutes of the HSR.[5]

Cutaneous manifestations of ISRs can be managed with topical lidocaine and ice.[73] Persistent ISR might benefit from topical corticosteroids.

Rapid Drug Desensitization

A proposed algorithm for the management of immediate HSR to mAbs can be found in **Fig. 2**.

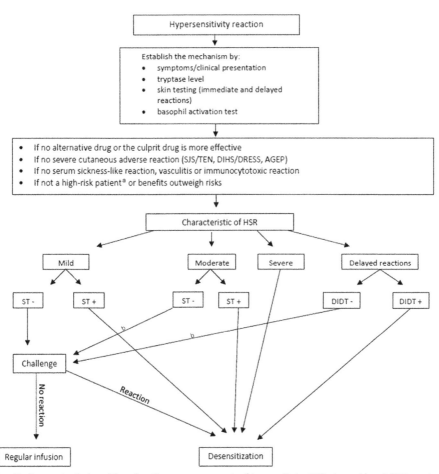

Fig. 2. Suggested algorithm for the management of immediate HSRs to mAbs. AGEP, acute generalized exanthematous pustulosis; DIDT, delayed-reading intradermal testing; DIHS, drug-induced hypersensitivity syndrome; DRESS, drug reaction with eosinophilia and systemic symptoms; SJS, Stevens-Johnson syndrome; ST, skin testing; TEN, toxic epidermal necrolysis. [a] High-risk patient is a relative contraindication: severe anaphylaxis, severe systemic diseases, use of beta-blockers, use of angiotensin-converting-enzyme inhibitor, pregnancy. [b] Assess comorbidities and comfort level for patient and doctor. (*Adapted from* Picard M, Pur L, Caiado J, et al. Risk stratification and skin testing to guide re-exposure in taxane-induced hypersensitivity reactions. J Allergy Clin Immunol 2016;137(4):1155; with permission.)

Patients who present immediate HSR to mAbs can be managed with RDD in a facility prepared to handle anaphylactic reactions and under the supervision of an allergist.

IgE-mediated HSRs are amenable to RDD, whereas IgG-mediated and cytokine release syndrome-type reactions can be managed with RDD depending on their severity.[27]

The standard RDD protocol to mAbs lasts 5.7 hours and consists of 12 steps and 3 solutions of 250 mL, administered sequentially. The first bag contains a solution with a 1/100 dilution; the second contains a 1/10 dilution, and the third concentration is calculated by subtracting the cumulative dose administered in steps 1 to 8 from the total target dose (**Table 4**). The final step is the longest and provides the highest dose. Tolerance acquired at the end of the protocol is transient; therefore, the procedure must be repeated at every mAb infusion.

Premedication is tailored according to the symptoms of the initial HSR. ASA and montelukast can be administered if flushing and bronchospasm occurred during the initial reaction, respectively. Acetaminophen can be administered if the patient presented fever during the initial reaction.[19,20]

A 16-step/4-bag protocol can be used for patients with an initial anaphylactic reaction to minimize risks.[20]

Breakthrough reactions might occur during RDD, most commonly during the last step,[19] and their occurrence prompts the interruption of the infusion. They present an incidence of 30% and are predominantly mild and less severe than the original HSR.[20] Although rare, anaphylactic reactions can occur and must always be treated with epinephrine. For milder reactions, treatment is based on the clinical presentation. HSR characterized by cutaneous signs and symptoms can benefit from antihistamines and corticosteroids: acetaminophen can be used in case of hyperthermia, ASA for flushing, meperidine for rigors, and montelukast and broncodilators for bronchospasm.

Switching the protocol to 16 steps/4 bags, reducing the rate of infusion, and infusing saline solution during RDD are valid measures to protect against breakthrough reactions.[20] The addition of prophylactic premedications before the step at which the patient reacted and, if unsuccessful, the inclusion of an additional step before the reaction step can also be tried.[20]

Rapid Drug Desensitization to Subcutaneous Monoclonal Antibodies

Severe injection site reactions and systemic reactions can occur following the administration of subcutaneous mAbs, and, in these cases, RDD can be a safe management option.[26]

Successful RDD protocols with weekly maintenance doses[26,30] as well as a rush desensitization protocol to adalimumab (2-hour duration) have been reported.[28] In the largest case series of adalimumab RDDs (n = 5), patients were successfully desensitized using 6 or 7 steps and maintained on weekly adalimumab injections for 3 months (which were subsequently spaced every other week).[26]

In addition to cases of ISR, Bavbek and colleagues[74] have described an immediate ISR to etanercept associated with whole-body urticaria and pruritus in a patient with ankylosing spondylitis presenting a positive intradermal test. A late-onset anaphylaxis has also been described on the fifth injection of etanercept, with a positive intradermal test. In both cases, patients underwent a 3-day RDD protocol and were maintained on weekly etanercept injections with cetirizine premedication.[26,74]

Two cases of ISR to etanercept presenting positive BATs were successfully treated with 8-step RDD protocols.[75]

Table 4
12-step/3-bag protocol for rapid drug desensitization to ofatumumab (total dose: 1000 mg)

Bag	Volume per Bag (mL)	Concentration (mg/mL)	Total Dose per Bag (mg)	Amount of Bag Infused (mL)
1	250	0.04	10	9.38
2	250	0.4	100	18.75
3	500	1.98425	992.125	500

Step	Bag	Rate (mL/h)	Time (min)	Volume Infused per Step (mL)	Cumulative Time (min)	Dose Administered with This Step (mg)	Cumulative Dose (mg)	Fold Increase per Step
1	1	2.5	15	0.63	15	0.025	0.025	0
2	1	5	15	1.25	30	0.05	0.075	2
3	1	10	15	2.5	45	0.1	0.175	2
4	1	20	15	5	60	0.2	0.375	2
5	2	5	15	1.25	75	0.5	0.875	2.5
6	2	10	15	2.5	90	1	1.875	2
7	2	20	15	5	105	2	3.875	2
8	2	40	15	10	120	4	7.875	2
9	3	10	15	2.5	135	4.9606	12.8356	1.24
10	3	20	15	5	150	9.9213	22.7569	2
11	3	40	15	10	165	19.8425	42.5994	2
12	3	80	361.875	482.5	526.88	957.4006	1000	2

Total infusion time: 8.78 h.

Cases of anaphylaxis to omalizumab successfully managed with RDD have been reported.[52] In both anaphylaxis cases, patients were desensitized using a 10-step protocol and kept on a weekly maintenance dose to avoid the loss of the desensitized state.

Challenge

The purpose of a graded challenge is to verify that a patient will not experience an immediate adverse reaction to a given drug. Except for suspected IgE-mediated HSR, if a reaction that occurred during an mAb infusion raises doubts of whether it presented an underlying allergic mechanism and its severity was low, a challenge might be a safe method of reexposure. The medication is therefore administered in a controlled manner to a patient who has a low likelihood of reacting to it.[27,76]

For mAb challenges, the initial infusion rate can be one-tenth of the recommended infusion rate. After 15 minutes, it can be reassessed and increased per manufacturer's instructions.[27]

SUMMARY

With the expansion of conditions that can be treated with mAbs, a concomitant increase in the prevalence of HSR associated with this drug class can be expected. The identification and management of such reactions are of extreme importance to secure and maintain the best treatment plan for patients. In this context, RDD presents as a safe method of reexposure to mAbs for selected patients, providing full-treatment doses while minimizing risks of anaphylactic reactions.

REFERENCES

1. Sebastian M, Kuemmel A, Schmidt M, et al. Catumaxomab: a bispecific trifunctional antibody. Drugs Today (Barc) 2009;45(8):589–97.
2. Kiewe P, Hasmüller S, Kahlert S, et al. Phase I trial of the trifunctional anti-HER2 x anti-CD3 antibody ertumaxomab in metastatic breast cancer. Clin Cancer Res 2006;12(10):3085–91.
3. Vultaggio A, Matucci A, Nencini F, et al. Drug-specific Th2 cells and IgE antibodies in a patient with anaphylaxis to rituximab. Int Arch Allergy Immunol 2012;159(3):321–6.
4. Chung CH, Mirakhur B, Chan E, et al. Cetuximab-induced anaphylaxis and IgE specific for galactose-alpha-1,3-galactose. N Engl J Med 2008;358(11):1109–17.
5. Galvão VR, Castells MC. Hypersensitivity to biological agents-updated diagnosis, management, and treatment. J Allergy Clin Immunol Pract 2015;3(2):175–85 [quiz: 186].
6. Finkelman FD, Khodoun MV, Strait R. Human IgE-independent systemic anaphylaxis. J Allergy Clin Immunol 2016;137(6):1674–80.
7. Van der Laken CJ, Voskuyl AE, Roos JC, et al. Imaging and serum analysis of immune complex formation of radiolabelled infliximab and anti-infliximab in responders and non-responders to therapy for rheumatoid arthritis. Ann Rheum Dis 2007;66(2):253–6.
8. Gamarra RM, McGraw SD, Drelichman VS, et al. Serum sickness-like reactions in patients receiving intravenous infliximab. J Emerg Med 2006;30(1):41–4.
9. Karmacharya P, Poudel DR, Pathak R, et al. Rituximab-induced serum sickness: a systematic review. Semin Arthritis Rheum 2015;45(3):334–40.
10. Yoshiki R, Nakamura M, Tokura Y. Drug eruption induced by IL-6 receptor inhibitor tocilizumab. J Eur Acad Dermatol Venereol 2010;24(4):495–6.

11. Cheifetz A, Mayer L. Monoclonal antibodies, immunogenicity, and associated infusion reactions. Mt Sinai J Med 2005;72(4):250–6.
12. Zeltser R, Valle L, Tanck C, et al. Clinical, histological, and immunophenotypic characteristics of injection site reactions associated with etanercept: a recombinant tumor necrosis factor alpha receptor: Fc fusion protein. Arch Dermatol 2001; 137(7):893–9.
13. Urosevic-Maiwald M, Harr T, French LE, et al. Stevens-Johnson syndrome and toxic epidermal necrolysis overlap in a patient receiving cetuximab and radiotherapy for head and neck cancer. Int J Dermatol 2012;51(7):864–7.
14. Lee S-S, Chu P-Y. Toxic epidermal necrolysis caused by cetuximab plus minocycline in head and neck cancer. Am J Otolaryngol 2010;31(4):288–90.
15. Lowndes S, Darby A, Mead G, et al. Stevens-Johnson syndrome after treatment with rituximab. Ann Oncol 2002;13(12):1948–50.
16. Ishida T, Ito A, Sato F, et al. Stevens–Johnson syndrome associated with mogamulizumab treatment of adult T-cell leukemia/lymphoma. Cancer Sci 2013; 104(5):647–50.
17. Luheshi G, Rothwell N. Cytokines and fever. Int Arch Allergy Immunol 1996; 109(4):301–7.
18. Suntharalingam G, Perry MR, Ward S, et al. Cytokine storm in a phase 1 trial of the anti-CD28 monoclonal antibody TGN1412. N Engl J Med 2006;355(10):1018–28.
19. Brennan PJ, Bouza TR, Hsu FI, et al. Hypersensitivity reactions to mAbs: 105 desensitizations in 23 patients, from evaluation to treatment. J Allergy Clin Immunol 2009;124(6):1259–66.
20. Sloane D, Govindarajulu U, Harrow-Mortelliti J, et al. Safety, costs, and efficacy of rapid drug desensitizations to chemotherapy and monoclonal antibodies. J Allergy Clin Immunol Pract 2016;4(3):497–504.
21. International Nonproprietary Names (INN) for biological and biotechnological substances. Available at: http://www.who.int/medicines/services/inn/BioRev2013.pdf. Accessed March 12, 2017.
22. REMICADE (infliximab) [package insert]. Philadelphia: Janssen Biotech, Inc; 2013.
23. Choquette D, Faraawi R, Chow A, et al. Incidence and management of infusion reactions to infliximab in a prospective real-world community registry. J Rheumatol 2015;42(7):1105–11.
24. O'Meara S, Nanda KS, Moss AC. Antibodies to infliximab and risk of infusion reactions in patients with inflammatory bowel disease: a systematic review and meta-analysis. Inflamm Bowel Dis 2014;20(1):1–6.
25. Matucci A, Pratesi S, Petroni G, et al. Allergological in vitro and in vivo evaluation of patients with hypersensitivity reactions to infliximab. Clin Exp Allergy 2013; 43(6):659–64.
26. Bavbek S, Ataman Ş, Akıncı A, et al. Rapid subcutaneous desensitization for the management of local and systemic hypersensitivity reactions to etanercept and adalimumab in 12 patients. J Allergy Clin Immunol Pract 2015;3(4):629–32.
27. Picard M, Galvão VR. Current knowledge and management of hypersensitivity reactions to monoclonal antibodies. J Allergy Clin Immunol Pract 2017;5(3):600–9.
28. Quercia O, Emiliani F, Foschi FG, et al. Adalimumab desensitization after anaphylactic reaction. Ann Allergy Asthma Immunol 2011;106(6):547–8.
29. Benucci M, Manfredi M, Demoly P, et al. Injection site reactions to TNF-alpha blocking agents with positive skin tests. Allergy 2008;63(1):138–9.

30. Bavbek S, Ataman Ş, Bankova L, et al. Injection site reaction to adalimumab: positive skin test and successful rapid desensitisation. Allergol Immunopathol (Madr) 2013;41(3):204–6.

31. SIMPONI® (golimumab) [package insert]. Philadelphia: Centocor Ortho Biotech, Inc; 2009.

32. Emery P, Fleischmann RM, Moreland LW, et al. Golimumab, a human anti-tumor necrosis factor alpha monoclonal antibody, injected subcutaneously every four weeks in methotrexate-naive patients with active rheumatoid arthritis: twenty-four-week results of a phase III, multicenter, randomized, double-blind, placebo-controlled study of golimumab before methotrexate as first-line therapy for early-onset rheumatoid arthritis. Arthritis Rheum 2009;60(8):2272–83.

33. Judson MA, Baughman RP, Costabel U, et al. Safety and efficacy of ustekinumab or golimumab in patients with chronic sarcoidosis. Eur Respir J 2014;44(5): 1296–307.

34. CIMZIA® (certolizumab pegol) [package insert]. Smyrna, GA: UCB, Inc; 2016.

35. Keystone E, Heijde DVD, Mason D, et al. Certolizumab pegol plus methotrexate is significantly more effective than placebo plus methotrexate in active rheumatoid arthritis: findings of a fifty-two–week, phase III, multicenter, randomized, double-blind, placebo-controlled, parallel-group study. Arthritis Rheum 2008;58(11): 3319–29.

36. Thompson LM, Eckmann K, Boster BL, et al. Incidence, risk factors, and management of infusion-related reactions in breast cancer patients receiving trastuzumab. Oncologist 2014;19(3):228–34.

37. Winkler U, Jensen M, Manzke O, et al. Cytokine-release syndrome in patients with B-cell chronic lymphocytic leukemia and high lymphocyte counts after treatment with an anti-CD20 monoclonal antibody (rituximab, IDEC-C2B8). Blood 1999; 94(7):2217–24.

38. Korycka-Wołowiec A, Wołowiec D, Robak T. Ofatumumab for treating chronic lymphocytic leukemia: a safety profile. Expert Opin Drug Saf 2015;14(12): 1945–59.

39. Taylor PC, Quattrocchi E, Mallett S, et al. Extended report: ofatumumab, a fully human anti-CD20 monoclonal antibody, in biological-naive, rheumatoid arthritis patients with an inadequate response to methotrexate: a randomised, double-blind, placebo-controlled clinical trial. Ann Rheum Dis 2011;70(12):2119.

40. Lemery SJ, Zhang J, Rothmann MD, et al. U.S. Food and Drug Administration approval: ofatumumab for the treatment of patients with chronic lymphocytic leukemia refractory to fludarabine and alemtuzumab. Clin Cancer Res 2010;16(17): 4331–8.

41. GAZYVA® (obinutuzumab) [package insert]. San Francisco (CA): Genentech, Inc; 2016.

42. Goede V, Fischer K, Busch R, et al. Obinutuzumab plus chlorambucil in patients with CLL and coexisting conditions. N Engl J Med 2014;370(12):1101–10.

43. Cook-Bruns N. Retrospective analysis of the safety of Herceptin immunotherapy in metastatic breast cancer. Oncology 2001;61(Suppl 2):58–66.

44. HERCEPTIN® (trastuzumab) [package insert]. San Francisco (CA): Genentech, Inc; 2011.

45. Sheu J, Hawryluk EB, Litsas G, et al. Papulopustular acneiform eruptions resulting from trastuzumab, a HER2 inhibitor. Clin Breast Cancer 2015;15(1):e77–81.

46. PERJETA® (pertuzumab) [package insert]. San Francisco (CA): Genentech, Inc; 2012.

47. González-de-Olano D, Morgado JM, Juárez-Guerrero R, et al. Positive basophil activation test following anaphylaxis to pertuzumab and successful treatment with rapid desensitization. J Allergy Clin Immunol Pract 2016;4(2):338–40.
48. XOLAIR® (omalizumab) [package insert]. San Francisco (CA): Genentech, Inc; 2010.
49. Price KS, Hamilton RG. Anaphylactoid reactions in two patients after omalizumab administration after successful long-term therapy. Allergy Asthma Proc 2007; 28(3):313–9.
50. Lieberman PL, Umetsu DT, Carrigan GJ, et al. Anaphylactic reactions associated with omalizumab administration: analysis of a case-control study. J Allergy Clin Immunol 2016;138(3):913–5.e2.
51. Limb SL, Starke PR, Lee CE, et al. Delayed onset and protracted progression of anaphylaxis after omalizumab administration in patients with asthma. J Allergy Clin Immunol 2007;120(6):1378–81.
52. Owens G, Petrov A. Successful desensitization of three patients with hypersensitivity reactions to omalizumab. Curr Drug Saf 2011;6(5):339–42.
53. O'Connell AE, Lee JP, Yee C, et al. Successful desensitization to brentuximab vedotin after anaphylaxis. Clin Lymphoma Myeloma Leuk 2014;14(2):e73–5.
54. DeVita MD, Evens AM, Rosen ST, et al. Multiple successful desensitizations to brentuximab vedotin: a case report and literature review. J Natl Compr Cancer Netw 2014;12(4):465–71.
55. Story SK, Petrov AA, Geskin LJ. Successful desensitization to brentuximab vedotin after hypersensitivity reaction. J Drugs Dermatol 2014;13(6):749–51.
56. Commins SP, Satinover SM, Hosen J, et al. Delayed anaphylaxis, angioedema, or urticaria after consumption of red meat in patients with IgE antibodies specific for galactose-alpha-1,3-galactose. J Allergy Clin Immunol 2009;123(2):426–33.
57. Commins SP, James HR, Kelly LA, et al. The relevance of tick bites to the production of IgE antibodies to the mammalian oligosaccharide galactose-α-1,3-galactose. J Allergy Clin Immunol 2011;127(5):1286–93.e6.
58. Dupont B, Mariotte D, Moldovan C, et al. Case report about fatal or near-fatal hypersensitivity reactions to cetuximab: anticetuximab IgE as a valuable screening test. Clin Med Insights Oncol 2014;8:91–4.
59. AVASTIN® (bevacizumab) [package insert]. San Francisco (CA): Genentech, Inc; 2016.
60. Gotlib V, Khaled S, Lapko I, et al. Skin rash secondary to bevacizumab in a patient with advanced colorectal cancer and relation to response. Anticancer Drugs 2006;17(10):1227–9.
61. Saif MW, Longo WL, Israel G. Correlation between rash and a positive drug response associated with bevacizumab in a patient with advanced colorectal cancer. Clin Colorectal Cancer 2008;7(2):144–8.
62. Ameen S, Entabi M, Lee N, et al. Adverse skin reactions following intravitreal bevacizumab injection. BMJ Case Rep 2011;2011 [pii:bcr0220102753].
63. Pezzuto A, Piraino A, Mariotta S. Lung cancer and concurrent or sequential lymphoma: two case reports with hypersensitivity to bevacizumab and a review of the literature. Oncol Lett 2015;9(2):604–8.
64. Rocchi V, Puxeddu I, Cataldo G, et al. Hypersensitivity reactions to tocilizumab: role of skin tests in diagnosis. Rheumatology 2014;53(8):1527–9.
65. REMOVAB® (catumaxomab), Fresenius, European Medicines Agency. 2016.
66. Brown SGA, Blackman KE, Heddle RJ. Can serum mast cell tryptase help diagnose anaphylaxis? Emerg Med Australas 2004;16(2):120–4.

67. Piva E, Chieco-Bianchi F, Krajcar V, et al. Adverse reactions in patients with B-cell lymphomas during combined treatment with rituximab: in vitro evaluation of rituximab hypersensitivity by basophil activation test. Am J Hematol 2012;87(11): E130–1.

68. Liew WK, Williamson E, Tang MLK. Anaphylaxis fatalities and admissions in Australia. J Allergy Clin Immunol 2009;123(2):434–42.

69. Simons FER, Ardusso LRF, Dimov V, et al. World Allergy Organization Anaphylaxis Guidelines: 2013 update of the evidence base. Int Arch Allergy Immunol 2013;162(3):193–204.

70. Mueller UR. Cardiovascular disease and anaphylaxis. Curr Opin Allergy Clin Immunol 2007;7(4):337–41.

71. Thomas M, Crawford I. Best evidence topic report. Glucagon infusion in refractory anaphylactic shock in patients on beta-blockers. Emerg Med J 2005;22(4): 272–3.

72. Lieberman P, Nicklas RA, Randolph C, et al. Anaphylaxis–a practice parameter update 2015. Ann Allergy Asthma Immunol 2015;115(5):341–84.

73. Feuerstein JD, Cheifetz AS. Miscellaneous adverse events with biologic agents (excludes infection and malignancy). Gastroenterol Clin North Am 2014;43(3): 543–63.

74. Bavbek S, Aydın O, Ataman S, et al. Injection-site reaction to etanercept: role of skin test in the diagnosis of such reaction and successful desensitization. Allergy 2011;66(9):1256–7.

75. De la Varga Martínez R, Gutiérrez Fernández D, Foncubierta Fernández A, et al. Rapid subcutaneous desensitization for treatment of hypersensitivity reactions to etanercept in two patients with positive basophil activation test. Allergol Int 2017; 66(2):357–9.

76. Joint Task Force on Practice Parameters, American Academy of Allergy, Asthma and Immunology, American College of Allergy, Asthma and Immunology, Joint Council of Allergy, Asthma and Immunology. Drug allergy: an updated practice parameter. Ann Allergy Asthma Immunol 2010;105(4):259–73.

77. Vultaggio A, Matucci A, Nencini F, et al. Anti-infliximab IgE and non-IgE antibodies and induction of infusion-related severe anaphylactic reactions. Allergy 2010;65(5):657–61.

78. Fréling E, Peyrin-Biroulet L, Poreaux C, et al. IgE antibodies and skin tests in immediate hypersensitivity reactions to infliximab in inflammatory bowel disease: impact on infliximab retreatment. Eur J Gastroenterol Hepatol 2015;27(10): 1200–8.

79. ENBREL (etanercept) [package insert]. Thousand Oaks (CA): Immunex Corp; 2013.

80. HUMIRA (adalimumab) [package insert]. Chicago (IL): Abbott Laboratories; 2008.

81. Grillo-López AJ, White CA, Varns C, et al. Overview of the clinical development of rituximab: first monoclonal antibody approved for the treatment of lymphoma. Semin Oncol 1999;26(5 Suppl 14):66–73.

82. ARZERRA (ofatumumab) [package insert]. Durham (NC): GlaxoSmithKline; 2011.

83. Chen K, Page JG, Schwartz AM, et al. False-positive immunogenicity responses are caused by CD20+ B cell membrane fragments in an anti-ofatumumab antibody bridging assay. J Immunol Methods 2013;394(1–2):22–31.

84. Guan M, Zhou Y-P, Sun J-L, et al. Adverse events of monoclonal antibodies used for cancer therapy. Biomed Res Int 2015;2015:428169.

85. Cox L, Platts-Mills TAE, Finegold I, et al. American Academy of Allergy, Asthma & Immunology/American College of Allergy, Asthma and Immunology Joint Task Force Report on omalizumab-associated anaphylaxis. J Allergy Clin Immunol 2007;120(6):1373–7.

86. Arora A, Bhatt VR, Liewer S, et al. Brentuximab vedotin desensitization in a patient with refractory Hodgkin's lymphoma. Eur J Haematol 2015;95(4):361–4.

87. Yamaguchi K, Watanabe T, Satoh T, et al. Severe infusion reactions to cetuximab occur within 1 h in patients with metastatic colorectal cancer: results of a nationwide, multicenter, prospective registry study of 2126 patients in Japan. Jpn J Clin Oncol 2014;44(6):541–6.

88. Cunningham D, Humblet Y, Siena S, et al. Cetuximab monotherapy and cetuximab plus irinotecan in irinotecan-refractory metastatic colorectal cancer. N Engl J Med 2004;351(4):337–45.

89. Siena S, Glynne-Jones R, Adenis A, et al. Reduced incidence of infusion-related reactions in metastatic colorectal cancer during treatment with cetuximab plus irinotecan with combined corticosteroid and antihistamine premedication. Cancer 2010;116(7):1827–37.

90. Sobrero AF, Maurel J, Fehrenbacher L, et al. EPIC: phase III trial of cetuximab plus irinotecan after fluoropyrimidine and oxaliplatin failure in patients with metastatic colorectal cancer. J Clin Oncol 2008;26(14):2311–9.

91. Keating K, Walko C, Stephenson B, et al. Incidence of cetuximab-related infusion reactions in oncology patients treated at the University of North Carolina Cancer Hospital. J Oncol Pharm Pract 2014;20(6):409–16.

92. O'Neil BH, Allen R, Spigel DR, et al. High incidence of cetuximab-related infusion reactions in Tennessee and North Carolina and the association with atopic history. J Clin Oncol 2007;25(24):3644–8.

93. George TJ, Laplant KD, Walden EO, et al. Managing cetuximab hypersensitivity-infusion reactions: incidence, risk factors, prevention, and retreatment. J Support Oncol 2010;8(2):72–7.

94. Steinke JW, Platts-Mills TAE, Commins SP. The alpha-gal story: lessons learned from connecting the dots. J Allergy Clin Immunol 2015;135(3):589–96 [quiz: 597].

95. ACTEMRA (tocilizumab) [package insert]. San Francisco (CA): Genentech, Inc; 2013.

96. Justet A, Neukirch C, Poubeau P, et al. Successful rapid tocilizumab desensitization in a patient with Still disease. J Allergy Clin Immunol Pract 2014;2(5):631–2.

Management of Children with Hypersensitivity to Antibiotics and Monoclonal Antibodies

Allison Eaddy Norton, MD[a],*, Ana Dioun Broyles, MD[b],*

KEYWORDS

- Pediatric drug allergy • Drug hypersensitivity • Allergy skin testing • Desensitization
- Antibiotic allergy • Monoclonal allergy • Drug provocation

KEY POINTS

- Testing in young children should not be avoided because of parental or physician fear of testing because it has been confirmed to be safe.
- Accurate diagnosis for both antibiotic allergy and monoclonal antibody allergy leads to better workup and management of these allergies.
- The range of hypersensitivity reactions that occur in monoclonal antibody allergy overlaps with antibiotic allergy but is also distinctly different.
- Graded challenges are the gold standard in diagnosis and have been proven to be safe in children.
- Desensitization should only be pursued if there are no alternatives and is contraindicated in drug reactions with severe skin disease.

INTRODUCTION

Proper management of drug allergy in children is based on accurate diagnosis. Unfortunately, there is a lack of understanding of drug allergy in this population as well as provider or parental fear of testing children, which can lead to incomplete workup and misdiagnosis. Overlabeling in antibiotic allergy is a huge health burden and leads to drug-resistant bacteria.[1] Overdiagnosis is rather common in children, likely because

Disclosure Statement: The authors have nothing to disclose.
[a] Division of Pediatric Pulmonary, Allergy and Immunology, Vanderbilt Children's Hospital, School of Medicine, 100 Oaks, 719 Thompson Lane, Nashville, TN 37204, USA; [b] Division of Allergy and Immunology, Boston Children's Hospital, Harvard Medical School, 300 Longwood Avenue, Boston, MA 02115, USA
* Corresponding authors.
E-mail addresses: Allison.norton@vanderbilt.edu (A.E.N.); ana.broyles@childrens.harvard.edu (A.D.B.)

Immunol Allergy Clin N Am 37 (2017) 713–725
http://dx.doi.org/10.1016/j.iac.2017.07.005
0889-8561/17/© 2017 Elsevier Inc. All rights reserved.

of the frequency of rashes that occur during an antibiotic course in a child and reluctance of testing to confirm allergy.[2,3] However, proper management should be based on a thorough history, in vitro testing (if available), in vivo testing, and if negative, drug challenge for delabeling because accurate diagnosis and management of the antibiotic allergic child are key factors in preventing children from carrying drug allergy labels that persist until adulthood.

It may also be difficult to determine the precise timing that a reaction begins in an infant or young child, making it challenging to ascertain immediate reactions from non-immediate reactions. Distinguishing the type of reaction is important because the workup and management vary depending on the timing and associated symptoms of the reaction. In addition, providers often choose avoidance over testing in children, although intradermal testing and drug challenge have been proven to be safe and well tolerated in children.[4,5]

Monoclonal antibodies are proteins, of human or murine origin, increasingly used in oncologic and autoimmune diseases in children. Their larger protein structure, as opposed to the small chemical structures of antibiotics, promotes immunogenicity and can elicit hypersensitivity reactions.[6,7]

This article focuses on the workup, management, and treatment of pediatric antibiotic and monoclonal antibody allergy.

EPIDEMIOLOGY

It is difficult to obtain a true incidence of drug allergy in the pediatric population.[8] Epidemiologic studies indicate that drug allergy affects more than 10% of children and adolescents, although community studies suggest that this number is grossly overestimated.[2] When these children undergo diagnostic studies, including skin testing or drug provocation testing (DPT), less than 10% are confirmed to be truly allergic to the suspected drug.[4,9,10]

Penicillin allergy is the most commonly reported drug allergy, with a prevalence rate of 5% to 10% in adults and children.[11–14] Amoxicillin has now replaced benzyl penicillin as the most frequently reported drug allergy in children.[15] Non–beta-lactam (BL) allergy is rare in children and estimated to affect 1% to 3% of this population. In regards to the most commonly reported reactions to non-BL drugs, sulfonamides are the most commonly reported, followed by macrolides.[16]

In contrast to antibiotic allergy, monoclonal antibody allergy is infrequently reported in children and is limited to case reports and case series.[6,7,17–19]

GENERAL PRINCIPLES

The general principles of drug allergy are based on the classic mechanisms initially described by Gell and colleagues[20] in 1968 and updated by Pichler in 2003 to include subtypes IVa to IVd as demonstrated in **Table 1**.[20–23] However, as new approaches to drug allergy have emerged, an additional classification based on precision medicine has recently been proposed. This newer classification is based on phenotype, endotypes, and biomarkers in drug allergy.[24]

Phenotypes are determined by specific clinical symptoms associated with timing from exposure to the culprit drug. Phenotypes are divided into the following 2 broad categories:

- Immediate-onset drug allergy: occurs within 1 to 6 hours of exposure to the drug and is associated with cutaneous, respiratory, gastrointestinal symptoms, or anaphylaxis.

Table 1
Gell and Coombs classification of reaction and management

Type of Reactions	Mechanism	Clinical Features	Timing	Testing	Management
Type I	Immediate or IgE-directed release of histamine and mediators via mast cells/basophils	Anaphylaxis, urticaria, angioedema, bronchospasm	Immediate: <1 h after ingestion of drug	Skin prick testing, serum-specific IgE, DPT	• Specific drug avoidance/cross-reacting drugs • Choose first-line alternative drugs if possible • Desensitization if alternative drugs cannot be used
Type II	Cytotoxic or antibody-dependent, hypersensitivity reactions	Drug-induced hemolytic anemia, thrombocytopenia, nephritis	1–2 wk after exposure[a]	Drug-specific antiplatelet antibodies	• Specific drug avoidance
Type III	Immune complex	Serum sickness, vasculitis	1–2 wk after exposure[a]	No testing	• Specific drug avoidance
Type IV: IVa IVb IVc IVd	Delayed or T-cell mediated	Benign delayed skin rashes: allergic contact dermatitis, maculopapular exanthema Severe cutaneous skin rashes: AGEP, FDE, EM, DRESS, and SJS/TEN	Nonimmediate: a few days to weeks after exposure	LTT, ELIspot; patch testing; delayed IDT, HLA screening	• Specific drug/class avoidance

Abbreviations: AGEP, Acute generalized exanthematous pustulosis; DRESS, drug reaction with eosinophilia and systemic symptoms; EM, erythema multiforme; FDE, fixed drug eruption; HLA, human leukocyte antigen; IDT, Intradermal testing; LTT, lymphocyte transformation testing; SJS/TEN, Stevens-Johnson syndrome/toxic epidermal necrolysis.

[a] May be sooner if there are preformed antibodies.

Data from Refs.[20–23]

- Delayed-onset drug allergy: presents within days to weeks after drug exposure with a wide range of clinical symptoms from maculopapular rash, urticaria and fixed drug eruption, to severe cutaneous adverse reactions (SCARs). Symptoms are not always isolated to one organ and may also affect the hepatic, renal, pulmonary, or hematologic system.

Endotypes are phenotypic subclasses associated with specific mechanisms of underlying disease. Endotypes for drug allergy are divided into the following categories:

- Immunoglobulin E (IgE)-mediated reactions
- T-cell–mediated reactions
- Pharmacologic interactions
- Genetic predispositions

Biomarkers used to distinguish disease in drug allergy vary depending on the phenotype and endotype and include the following:

- Skin prick testing and serum-specific IgE (immediate hypersensitivity testing)
- Basophil activation testing and basophil histamine release assay (immediate hypersensitivity testing)
- Mediators (ie, tryptase)
- Cells (ie, lymphocyte transformation testing in T-cell–mediated disease, granulysin, and granzyme B in Stevens-Johnson syndrome [SJS])
- Patch testing (useful in maculopapular exanthems, fixed drug eruptions, acute generalized exanthematous pustulosis [AGEP], and potentially in drug reaction with eosinophilia and systemic symptoms [DRESS], and SJS in specific drugs)
- HLA markers (ie, HLA–B*57:01 in abacavir drug hypersensitivity)

RISK FACTORS

Risk factors for drug allergy include structures inherent within the drug itself as well as the host. Some drugs are better than others at inducing immunologic reactions.

Drug-related risk factors include the following:

- Ability to act as a hapten
- Ability to act as a pro-hapten
- Ability to bind covalently to immune receptors (p-i concept)[23,25,26]

The hapten and pro-hapten concept explains how drugs and other small molecular weight proteins (<1000 D) like antibiotics can become immunogenic. Haptens are small chemically reactive compounds that bind to proteins or peptides, enabling them to stimulate an immune response. Pro-haptens are not immunogenic until they are modified chemically into haptens. Both haptens and pro-haptens can stimulate the immune system either innately or specifically.

The hapten theory does not explain how proteins such as monoclonal antibodies or carbohydrate substances can be immunogenic.[27] The p-i concept is a direct pharmacologic interaction of drugs with immune receptors. The p-i concept explains how a drug directly stimulates the immune system without modification or processing.

In addition to the drug structure, it is known that route, dose, duration, and repeated exposure are known risk factors. For example, a drug given parenterally is known to be more sensitizing compared with a dose administered orally.[28]

Host risk factors in children include specific genetic polymorphisms and previous drug reactions to unrelated drugs or multiple drug allergy syndrome.[28,29] It is really not known if sex, age, and atopy are risk factors for the development of drug allergy in children. In a large retrospective study by Ponvert and colleagues,[30] in the 1865 children with suspected BL allergy that were evaluated, sex, age, and atopy were not risk factors.

Very few studies have evaluated risk factors for drug allergy in children. It is not known whether family history of drug allergy actually predisposes one to drug allergy. However, one study of Turkish children evaluated 97 subjects aged 8 months to 18 years with a history of immediate or nonimmediate drug allergy. Children with confirmed drug allergy by skin testing or patch testing in this study were 4.4% more likely to have a family history of drug allergy. In addition, children with index reactions that were supported by strong histories were 3.5 times more likely to have a confirmed drug allergy than those with vague histories of reaction.[31]

CLINICAL FEATURES

Clinical features of drug allergy vary depending on the immunologic mechanisms of the reaction. Immediate-onset reactions typically occur within 1 to 6 hours of exposure to the drug, whereas nonimmediate or delayed-onset reactions, depending on severity, can occur within hours to weeks after treatment with the drug.[27]

Immediate-onset reactions (<6 hours) can be divided into IgE-mediated reactions and non-IgE-mediated reactions (anaphylactoid or pseudoallergic). Clinical features associated with immediate reactions include urticaria, angioedema, bronchospasm, gastrointestinal symptoms, or anaphylaxis.

Nonimmediate reactions to drugs can also vary in clinical features, timing, and severity depending on the immunologic mechanism.[27]

Clinical reactions to monoclonal antibodies vary by drug and range from acute idiosyncratic infusion reactions, rash, anaphylaxis, to serum sickness.[32] They are classified as immediate or nonimmediate, based on timing of reaction. Immediate reactions have recently been described by 3 mechanisms, as discussed below, although mixed reactions can occur.[7]

Cytokine Release Syndrome

Cytokine release syndrome typically occurs immediately upon first exposure to a monoclonal antibody and can be characterized by flushing, dyspnea, fever, hypotension/hypertension, chest/back pain, throat tightness, dizziness, and gastrointestinal symptoms.[7] In some cases, death has even occurred.[33] These clinical symptoms are a result of complement or antibody-mediated cell destruction. Management includes slowing the infusion rate and using premedication, such as corticosteroids and acetaminophen.[7]

Immunoglobulin E-Mediated Reactions

IgE-mediated reactions typically require prior exposure, although some monoclonal antibodies such as cetuximab are known to elicit reactions on first exposure via preformed antibodies.[7] Symptoms can range from typical IgE-mediated symptoms and anaphylaxis to atypical symptoms like fevers and chills. Serum tryptase levels may be elevated. Management includes skin testing with nonirritating concentrations. If testing is positive, desensitization should be considered.[7] Because the predictive value of skin testing is not known, desensitization may be attempted in cases with negative skin testing depending on the clinical history.

IgG-Mediated Reactions

Immunoglobulin G or IgG-mediated reactions typically require prior exposure. Symptoms vary but clinically may appear like IgE-mediated reactions or may present as reduced efficacy through increased clearance or by blocking antibody binding sites.[7]

The most common nonimmediate symptoms reported with monoclonal antibodies are serum sickness-like reaction. These reactions typically require prior exposure, but have been reported to occur on first exposure as well. Some reactions that occur several hours after drug exposure may be IgE mediated, especially if they were administered subcutaneously.[7]

DIFFERENTIAL DIAGNOSIS AND CROSS-REACTIVITY

Differential diagnosis for drug reactions in children depends upon the immunologic basis of the reaction. However, drug reaction in children is often confused with symptoms that accompany a viral illness (**Tables 2** and **3**).[5,34]

Knowledge of cross-reactivity is important in the management of a pediatric antibiotic allergy. Cross-reactivity is well studied within BL drugs but less understood with non-BL antibiotics. Patients with penicillin allergy rarely react to cephalosporins, typically 2%, unless the 2 antibiotics share a particular side chain that arises from the BL ring, called the R1 side chain. When a penicillin-allergic patient is administered a cephalosporin with identical R1 side chains, the risk for allergic reaction increases by 30%.[35] Therefore, when choosing an alternative drug for a penicillin-allergic child, a provider should choose a BL with a different side chain. Penicillin-allergic patients have a rare chance of reactivity to carbapenems and aztreonam, lower than 1%.[36,37] Thus, these drugs can be used safely in a penicillin-allergic child. Macrolides and quinolones are known to have some cross-reactivity within their own groups; therefore, patients allergic to these drugs should choose another class of drugs for treatment.[2,38]

DIAGNOSTIC TESTING

Studies indicate that clinical history alone is a poor indicator of allergic status. Skin testing or DPT are imperative for confirmation of drug allergy and should be considered, even in young children.[9]

Skin testing protocols for BL drugs, in particular penicillin, have been well established, but not for non-BL drugs. However, there are published data regarding nonirritating concentrations on several antibiotics.[39,40] Testing for BL drugs should always include PRE-PEN (benzylpenicilloyl polylysine), minor determinants, and ampicillin/amoxicillin. When skin testing is negative, one must undergo DPT to delabel the drug allergy.[39]

Table 2 Differential diagnosis of immediate reactions	
Non-IgE-mediated (pseudoallergic/anaphylactoid)	Anaphylaxis IgE-mediated reaction
IgE-mediated	Food allergy Venom allergy Idiopathic urticaria and angioedema Idiopathic anaphylaxis Non–IgE-mediated reaction

Data from Atanaskovic-Markovic M, Gaeta F, Medjo B, et al. Non-immediate hypersensitivity reactions to beta-lactam antibiotics in children—our 10-year experience in allergy work-up. Pediatr Allergy Immunol 2016;27(5):533–8; and Caubet JC, Kaiser L, Lemaitre B, et al. The role of penicillin in benign skin rashes in childhood: a prospective study based on drug rechallenge. J Allergy Clin Immunol 2011;127(1):218–22.

Table 3	
Differential diagnosis of delayed drug reactions	
Delayed drug reaction	Viral exanthem
	IgE-mediated drug allergy
	Early DRESS or SJS/TEN
SJS/TENS	Erythema multiforme
	Bullous skin diseases
	Fixed drug eruption
	DRESS
DRESS	Delayed drug rash
	Early SJS/TEN
	Severe eczema or psoriasis
AGEP	Pustular psoriasis
	Bullous impetigo
	Subcorneal pustular dermatosis
	DRESS
Serum sickness–like reaction	Vasculitis
	Rheumatic fever

Data from Atanaskovic-Markovic M, Gaeta F, Medjo B, et al. Non-immediate hypersensitivity reactions to beta-lactam antibiotics in children—our 10-year experience in allergy work-up. Pediatr Allergy Immunol 2016;27(5):533–8; and Caubet JC, Kaiser L, Lemaitre B, et al. The role of penicillin in benign skin rashes in childhood: a prospective study based on drug rechallenge. J Allergy Clin Immunol 2011;127(1):218–22.

Monoclonal antibodies have much higher molecular weights; therefore, skin testing is more diagnostic compared with drugs that are small molecular weight or haptens.[41] Although skin testing to monoclonal antibodies has not been standardized, nonirritating concentrations have been published. Skin prick testing strengths vary depending on the monoclonal antibody but are typically tested at full strength. Intradermal testing can be done at 1:100 dilution, and if negative, proceed to 1:10.[7,32]

Selection of testing is based upon the type of reaction that occurred:

- Immediate drug allergy (based on timing and IgE-mediated symptoms):
  ○ Skin prick testing and intradermal testing to the drug, with nonirritating concentrations.
  ○ If testing is negative and there is a history of a mild reaction, then the allergist should consider DPT even in young children.
  ○ If testing is positive, clinical scenario does not allow testing because of time pressure, or history is suggestive of a more severe or potentially anaphylactic type reaction, the allergist should recommend avoidance of drug and any possible cross-reacting drug. Desensitization may be considered if no alternate treatment is available or the drug is first-line treatment.
- Nonimmediate or delayed drug allergy:
  ○ Consider delayed intradermal testing to a nonirritating concentration of the culprit drug.[42]
  ○ If testing is negative or challenge is deemed low risk, the allergist should seek DPT and delabel.
  ○ If testing is positive, the allergist should recommend avoidance or could consider DPT, only if index reaction was not severe. Desensitization may be considered in some cases.

- SCARs, such as DRESS syndrome, SJS, and toxic epidermal necrolysis (TEN):
  - No widely used commercially available testing.
  - Lymphocyte transformation testing (LTT) and Elispot are novel testing, but not commercially available.
  - DPT and desensitization are contraindicated.

DRUG CHALLENGE AND DESENSITIZATION

The gold standard for diagnosis of drug allergy is drug challenge or DPT. DPT in the form of single-dose challenge or graded challenge has been demonstrated to be well tolerated in children and is a diagnostic measure/delabeling strategy as opposed to desensitization, which is a therapeutic measure for safe administration of a drug in children who are known to be allergic to that drug.[4,30,43] Both DPT and desensitization should be done in an appropriate medical setting with continual monitoring and equipped with staff and medical equipment capable of treating anaphylaxis, should it occur.[28]

The literature demonstrates that testing with BL drugs with skin testing followed by DPT in even large groups of children suspected of drug allergy yields small numbers of children who are proven allergic. Results from recent studies in children are summarized in **Table 4**.[4,5,30,43–45]

When DPT exceeds 4 steps, downregulation of mast cells may occur, resulting in desensitization rather than challenge. A single- or multidose challenge with 2 to 3 steps alternatively can be used to confirm or deny allergy without the untoward consequence of desensitization.[28]

There are published reports on desensitization in pediatrics to both BL and non-BL drugs.[46,47] In general, drug desensitization protocols for children differ little from those in adults with the exception of the cumulative dose, because the drug goal is typically weight based.[48] **Table 5** is an example of the commonly used 12-step desensitization protocol.

Monoclonal antibodies are often life saving or disease modifying, leaving allergic patients little options for alternatives, other than desensitization. Desensitization to

Table 4				
Confirmation of drug allergy to antibiotics via drug provocation testing				
Publication	Culprit Drugs	Age of Subjects	Timing of Drug Reaction	Confirmed Allergy (No. of Positive Skin Prick Testing ± DPT/%)
Atanaskovic-Markovic et al,[5] 2016	BL	1–18 y	Nonimmediate	7.4% of 1026 subjects
Mill et al,[43] 2016	Amoxicillin	Median age 1.7 y	Immediate Nonimmediate	5.9% (48/818)
Moral et al,[44] 2011	BL	Mean age 6.7 y	Nonimmediate	1/50
Ponvert et al,[30] 2011	BL	4 mo–17 y	Immediate Nonimmediate	7.7% (111/1431)
Vezir et al,[4] 2014	BL	Median age of 4.3 y	Nonimmediate	4/119
Zambonino et al,[45] 2014	BL	1–14 y	Immediate Nonimmediate	7.92% (62/783)

Data from Refs.[4,5,30,43–45]

Table 5					
Desensitization to antibiotics (example ampicillin)					
	Ampicillin	**Target 1000 mg**			
Full dose	**1000.0**	**mg**	**IV Q6**		**Total mg to be injected in each bottle**[a]
Solution 1	250	cc of	0.040	mg/mL	10.000
Solution 2	250	cc of	0.400	mg/mL	100.000
Solution 3	250	cc of	3.969	mg/mL	992.130
Step	**Solution**	**Rate (cc/h)**	**Time (min)**	**Administered Dose (mg)**	**Cumulative Dose (mg)**
1	1	2	15	0.0200	0.0200
2	1	5	15	0.0500	0.0700
3	1	10	15	0.1000	0.1700
4	1	20	15	0.2000	0.3700
5	2	5	15	0.5000	0.8700
6	2	10	15	1.0000	1.8700
7	2	20	15	2.0000	3.8700
8	2	40	15	4.0000	7.8700
9	3	10	15	9.9213	17.7913
10	3	20	15	19.8426	37.6339
11	3	40	15	39.6852	77.3191
12	3	75	186	922.6809	1000.0000
	Total time =		351	minutes	

[a] Note to pharmacy: The total milligrams injected is more than the final dose because solutions 1 and 2 are not completely infused.

Data from Brennan PJ, Rodriguez Bouza T, Hsu FI, et al. Hypersensitivity reactions to mAbs: 105 desensitizations in 23 patients, from evaluation to treatment. J Allergy Clin Immunol 2009;124(6):1259–66.

monoclonal antibodies has been reported mostly for adults, but there are successful desensitizations in children as well.[6,7,49] The desensitization protocols to monoclonal antibodies use the 12-bags protocol, similar to antibiotic protocol in **Table 5**, and have been described by Brennan and colleagues.[32] This same procedure can be used in children but may need to be modified based on weight and reaction, as described by Dilley and colleagues[6] for rituximab allergy (**Table 6**).[32]

Desensitization should only be pursued in a child if there are no alternative drugs available for the care of the child. Desensitization is time consuming and costly, but safe in children. Desensitization and graded challenge should never be performed in children with a history of severe T-cell–mediated drug reaction such as TEN/SJS or DRESS.[28]

FUTURE CONSIDERATIONS

Management of drug allergy in children depends on accurate diagnosis of drug allergy that can lead to appropriate testing depending on the type of reaction that occurred. New classifications based on phenotypes and endotypes may lead to more individualized treatments for drug allergy in the future. Testing young children should not be avoided because of parental or physician fear of testing because it has been confirmed to be safe in the pediatric populations and would help to address overlabeling. Monoclonal antibody allergy is likely to increase as more of these products

Table 6
Protocol for desensitization to monoclonal antibodies in children (example rituximab)

Name of medication:	*Rituximab*	
Target Dose (mg)		225.0
Standard volume per bag (mL)		250
Final rate of infusion (mL/hr)		30

Calculated final concentration (mg/mL)	0.9
Standard time of infusion (minutes)	187.5

					Total mg per bag
Solution 1	250	mL of	0.009	mg/mL	2.250
Solution 2	250	mL of	0.090	mg/mL	22.500
Solution 3	250	mL of	0.896	mg/mL	224.115

*** PLEASE NOTE *** The total volume and dose dispensed are more than the final dose given to patient because many of the solutions are *not completely infused*

Step	Solution	Rate (mL/hr)	Time (min)	Volume infused per step (mL)	Dose administered with this step (mg)	Cumulative dose (mg)
1	1	1.0	15	0.25	0.0023	0.0023
2	1	2.5	15	0.63	0.0056	0.0079
3	1	5.0	15	1.25	0.0113	0.0191
4	1	10.0	15	2.50	0.0225	0.0416
5	2	2.5	15	0.63	0.0563	0.0979
6	2	5.0	15	1.25	0.1125	0.2104
7	2	10.0	15	2.50	0.2250	0.4354
8	2	20.0	15	5.00	0.4500	0.8854
9	3	5.0	15	1.25	1.1206	2.0059
10	3	10.0	15	2.50	2.2411	4.2471
11	3	20.0	15	5.00	4.4823	8.7294
12	3	30.0	482.5	241.25	216.2706	225.0000

Total time (minutes) = 647.5 = 10.79 h

Data from Dilley MA, Lee JP, Platt CD, et al. Rituximab desensitization in pediatric patients: results of a case series. Pediatr Allergy Immunol Pulmonol 2016;29(2):91–4; and Brennan PJ, Rodriguez Bouza T, Hsu FI, et al. Hypersensitivity reactions to mAbs: 105 desensitizations in 23 patients, from evaluation to treatment. J Allergy Clin Immunol 2009;124(6):1259–66.

become available on the market with pediatric indications. Accurate diagnosis for both antibiotic allergy and monoclonal antibody allergy leads to better workup and management of these allergies.

REFERENCES

1. Macy E, Contreras R. Health care use and serious infection prevalence associated with penicillin "allergy" in hospitalized patients: a cohort study. J Allergy Clin Immunol 2014;133(3):790–6.
2. Esposito S, Castellazzi L, Tagliabue C, et al. Allergy to antibiotics in children: an overestimated problem. Int J Antimicrob Agents 2016;48(4):361–6.
3. Bass JW, Crowley DM, Steele RW, et al. Adverse effects of orally administered ampicillin. J Pediatr 1973;83(1):106–8.
4. Vezir E, Erkocoglu M, Civelek E, et al. The evaluation of drug provocation tests in pediatric allergy clinic: a single center experience. Allergy Asthma Proc 2014;35: 156–62.

5. Atanaskovic-Markovic M, Gaeta F, Medjo B, et al. Non-immediate hypersensitivity reactions to beta-lactam antibiotics in children - our 10-year experience in allergy work-up. Pediatr Allergy Immunol 2016;27(5):533–8.

6. Dilley MA, Lee JP, Platt CD, et al. Rituximab desensitization in pediatric patients: results of a case series. Pediatr Allergy Immunol Pulmonol 2016;29(2):91–4.

7. Picard M, Galvao VR. Current knowledge and management of hypersensitivity reactions to monoclonal antibodies. J Allergy Clin Immunol Pract 2017;5(3):600–9.

8. Thong B, Tan TC. Epidemiology and risk factors for drug allergy. Br J Clin Pharmacol 2011;71(5):684–700.

9. Fox SJ, Park MA. Penicillin skin testing is a safe and effective tool for evaluating penicillin allergy in the pediatric population. J Allergy Clin Immunol Pract 2014; 2(4):439–44.

10. Rebelo Gomes E, Fonseca J, Araujo L, et al. Drug allergy claims in children: from self-reporting to confirmed diagnosis. Clin Exp Allergy 2008;38(1):191–8.

11. Solensky R. Allergy to β-lactam antibiotics. J Allergy Clin Immunol 2012;130(6): 1442-2.e5.

12. Le J, Nguyen T, Law AV, et al. Adverse drug reactions among children over a 10-year period. Pediatrics 2006;118(2):555–62.

13. Ibia EO, Schwartz RH, Wiedermann BL. Antibiotic rashes in children: a survey in a private practice setting. Arch Dermatol 2000;136(7):849–54.

14. Romano A, Caubet J-C. Antibiotic allergies in children and adults: from clinical symptoms to skin testing diagnosis. J Allergy Clin Immunol Pract 2014;2(1):3–12.

15. Caubet JC, Eigenmann PA. Managing possible antibiotic allergy in children. Curr Opin Infect Dis 2012;25(3):279–85.

16. Kuyucu S, Mori F, Atanaskovic-Markovic M, et al. Hypersensitivity reactions to non-betalactam antibiotics in children: an extensive review. Pediatr Allergy Immunol 2014;25(6):534–43.

17. Caimmi SM, Caimmi D, Riscassi S, et al. A new pediatric protocol for rapid desensitization to monoclonal antibodies. Int Arch Allergy Immunol 2014; 165(3):214–8.

18. Hong DI, Dioun AF. Indications, protocols, and outcomes of drug desensitizations for chemotherapy and monoclonal antibodies in adults and children. J Allergy Clin Immunol Pract 2014;2(1):13–9 [quiz: 20].

19. O'Connell AE, Lee JP, Yee C, et al. Successful desensitization to brentuximab vedotin after anaphylaxis. Clin Lymphoma Myeloma Leuk 2014;14(2):e73–5.

20. Gell P, Coombs R, Lachmann P. Classification of allergic reactions for clinical hypersensitivity disease. In: Gell PGH, Coombs RPA, editors. Clinical aspects of immunology. Oxford (United Kingdom): Blackwell Scientific Publications; 1968. p. 575–9.

21. Trubiano J, Phillips E. Antimicrobial stewardship's new weapon? A review of antibiotic allergy and pathways to 'de-labeling'. Curr Opin Infect Dis 2013;26(6): 526–37.

22. Aung AK, Haas DW, Hulgan T, et al. Pharmacogenomics of antimicrobial agents. Pharmacogenomics 2014;15(15):1903–30.

23. Pichler WJ. Delayed drug hypersensitivity reactions. Ann Intern Med 2003;139(8): 683–93.

24. Muraro A, Lemanske RF, Castells M, et al. Precision medicine in allergic disease - food allergy, drug allergy, and anaphylaxis-PRACTALL document of the European Academy of Allergy and Clinical Immunology and the American Academy of Allergy, Asthma & Immunology. Allergy 2017;72(7):1006–21.

25. Schneck J, Fagot J-PP, Sekula P, et al. Effects of treatments on the mortality of Stevens-Johnson syndrome and toxic epidermal necrolysis: a retrospective study on patients included in the prospective EuroSCAR Study. J Am Acad Dermatol 2008;58(1):33–40.

26. Pichler WJ, Beeler A, Keller M, et al. Pharmacological interaction of drugs with immune receptors: the p-i concept. Allergol Int 2006;55(1):17–25.

27. Demoly P, Adkinson NF, Brockow K, et al. International consensus on drug allergy. Allergy 2014;69(4):420–37.

28. Joint Task Force on Practice Parameters, American Academy of Allergy, Asthma and Immunology, American College of Allergy, Asthma and Immunology, Joint Council of Allergy, Asthma and Immunology. Drug allergy: an updated practice parameter. Ann Allergy Asthma Immunol 2010;105(4):259–73.

29. Dioun A. Management of multiple drug allergies in children. Curr Allergy Asthma Rep 2012;12(1):79–84.

30. Ponvert C, Perrin Y, Bados-Albiero A, et al. Allergy to betalactam antibiotics in children: results of a 20-year study based on clinical history, skin and challenge tests. Pediatr Allergy Immunol 2011;22(4):411–8.

31. Arikoglu T, Aslan G, Batmaz S, et al. Diagnostic evaluation and risk factors for drug allergies in children: from clinical history to skin and challenge tests. Int J Clin Pharm 2015;37(4):583–91.

32. Brennan PJ, Bouza T, Hsu IF, et al. Hypersensitivity reactions to mAbs: 105 desensitizations in 23 patients, from evaluation to treatment. J Allergy Clin Immunol 2009;124(6):1259–66.

33. Seifert G, Reindl T, Lobitz S, et al. Fatal course after administration of rituximab in a boy with relapsed all: a case report and review of literature. Haematologica 2006;91(6 Suppl):Ecr23.

34. Caubet JC, Kaiser L, Lemaitre B, et al. The role of penicillin in benign skin rashes in childhood: a prospective study based on drug rechallenge. J Allergy Clin Immunol 2011;127(1):218–22.

35. Romano A, Gaeta F, Arribas Poves MF, et al. Cross-reactivity among beta-lactams. Curr Allergy Asthma Rep 2016;16(3):24.

36. Atanaskovic-Markovic M, Gaeta F, Gavrovic-Jankulovic M, et al. Tolerability of imipenem in children with IgE-mediated hypersensitivity to penicillins. J Allergy Clin Immunol 2009;124(1):167–9.

37. Romano A, Gaeta F, Valluzzi RL, et al. Cross-reactivity and tolerability of aztreonam and cephalosporins in subjects with a T cell-mediated hypersensitivity to penicillins. J Allergy Clin Immunol 2016;138(1):179–86.

38. Scherer K, Bircher AJ. Hypersensitivity reactions to fluoroquinolones. Curr Allergy Asthma Rep 2005;5(1):15–21.

39. Brockow K, Garvey LH, Aberer W, et al. Skin test concentrations for systemically administered drugs – an ENDA/EAACI Drug Allergy Interest Group position paper. Allergy 2013;68(6):702–12.

40. Empedrad R, Darter AL, Earl HS, et al. Nonirritating intradermal skin test concentrations for commonly prescribed antibiotics. J Allergy Clin Immunol 2003;112(3):629–30.

41. Khan DA. Hypersensitivity and immunologic reactions to biologics: opportunities for the allergist. Ann Allergy Asthma Immunol 2016;117(2):115–20.

42. Atanaskovic-Markovic M, Caubet J-C. Management of drug hypersensitivity in the pediatric population. Expert Rev Clin pharmacol 2016;9(10):1341–9.

43. Mill C, Primeau MN, Medoff E, et al. Assessing the diagnostic properties of a graded oral provocation challenge for the diagnosis of immediate and nonimmediate reactions to amoxicillin in children. JAMA Pediatr 2016;170(6):e160033.
44. Moral L, Garde J, Toral T, et al. Short protocol for the study of paediatric patients with suspected betalactam antibiotic hypersensitivity and low risk criteria. Allergol Immunopathol (Madr) 2011;39(6):337–41.
45. Zambonino MA, Corzo JL, Munoz C, et al. Diagnostic evaluation of hypersensitivity reactions to beta-lactam antibiotics in a large population of children. Pediatr Allergy Immunol 2014;25(1):80–7.
46. Cernadas JR. Desensitization to antibiotics in children. Pediatr Allergy Immunol 2013;24(1):3–9.
47. Turvey SE, Cronin B, Arnold AD, et al. Antibiotic desensitization for the allergic patient: 5 years of experience and practice. Ann Allergy Asthma Immunol 2004;92(4):426–32.
48. de Groot H, Mulder WM. Clinical practice: drug desensitization in children. Eur J Pediatr 2010;169(11):1305–9.
49. Puchner TC, Kugathasan S, Kelly KJ, et al. Successful desensitization and therapeutic use of infliximab in adult and pediatric Crohn's disease patients with prior anaphylactic reaction. Inflamm Bowel Dis 2001;7(1):34–7.

Aspirin and Nonsteroidal Antiinflammatory Drugs Hypersensitivity and Management

 CrossMark

Brian Modena, MD, Andrew A. White, MD*,
Katharine M. Woessner, MD

KEYWORDS

- Aspirin • Nonsteroidal antiinflammatory drugs • Chronic spontaneous urticaria
- Aspirin-exacerbated respiratory disease • Desensitization • Oral challenge

KEY POINTS

- Hypersensitivity reactions to aspirin and nonsteroidal antiinflammatory drugs (NSAIDs) are common, and the allergist must carefully elicit the history when these drugs could be the cause.
- Desensitization protocols are an option for most causes of hypersensitivity reactions. Oral challenges can be equally useful to identify safe alternatives.
- Cyclooxygenase-2–specific medications are often well-tolerated in the NSAID- or aspirin-allergic patient.

INTRODUCTION

Nonsteroidal antiinflammatory drugs (NSAIDs) are a group of pharmaceuticals primarily used for analgesic purposes with the exception of acetylsalicylic acid (aspirin [ASA]) whose primary use is for its antiplatelet effect. The availability of these medications over the counter, combined with their often first-line use in most types of pain and fever, make them one of the most popular classes of medications used worldwide. The use of ASA for primary and secondary prevention of cardiovascular disease significantly increases the global use of this medication class. In 2005, 19.3% of adult Americans took ASA daily or every other day.[1] Although the prevalence of hypersensitivity to NSAIDs may be low, the sheer volume of use and exposure makes

The authors have nothing to disclose.
Division of Allergy, Asthma and Immunology, Scripps Clinic, 3811 Valley Centre Drive, S99, San Diego, CA 92130, USA
* Corresponding author.
E-mail address: White.andrew@scrippshealth.org

Immunol Allergy Clin N Am 37 (2017) 727–749
http://dx.doi.org/10.1016/j.iac.2017.07.008
0889-8561/17/© 2017 Elsevier Inc. All rights reserved.

consultation to the allergist for a reaction to one of these medications a relatively common occurrence.

The existence of several types of hypersensitivity reactions can make the approach to these patients somewhat challenging. Yet, hypersensitivity reactions can be most effectively compartmentalized into pharmacologic (secondary to cyclooxygenase-1 [COX-1] inhibition) or a specific (likely IgE) mediated effect. The presence of reactions to more than one structurally dissimilar NSAID will greatly inform the clinician to the presence of a COX-1 based hypersensitivity reaction.

Several specific reaction phenotypes have been described[2] and will are outlined below, and discussed throughout the article in finer detail.

1. *NSAID-exacerbated cutaneous disease (NECD)*: Sensitivity to all COX-1–inhibiting NSAIDs in the setting of active chronic spontaneous urticaria (pharmacologic effect of COX-1 inhibition).
2. *NSAID-induced urticaria/angioedema (NIUA)*: These patients have no underlying chronic urticaria, but experience cutaneous symptoms with all COX-1–inhibiting NSAIDs.
3. *Single NIUA, anaphylaxis, or both*: Patients experience cutaneous or systemic anaphylactic reactions isolated to a single NSAID.
4. *ASA-exacerbated respiratory disease (AERD)*: A complex pharmacologic effect of COX-1 inhibition leading to primary respiratory hypersensitivity reactions. This occurs with all COX-1–inhibiting NSAIDs.
5. *Non–mast cell–related* (drug rash with eosinophilia and systemic symptoms, aseptic meningitis etc): These involve immune reactions do not depend on mast cell involvement and will not be specifically addressed further.

As would be true for any consultation for a drug allergy, the differentiation of immunologic hypersensitivity from adverse drug effect becomes paramount. NSAIDs are well-known for effects on the gastrointestinal tract. These reactions can vary from annoying to severe, with severe gastritis potentially being inaccurately labeled as an "allergy" in the electronic health record.[3]

NONSTEROIDAL ANTIINFLAMMATORY DRUG HYPERSENSITIVITY ENDOTYPES AND MECHANISMS

ASA had been in clinical use since 1899 when Bayer began marketing it. Yet, it was not until John Vane published the first study of prostaglandin inhibition by ASA in 1971[4] that the pharmacology of NSAIDs became defined. The ensuing decades saw significant progress to the point we are today with numerous COX-1 and COX-2 selective agents on the market. Nonspecific NSAIDs can have action at both COX-1 and COX-2. COX-1 has a constitutive "housekeeping" function in endothelium, kidney, and stomach as well as other locations.[5] Yet, it most likely that the benefits of the NSAID class are related to the effect on COX-2, which is an inducible enzyme at the site of inflammation. COX-2 inhibition can decrease localized prostaglandin formation therefore improving pain and swelling. It is now felt likely the most common side effects of NSAIDs (gastritis, increased thrombosis potential, etc) are related to the NSAID effects on COX-1.

One potential pitfall for the clinician might be to dichotomize this class of drugs into COX-1 versus COX-2 inhibitors. Although this fits into the general paradigm of hypersensitivity reaction phenotypes that can be seen, it also may be overly simplified. A better understanding of NSAID function in and around COX-1 and COX-2 might help to inform reaction phenotypes that do not also fit into a classic pattern. In that regard, 4 broad groups have been described within the NSAID family (**Box 1**). First, there are compounds that produce full inhibition of both COX-1 and COX-2 with poor selectivity. Second are compounds that fully inhibit COX-1 and COX-2 with preferential COX-2 activity. A third group strongly inhibits COX-2 with minimal activity at COX-1, and finally, there are compounds that only weakly act at both COX 1 and COX-2.[5]

PREVALENCE

It is somewhat difficult to pinpoint a precise NSAID hypersensitivity prevalence estimate because the various subtypes of hypersensitivity discussed make it challenging to identify in the general population. Furthermore, some reactions only occur within a specific defined disease population (AERD in nasal polyposis and NECD in chronic urticaria), making it less relevant to describe global prevalence. Yet, with millions of Americans using an NSAID on a regular basis, it is important to understand the scope of the problem that allergists encounter. In nearly all subtypes of drug allergy, NSAIDs are a common cause.

In a Latin American study, of confirmed cases of drug-induced anaphylaxis, 57.8% were secondary to an NSAID.[6] In 806 patients with adverse drug reactions, anaphylaxis was identified in 14.5%. NSAIDs represented the most frequent cause.[7] In

---

Box 1
List of NSAIDs classified by effects on COX-1 and COX-2

NSAIDs that fully inhibit COX-1 and COX-2
  Aspirin
  Piroxicam
  Sulindac
  Ibuprofen
  Ketorolac
  Naproxen
  Ketoprofen
  Indomethacin
  Diclofenac

Preferential COX-2 inhibitors with partial COX-1 inhibition
  Etodolac
  Meloxicam
  Nimesulide[a]
  Nabumetone

Primary COX-2 inhibitors with little action at COX-1
  Rofecoxib[a]
  Etoricoxib[a]
  Valdecoxib[a]
  Lumiracoxib[a]
  Celecoxib

Weak inhibitors of both COX-1 and COX-2
  5-ASA
  Acetaminophen
  Diflunisal
  Sulfasalazine

Abbreviations: COX, cyclooxygenase; NSAIDs, nonsteroidal antiinflammatory drugs.

  [a] Not available in the United States.

cutaneous drug reactions in the outpatient clinic, NSAIDs were the second most common cause behind antimicrobials.[8] NSAID induced adverse cutaneous drug reactions in Chinese inpatients caused 18.5% of all drug induced reactions and were the third most common behind antimicrobials and radiocontrast media.[9]

Ortiz-Sanjuán and colleagues[10] evaluated 239 patients with drug-induced cutaneous vasculitis and identified the cause as NSAIDs in 10% (second only to beta-lactams). In Brazil, 10.5% of severe cutaneous adverse reactions were secondary to analgesic or antiinflammatory drugs.[11]

It would seem that, globally, in any case of a suspected hypersensitivity reaction, a specific and focused history on NSAID exposure is imperative. The fact that many of these medications are available over the counter and will not necessarily show up on pharmacy or medical records adds to the importance of inquiring specifically about these medications.

NONSTEROIDAL ANTIINFLAMMATORY DRUG-EXACERBATED CUTANEOUS DISEASE

Patients with chronic spontaneous urticaria who experience an exacerbation of their underlying urticaria and/or angioedema with COX-1 inhibitors are defined as having NECD.[12]

Clinical Presentation of Nonsteroidal Antiinflammatory Drug-exacerbated Cutaneous Disease

In patients with chronic spontaneous urticaria, approximately 12% to 30% will experience an exacerbation of their urticaria and/or angioedema with minutes to hours of exposure to COX-1–inhibiting NSAIDs.[13,14] As seen in AERD, individuals with NECD react to all COX-1–inhibiting NSAIDs and, despite avoidance of NSAIDs, the underlying disease process continues (ie, avoidance of COX-1-inhibiting NSAIDs will not ameliorate their chronic urticaria).[15] In general, the highly selective COX-2 inhibitors are well-tolerated.[16,17] The sensitivity to NSAIDs can fluctuate over time and, in general, during periods of remission of their chronic urticaria, all NSAIDs are well-tolerated.[18]

Diagnosis of Nonsteroidal Antiinflammatory Drug-exacerbated Cutaneous Disease

The single criterion for diagnosing NECD is flare of their underlying chronic urticaria with NSAID exposure.

Controversy

For the patient who has chronic urticaria and needs an NSAID, determining whether or not they will tolerate one necessitates conducting a challenge. There are many variables that can lead to worsening urticaria in chronic urticaria, such as viral infections, physical factors, and hormones, thus making it difficult to rely on history for making the diagnosis of NECD. Therefore, oral ASA challenge is the gold standard for making the diagnosis. The European guidelines recommend doing a 2-day placebo controlled ASA challenge after the patient has been without any eruption for 1 to 2 weeks.[19] A problem with that approach is that their chronic urticaria will be in remission and they may no longer be reactive.[18] Another approach would be to withdraw the patient from antihistamines to do the challenge; however, the interpretation of the challenge is complicated by the question as to whether the ASA triggered the urticarial flare or was it the withdrawal of the antihistamines. Taking an example from a study looking at food additives in chronic urticaria, using the minimum effective dose of antihistamine to control the urticaria but still having some symptoms, an NSAID challenge can be performed while the urticaria is active.[20]

Management of Nonsteroidal Antiinflammatory Drug-exacerbated Cutaneous Disease

Avoidance of NSAIDs is the cornerstone of management of NECD. The highly selective COX-2 inhibitors are generally well-tolerated in this patient population.[16,17] When the chronic urticaria is quiescent, the majority of patients will be able to once again tolerate the COX-1–inhibiting NSAIDs. Often these patients and their providers believe they are hypersensitive to NSAIDs going forward and they unnecessarily avoid these medications. It is useful to rechallenge with ASA once the chronic urticaria is not active. Some patients with chronic urticaria have relapses episodically; it is likely that their sensitivity to NSAIDs will recur with subsequent flares of chronic urticaria.

Nonsteroidal Antiinflammatory Drug-exacerbated Cutaneous Disease and the Role of Aspirin Desensitization

If there is a need for ASA in chronic urticaria for cardioprotective reasons, the 81-mg dose is often below the provoking dose for exacerbating urticaria.[21] Therefore, it is worth challenging with 40.5 mg of ASA on their maintenance dose of chronic urticaria therapy and repeat in 90 minutes. If tolerated, start ASA 81 mg/d[22] (**Fig. 1**).

If they react to ASA, it is the authors' clinical experience that ASA desensitization is rarely successful in patients with NECD. Simon[23] reported attempts to desensitize 25 patients to ASA with a history of chronic urticaria and NECD. These patients developed marked worsening of urticaria, not responsive to antihistamines, and required

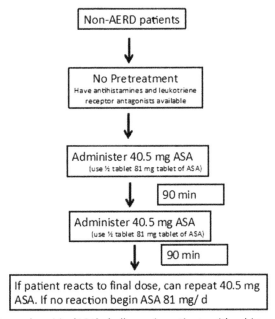

Fig. 1. Protocol for oral aspirin (ASA) challenge in patients with a history of cutaneous reactions to nonsteroidal antiinflammatory drugs. to get to 81 mg antiplatelet dose. Symptoms should be treated with antihistamines; if severe symptoms occur, treat and repeat the dose. Once tolerant can start 81 mg/d of aspirin. AERD, aspirin-exacerbated respiratory disease. (*From* White AA, Stevenson DD, Woessner KM, et al. Approach to patients with aspirin hypersensitivity and acute cardiovascular emergencies. Allergy Asthma Proc 2013;34(2):141; with permission.)

prednisone. Rechallenge with ASA met with the same reaction.[23] There are several case reports of successful desensitization to ASA in NECD, but these are isolated reports suggesting that attempts to desensitize even with high-dose antihistamines are not successful in the majority of cases.[24,25]

NONSTEROIDAL ANTIINFLAMMATORY DRUG-INDUCED URTICARIA/ANGIOEDEMA

These patients have no underlying chronic skin disease but develop urticaria and/or angioedema within minutes to hours after ingesting COX-1 inhibiting NSAIDs. NSAID-induced angioedema (often periorbital) without urticaria can be seen sometimes developing up to 24 hours after exposure.[26–28] It was originally suggested that NIUA was a precursor to developing chronic urticaria, preceding its development by years.[29] However, a more recent study found that the percentage of patients with NIUA who developed chronic urticaria was not different from that among healthy control subjects.[30] Patients with NIUA react to chemically unrelated COX-1 inhibitors, suggesting the pathogenesis is due to COX-1 inhibition, similar to AERD.

Diagnosis of Nonsteroidal Antiinflammatory Drug-induced Urticaria/Angioedema

A history of skin reactions to at least 2 chemically unrelated NSAIDs in patients without underlying chronic cutaneous disease have a high likelihood of having NIUA.[28,30] If the history is not clear, then an oral challenge with ASA is recommended to confirm the diagnosis of a cross-reactive type of NSAID hypersensitivity as well as to differentiate it from single NIUA.[31]

Management of Nonsteroidal Antiinflammatory Drug-induced Urticaria/Angioedema

If no NSAIDs are required, a simple management strategy is avoidance of strong COX-1 inhibitors. In general, the highly selective COX-2 inhibitors and weak COX-1 inhibitors (acetaminophen and paracetamol) are well-tolerated.[16,17]

Aspirin Desensitization in Nonsteroidal Antiinflammatory Drug-Induced Urticaria/Angioedema

Unlike NECD, if ASA or other NSAIDs are required, these patients can undergo successful desensitization[21,22,32] (see **Fig. 1**; **Fig. 2**). The clinical experience of the authors' is that these desensitizations can sometimes be challenging and may require multiple days to be successful. The addition of antihistamines and antileukotrienes are helpful until tolerance is established. As with AERD, when desensitized with ASA, they are cross-desensitized to all COX-1–inhibiting NSAIDs, which can be maintained with daily dosing.

A recent longitudinal study by Doña and colleagues[33] found that 63% of patients lost their sensitivity to NSAIDs and could tolerate them at 72 months after the last reaction. This stresses the importance of reassessment periodically to prevent the unnecessary avoidance of ASA or other NSAIDs.

SINGLE NONSTEROIDAL ANTIINFLAMMATORY DRUG-INDUCED URTICARIA/ANGIOEDEMA, ANAPHYLAXIS, OR BOTH

This NSAID hypersensitivity classification is characterized by wheals, angioedema and/or anaphylaxis triggered by a single NSAID or by 2 or more NSAIDs with a similar chemical structure.[34] Any of the following clinical manifestations may be observed after oral, topical, or injected exposure to a single NSAID: urticaria, angioedema, laryngeal edema, generalized pruritus, rhinitis, bronchospasm, anaphylaxis, and even

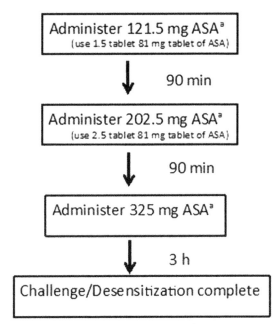

Fig. 2. Protocol for increasing the aspirin (ASA) dose from 81 mg to 325 mg. Symptoms should be treated if they occur. [a] If severe symptoms occur at any dose, that dose should be repeated before proceeding to final dose. (*From* White AA, Stevenson DD, Woessner KM, et al. Approach to patients with aspirin hypersensitivity and acute cardiovascular emergencies. Allergy Asthma Proc 2013;34(2):142; with permission.)

death can occur.[35,36] Reactions to a single NSAID are seen most commonly with the pyrazolone class followed by acetaminophen, paracetamol, diclofenac, and ibuprofen.[37–41]

Diagnosis of Single Nonsteroidal Antiinflammatory Drug-Induced Urticaria/Angioedema

Diagnosing single NSAID reactors can be challenging. With the exception of pyrazolones, there are no standardized skin tests or in vitro assays. Relying on the patient 's history is unreliable, as was shown in a study by Viola and colleagues,[42] in which they assessed NSAID hypersensitivity in 275 patients with a history of an NSAID reaction with provocation tests. Despite a history of reacting to an NSAID, 77.8% of their subjects tolerated that NSAID in an oral challenge (patients with AERD were excluded).[42]

In the absence of a reliable in vitro test, an accurate diagnosis depends on a careful history and oral drug challenge and provocation testing. In patients with a history of anaphylaxis or a very severe reaction, an oral provocation test with the suspect drug should almost never be performed because alternative NSAIDs are readily available.[34]

Management of Single Nonsteroidal Antiinflammatory Drug-Induced Urticaria/Angioedema

Once the culprit NSAID is identified in single NSAID reactors, management involves avoidance of that drug and others that are chemically related (**Box 2**). Desensitization is not recommended because the multiple other NSAID alternatives on the market

---

Box 2
List of NSAIDs classified by physical structure

Enolic acids

Oxicams
  Piroxicam (Feldene)

Pyrazoles
  Phenylbutazone (Butazolidin)
  Oxyphenbutazone (Tandearil)

Carboxylic acids

Salicylates
  Acetylsalicylic acid (aspirin)
  Salsalate (Disalcid)
  Difunisal (Dolobid)
  Choline salicylate (Trilisate)

Acetic acids
  Indomethacin (Indocin)
  Etodolac (Lodine)
  Sulindac (Clinoril)
  Tometin (Tolectin)
  Zomepirac (Zomax)
  Diflofenac (Voltaren)

Fenamates
  Meclofenamate (Meclomen)
  Mefenamic acid (Ponstel)

Pyrrolo-pyrrole
  Ketorolac tromethamine (Toradol)

Propionic acids
  Ibuprofen (Motrin, Rufen)
  Naproxen (Naprosyn)
  Naproxen sodium (Anaprox)
  Benoxaprofen (Oraflex)
  Fenoprofen (Nalfon)
  Ketoprofen (Orodis)

Abbreviation: NSAIDs, nonsteroidal antiinflammatory drugs.

---

make substitution of a COX-2 or structurally dissimilar NSAID a better option in almost all cases.

ASPIRIN-EXACERBATED RESPIRATORY DISEASE
Clinical Characteristics

AERD, a specific subtype of chronic rhinosinusitis and asthma, is characterized by chronic eosinophilic sinonasal and lower airway inflammation with severe and recurrent nasal polyposis, asthma, and acute exacerbations of upper and lower respiratory symptoms when exposed to ASA or other COX-1–inhibiting NSAIDs. AERD occurs in roughly 7% of asthmatics, although the prevalence is 1 in 8 of those with severe asthma. It occurs in roughly 9% of patients with chronic rhinosinusitis, and one-third of those with asthma and nasal polyposis.[43]

A recent survey of 190 participants with AERD showed that the impact of AERD on quality of life is substantial.[44] Using a scale of 1 (mild) to 9 (severe), the mean score was 6, with roughly 28% of patients reporting either an 8 or 9. When asked to identify the one aspect that most reduced their quality of life, chronic nasal symptoms and anosmia were most common, reported in 43% and 39% of respondents, respectively. Further, 87% and 89% of patients reported that chronic nasal symptoms and a decreased sense of smell decreased their quality of life, which compared with only 65% reported chronic asthma symptoms.

It is increasingly recognized that alcohol ingestion also induces respiratory symptoms in patients with AERD. A survey of 59 patients with AERD (confirmed by a positive reaction to a supervised ASA challenge) found that 75% reported upper respiratory reactions (rhinorrhea or nasal congestion) and 51% reported lower respiratory reactions (wheezing or dyspnea) with ingestion of only a few sips of alcohol.[45] Overall, 83% of patients with AERD reported alcohol-induced respiratory symptoms, compared with 43% of patients with ASA-tolerant asthma and 43% of patients with nasal polyps (with ASA tolerance). The etiology of this phenomenon is yet to be elucidated, but the authors theorize that alcohol-induced reactions occur by altered production or metabolism of cysteinyl leukotrienes, the putative mediators of ASA-induced reactions.

Not only are daily symptoms contributing to the morbidity of AERD, but the aggressive nature of the inflammation tends toward more severe outcomes in both the upper and lower airways. Patients with AERD are at a 10-fold greater risk for sinus surgery and have much higher rates of recurrence 6 months after surgery.[46] In terms of lower airway involvement, patients with AERD are much more likely to have persistent airflow limitation, to have been intubated for asthma, to have had an asthma exacerbation in the past year, and to require systemic corticosteroids when compared with ASA-tolerant asthmatics.[47–49]

Pathogenesis of Aspirin-Exacerbated Respiratory Disease

The etiology of AERD is incompletely understood. AERD occurs typically in adulthood. Nasal and sinus symptoms typically precede lower airway disease, and the development of pulmonary symptoms is believed to indicate disease progression. Thus, the development of AERD is possibly the result of a combination of environmental insults and airway changes, likely in individuals with a yet-to-identified genetic susceptibility.

The molecular pathophysiology is characterized by an imbalance in proinflammatory and antiinflammatory mediators of the arachidonic acid signaling pathway. Particularly, the overproduction of inflammatory cysteinyl leukotrienes LTC_4, LTD_4, and LTE_4, which are potent inducers of mucous production, bronchospasm, and airway edema,[50] and a reduction in the antiinflammatory prostaglandin E2 (PGE_2) are believed to have central roles.

Mast Cells

Mast cell activation and marked tissue eosinophilia characterize airway inflammation in AERD. Degranulated mast cells are readily found in nasal polyps,[51,52] and their presence does not depend on allergic sensitization.[53] Administration of ASA has shown to acutely increase mast cell granule contents (ie, tryptase and histamine) and eicosanoid mediators (ie, PGD_2) in the nasal passage.[54–56] As a result, mast cell degranulation is believed to contribute to the acute symptoms of an ASA reaction. Supportively, mast cell–stabilizing medications, such as cromolyn sodium, have shown to prevent ASA-induced bronchoconstriction.[57,58]

The mechanisms by which COX-1 inhibiting medications trigger mast cell degranulation are unknown, but likely involve reduction in PGE_2, an inhibitor of mast cell degranulation. AERD airway mast cells produce diminished levels of PGE_2 at baseline.[59,60] A further reduction of PGE_2 by COX-1 inhibition is likely central to the pronounced mast cell degranulation.[59,61]

Additionally, activated mast cells are responsible for the production of prostaglandin D2 (PGD_2), a proinflammatory arachidonic acid metabolite overrepresented in AERD airways at baseline and further increased during an ASA challenge reaction.[55,62–64] PGD_2 causes airway bronchoconstriction and nasal congestion by dilatation of sinusoid vessels, which occurs mechanistically by increases in cyclic adenosine monophosphate tissue levels.[63,65] PGD_2 mediates chemotaxis of eosinophils and newly described ILC2b.[66,67] PGD_2 activates T2-delineated T cells, basophils, and monocytes via the CRTH2 receptor.[68] Finally, a failure of ASA desensitization has been recently associated with markedly higher levels of basal urine PGD_2 metabolite, termed PGD-M.[64]

Eosinophils

Eosinophils comprise more than 60% of nasal polyp cell population, and can be found in mostly between the thickened basement membrane and epithelial cells.[51] Patients with AERD have higher sinonasal and lower airway eosinophilia than patients with chronic rhinosinusitis with nasal polyps alone.[51] Mast cells contribute to eosinophil chemotaxis into the airways by secretion of eosinophil chemoattractant factors eotaxin and IL-5,[69] providing a link between mast cell degranulation/activation and eosinophil infiltration, and perhaps the first step in polyp formation. Eosinophils alternatively act on mast cells, and the 2 cell types act reciprocally to guide and enhance each other's function, something that has recently been termed the "allergic effector unit.[70]"

Notwithstanding the paradigm that mast cells and eosinophils conspire to produce AERD airway inflammation, several studies have shown that it is the intensity of eosinophil infiltration of the sinuses and lungs, and not the presence of mast cells, that distinguishes AERD from ASA-tolerant asthma.[71,72] Like mast cells, PGE_2 acts through receptor EP2 to inhibit eosinophil activation.[72] PGE_2 production is suppressed, and expression of its receptor EP2 is diminished in AERD. COX-1–inhibiting enzymes further suppress PGE_2 production, overcoming inhibition thresholds of eosinophils.[72] The breakthrough release of the PGE_2 'brake' leads to a surge in cysteinyl leukotriene secretion by airway eosinophils, which mechanistically occurs by a dramatic upregulation in leukotriene C4 synthase.[73] Platelets that are adherent to eosinophils in the inflammatory milieu and other leukocytes also express LTC_4 synthase and contribute to the surge in leukotriene production.[74] Further, there is recent evidence that impaired granulocyte protein kinase A synergizes with adherent platelets to dysregulate PGE_2-dependent suppression of 5-lipoxygenase activity.[75]

As an alternative explanation to mast cell degranulation, this surge in cysteinyl leukotrienes produced by platelets and eosinophils is theorized to be the primary driver of bronchospasm. Supportively, drugs that inhibit leukotrienes are shown to increase FEV_1 after 6 weeks of therapy,[76] and blunt the decrease in FEV_1 in response to ASA ingestion.[77] Of note, mast cells in AERD have shown to modestly express LTC4 synthase,[73] and are thought to be unlikely contributors to the "leukotriene surge."[72] Yet, in 30 patients with ASA-tolerant asthma, it was mucosal mast cells, and not eosinophils, that were the dominate cells containing LTC4 synthase.[78]

Tissue Remodeling

Nasal polyps are edematous and fibromatous structures surrounded by a thick basement membrane, and demonstrate high rates of extracellular matrix breakdown and tissue remodeling. Nasal polyp tissues express high levels of matrix metalloproteinases (MMPs).[79,80] Matrix metalloproteinase-9 is secreted by activated mast cells with levels paralleling eosinophil cationic protein, an eosinophil matrix protein, and its activity upregulated by the presence of mast cell enzymes tryptase and chymase.[81]

The growth factor transforming growth factor-beta, which is secreted by mast cells, eosinophils, macrophages, and epithelial cells, causes fibroblastic proliferation, collagen production, and nasal polyp fibroblast expression of vascular endothelial growth factor.[82] Transforming growth factor-beta enhances eosinophilic inflammation by augmentation of eotaxin production.[83,84]

PGE_2, which has demonstrated an antiproliferative effect on nasal fibroblasts via the E prostanoid (EP2) receptor, may play a second important role in the prevention of nasal polyp growth. AERD nasal fibroblasts have demonstrated decreased expression of EP2 receptors and the ability to resist the antiproliferative effect of PGE_2.[85] Providing evidence that environmental insults and influences are responsible for development of AERD by way of epigenetic modification of DNA, histone acetylation at the EP2 promotor site has been shown to correlate with EP2 messenger RNA levels.

Aspirin Challenges and Diagnosis of Aspirin-Exacerbated Respiratory Disease

AERD reactions are prototypically described as acute worsening of upper and lower airway symptoms, most often an increase in nasal congestion with accompanying shortness of breath, wheezing and/or chest tightness within 2 to 3 hours of ingesting ASA of other NSAIDs. NSAID reactions are not mediated by IgE, and are believed to result from a chemical imbalance in arachidonic acid metabolites. Individual responses to NSAIDs can vary from mild pruritus and nasal congestion to life-threatening acute asthma exacerbation, with reaction characteristics and severity are dependent on intrinsic and extrinsic factors not yet fully understood.

A positive provocation challenge to ASA or NSAIDs in an individual with nasal polyposis and asthma makes the diagnosis of AERD. To date, there are no validated biomarkers to make the diagnosis.[86] Only 43% of ASA challenges result in bronchial reactions in those suspected to have AERD,[87] and the sensitivity is only 45% to 69% when a positive response is defined as decrease in the FEV_1 of 20% or greater.[88–92] Further, with the increased use inhaled corticosteroids and leukotriene-modifying drugs before drug challenges and the transition to intranasal ketorolac with modified oral ASA challenge as a safe alternative to an oral ASA challenges, the number and severity of bronchial reactions and extrapulmonary reactions has decreased significantly.[92–94]

Several recent studies have proposed a decrease in the FEV_1 of 15% or greater as a new diagnostic criterion for ASA positive response. The lowered criterion seems to improve sensitivity while maintaining a satisfactory specificity. Yet, if this criterion were used alone to make the diagnosis, it would miss many "reactors"; an estimated 65% of individuals reportedly experience eye and/or nasal symptoms alone.

Peak nasal inspiratory flow is another measure that has been used to quantify nasal reactions, where a decrease of greater than 25% is highly specific for a positive reactions.[90] Like the use of spirometry, peak nasal inspiratory flow is not sensitive and neglects other symptoms that indicate a positive allergic response, such as tearing, rhinorrhea, or pruritus. As a result, the determination of a positive challenge still depends on the clinical judgment of the supervising physician.

Recently, a composite score termed the 10-Symptom AERD Composite Score, based on patient yes or no responses to the presence of 10 clinical symptoms, has been developed to aid physicians in quantifying subjective complaints during an ASA challenge. Specifically, 1 point is awarded for each yes response to nasal congestion, runny nose, itchy nose, sneezing, itchy or watery eyes, itchy tongue or mouth, throat tightness, and wheezing or chest tightness. Although not validated on an external cohort, an additive score of 5 or greater was moderately sensitive and highly specific in an internal cohort of 115 suspected patients with AERD.[95]

Aspirin Desensitization for Aspirin-exacerbated Respiratory Disease

There are several methods described for ASA desensitization. The general recommendations for any patient undergoing ASA desensitization for AERD include ensuring that the underlying asthma is well-controlled before commencing the desensitization and using a leukotriene modifier drug during the desensitization unless there is a contraindication. It would seem obvious that an unstable asthmatic patient should not undergo a desensitization, which could worsen asthma further. This caution sometimes means that a patient requires a step up in asthma management or even a systemic corticosteroid burst before the desensitization. The use of leukotriene modifier drugs during the desensitization have been shown to have a significant effect on blunting the asthmatic reaction while preserving the upper airway reaction in most patients, allowing for the desensitization to serve a diagnostic purpose in those patients where the diagnosis of AERD is in doubt.[94,96]

Initial desensitization protocols were often spread out over an entire week. When done exclusively under a research protocol, the first day generally included placebo challenges only to ensure stable airways. In the past decade, the desensitization setting has migrated to the outpatient and nonresearch setting. This change has generated interest in accelerating the desensitization, while preserving the excellent safety record of ASA desensitization. Lee and colleagues[92] described the use of nasal ketorolac in an effort to diminish lower respiratory reactions and increase the speed of the desensitization (**Table 1**). Many institutions use an oral ASA protocol with approximately 90-minute dosing intervals. Both the nasal ketorolac and the oral ASA protocols involved more than 1 clinic day to accomplish; with most patients finishing on day 2 and some on the third day. Chen and colleagues[91] describe an hourly dose escalation protocol that allows those patients with a completely negative challenge to be completed on the first day. Even in this protocol, many patients needed to return on the second day to complete the protocol. Overall, there are several published protocols describing successful ASA desensitization in patients with AERD.

COX-2 INHIBITORS

COX-2 inhibitors have been available throughout the world primarily for use as analgesic and antiinflammatory agents. Initially, the lack of safety data in COX-1–hypersensitive patients and warning labels from the US Food and Drug Administration (which are still present) raised the specter of possible cross-reactivity in NSAID-hypersensitive patients. Yet, mechanistically, the COX-2 inhibitors would not be expected to cause a problem in COX-1 reactors. Because, by definition, the COX-2 inhibitors have little to no activity at COX-1 and are structurally dissimilar, it became a logical conclusion that COX-2 agents would provide an alternative to narcotics in COX-1–sensitive patients. Numerous studies have now shown this to be the case in both AERD and NECD.[17,97,98] In a metaanalysis of blinded, placebo-controlled clinical trials, there was no respiratory reactivity seen in AERD upon selective COX-2 challenge.[99] With selective NSAIDs (weak COX-1 activity at higher doses), approximately 1 in 13 patients with AERD reacted[99] (curiously, a small number of COX-2 induced reactions are reported in COX-1 reactors). Bobolea and colleagues[100] report a case of

Table 1	
Nasal ketorolac and oral aspirin challenge protocol	
Time	**Dose[a]**
Day 1	
8:00 AM	1 spray ketorolac (1 spray in 1 nostril)
8:30 AM	2 sprays ketorolac (1 each nostril)
9:00 AM	4 sprays ketorolac (2 each nostril)
9:30 AM	6 sprays ketorolac (3 each nostril)
10:30 AM	60 mg aspirin
12:00 PM	60 mg aspirin
3:00 PM	Discharge patient
Day 2	
8:00 AM	150 mg aspirin
11:00 AM	325 mg aspirin[b]
2:00 PM	Discharge patient

[a] (1) Spirometry (FEV_1) and objective clinical evaluation should be performed before each dose. (2) Treat reactions appropriately and wait until symptoms resolve. (a) Reactions are classified as follows: (i) Nasoocular. (ii) Nasoocular with ≥15% decline in FEV_1 ("Classic reaction"). (iii) Lower respiratory reaction [≥20% decline in FEV_1]. (iv) Laryngospasm with or without (i), (ii), or (iii). (v) Systemic reaction (urticaria, gastrointestinal symptoms, hypotension). (3) Aspirin desensitization: (a) After reactions are treated and resolve, continue next scheduled ketorolac dose OR repeat oral provoking aspirin dose. (b) Desensitization is complete after 325 mg of aspirin. (c) Patient should take 650 mg of aspirin that evening then continue 650 mg twice daily as their continuous aspirin dose until further instructed. *Preparing nasal ketorolac*: (1) Take ketorolac (60 mg/2 mL) and mix with preservative-free normal saline (2.75 mL). (2) Place combined solution in a nasal spray bottle (one that delivers 100 μL/actuation). (3) Prime with 5 sprays before use. Each spray will now actuate 1.26 mg of ketorolac solution. (4) Patient should tilt head down during sprays and sniff gently to avoid swallowing solution.
[b] If no reaction occurs within 3 hours after 325 mg dose, consider it a negative challenge.
Adapted from Lee RU, White AA, Ding D, et al. Use of intranasal ketorolac and modified oral aspirin challenge for desensitization of aspirin-exacerbated respiratory disease. Ann Allergy Asthma Immunol 2010;105(2):132; with permission.

an individual with respiratory reactions to high-dose NSAIDs and 2 different COX-2 inhibitors, despite being on low-dose ASA (100 mg) for antiplatelet effect. The authors hypothesize that COX-2 inhibitors, which might have a gradual effect on total body PGE_2 levels,[101] might be more likely to cause acute symptoms in patients with a chronically low PGE_2 from low-dose ASA. Indeed, recent studies demonstrate the central involvement of COX-2 in the pathophysiology of AERD.[102] Although there is no clear mechanism to explain this phenomenon, the presence of these rare dual reactors suggests that most COX-1 reactive patients should receive the first dose of a COX-2 inhibitor under observation in the office.

SALICYLATES

There is no known cross-reactivity between salicylates and NSAIDs. The potential concern for reactivity likely comes from the common salicylate component of acetyl salicylic acid (ASA) and other nonacetylated salicylates. This issue tends to emerge in the clinical setting when a patient has a history of NSAID hypersensitivity and is a candidate for a salicylate compound for an autoimmune indication. Direct challenges with salicylates in AERD subjects were tolerated in all.[103–105]

CHILDREN

Clearly, far less is known regarding hypersensitivity reactions to NSAIDs in pediatric patients. The general approach to categorizing reactions would be similar to that of adults, with the main exception being that AERD does not occur in young children. Although there are rare case reports of AERD in the pediatric age group, even those are primarily in the teenage years.[106,107] In challenge studies of children with a history of NSAID hypersensitivity, the reaction could be confirmed in only one-third to two-thirds (31% to 68%).[108–110] As in adults, it seems that clinical history is insufficient to make the diagnosis, and drug provocation studies are likely necessary to truly confirm the diagnosis. In children with a negative provocative challenge, 12% reported subsequent NSAID reactivity, including several cases that were subsequently proven upon reevaluation.[111] It is important to note that several studies point out that there are a group of children with NSAID reaction patterns that cannot be explained by our current mechanistic understanding of these reactions.[109,112]

Chronic Urticaria

In pediatric patients with chronic urticaria, single-blinded, placebo-controlled challenges identified 24% reacting to ASA in the daily or near daily hive group, and in only 1 in 10 of the recurrent urticaria group (urticaria 2–4 days per week).[113]

Respiratory Reactions

Interestingly, a small group of pediatric patients have been described with respiratory reactions to NSAIDs. This number is 2% of all asthmatics,[114] although a much earlier study suggested that as many as 28% might be ASA intolerant with respiratory reactions.[115] It seems unlikely that these subjects had the clinical phenotype of AERD, making reactivity at this level hard to explain. Perhaps differences in asthma control over the decades could explain either true or perceived reactivity to NSAIDs in these patients. Larger challenge studies include cutaneous, respiratory, and anaphylaxis reactions; therefore, it seems that some children are prone to respiratory reactions (whether or not they have asthma).[116] In general, the limited literature on this subject would suggest that drug provocation challenges are necessary and safe in children. Most pediatric reactors react to more than 1 drug.[117] Cross-reactions to paracetamol are not unusual (10%).[116]

COMMON CLINICAL SCENARIOS

There are a few common situations that merit specific discussion. These are situations that emerge in the literature repeatedly and are also the most common clinical questions posed to the authors by referring providers.

Emergent Need for Aspirin in Acute Coronary Syndrome

First is the acute need for ASA in the cardiac care unit in a patient with a history of an ASA or NSAID reaction. This is a logistical challenge for the allergist, frequently involving a vague and remote history of NSAID reactivity. Fortunately, there now are several studies addressing this issue. The main limitation of all of these studies is the inability to prove the patient truly has hypersensitivity. Thus, desensitization protocols proceed under the assumption that the patient has ongoing hypersensitivity. The tremendous success of these protocols should not be used as a diagnosis of NSAID reactivity unless the patient clearly has a reaction during the procedure. Many times, in the acute setting in the coronary care unit, the medical need for ASA outweighs the desire to make an accurate diagnosis.

The literature clearly supports the safety of performing one of the various desensitization protocols that have been published.[21,118–120] Although previous studies were generally just small case series, a large multicenter prospective trial involving 330 patients provides convincing evidence that it is safe to perform ASA desensitization in the acute setting.[121] When reactions occur, they are mild and easy to treat. The authors' experience is that most of these cases can be approached with a graded ASA challenge in the cardiac care unit (see **Figs.** 1and 2; **Fig. 3**). This allows a more accurate determination of ongoing hypersensitivity, while also allowing the timely administration of ASA.

It is critical to point out that a patient with a high suspicion of AERD who requires ASA presents a different challenge. This patient should not undergo a rapid desensitization, because these protocols are not studied in the acute setting. A rapid desensitization would likely lead to more severe asthma and a potentially more dangerous situation in a patient recovering from a cardiac event. The initial consultation in the coronary care unit should identify anosmia, history of asthma, and types of NSAID reactions, which would help to raise the suspicion for AERD.

Need Assessment of Nonsteroidal Antiinflammatry Drug Hypersensitivity for Pain Management Options

The other common clinical situation is a patient with a history of an NSAID reaction in the past who wants to know what they can take for pain. Generally, these patients

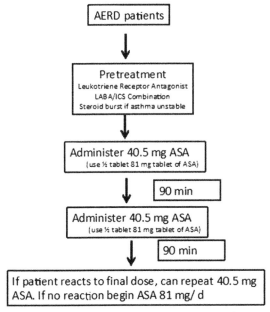

Fig. 3. Protocol that could be used in the acute hospital setting for a patient with aspirin-exacerbated respiratory disease (AERD) needing desensitization emergently owing to acute coronary syndrome. Be prepared to treat respiratory reactions: bronchodilators, antihistamines, and so on. Typical provoking dose between 60 and 100 mg in AERD. ASA, aspirin. (*From* White AA, Stevenson DD, Woessner KM, et al. Approach to patients with aspirin hypersensitivity and acute cardiovascular emergencies. Allergy Asthma Proc 2013;34(2):141; with permission.)

present with a history of a cutaneous reaction or systemic anaphylaxis symptoms. Many times, the patient and referring provider are unaware that a COX-2 inhibitor could be an option. Office challenge with a COX-2 is recommended because there are rare cases of reactivity, but in general COX-2 inhibitors are well-tolerated and provide an adequate solution for intermittent pain relief. The next step would be to address whether the reaction is cross-reactive or not. Cross-reactivity reactions can present a challenge, because there become few options for the patient to take. There are reports that premedication with antihistamines could allow tolerance in some patients.[122] Desensitization could be attempted, but would require daily administration to maintain desensitization, a circumstance that might not be necessary or valuable in a patient who only needs intermittent use.

SUMMARY

The successful approach to NSAID hypersensitivity can be distilled down to 2 critical elements: the ability to obtain a history that points toward a specific NSAID reactivity pattern and the willingness to perform targeted graded dose challenges. The literature supports these as safe and extremely useful in guiding the use of pain medications, antiplatelet ASA, or therapeutic ASA in AERD.

REFERENCES

1. Soni A. Aspirin use among the adult U.S. noninstitutionalized population with and without indicators of heart disease. Brief #179-Medical Expenditure Panel Survey. Rockville (MD): Agency for Healthcare Research and Quality; 2005.
2. Gollapudi RR, Teirstein PS, Stevenson DD, et al. Aspirin sensitivity - Implications for patients with coronary artery disease. JAMA 2004;292(24):3017–23.
3. Feng CH, White AA, Stevenson DD. Characterization of aspirin allergies in patients with coronary artery disease. Ann Allergy Asthma Immunol 2013;110(2): 92–5.
4. Vane JR. Inhibition of prostaglandin synthesis as a mechanism of action for aspirin-like drugs. Nat New Biol 1971;231(25):232–5.
5. Warner TD, Giuliano F, Vojnovic I, et al. Nonsteroid drug selectivities for cyclo-oxygenase-1 rather than cyclo-oxygenase-2 are associated with human gastrointestinal toxicity: a full in vitro analysis. Proc Natl Acad Sci U S A 1999;96(13): 7563–8.
6. Jares EJ, Baena-Cagnani CE, Sánchez-Borges M, et al. Drug-induced anaphylaxis in Latin American Countries. J Allergy Clin Immunol Pract 2015;3(5):780–8.
7. Aun MV, Blanca M, Garro LS, et al. Nonsteroidal anti-inflammatory drugs are major causes of drug-induced anaphylaxis. J Allergy Clin Immunol Pract 2014;2(4): 414–20.
8. Drago F, Cogorno L, Agnoletti AF, et al. A retrospective study of cutaneous drug reactions in an outpatient population. Int J Clin Pharm 2015;37(5):739–43.
9. Tian XY, Liu B, Shi H, et al. Incidence of adverse cutaneous drug reactions in 22,866 Chinese inpatients: a prospective study. Arch Dermatol Res 2015; 307(9):829–34.
10. Ortiz-Sanjuán F, Blanco R, Hernández JL, et al. Drug-associated cutaneous vasculitis: study of 239 patients from a single referral center. J Rheumatol 2014;41(11):2201–7.
11. Grando LR, Schmitt TA, Bakos RM. Severe cutaneous reactions to drugs in the setting of a general hospital. An Bras Dermatol 2014;89(5):758–62.

12. Kowalski ML, Makowska JS, Blanca M, et al. Hypersensitivity to nonsteroidal anti-inflammatory drugs (NSAIDs) - classification, diagnosis and management: review of the EAACI/ENDA and GA2LEN/HANNA. Allergy 2011;66(7):818–29.

13. Szczeklik A, Gryglewski RJ, Czerniawska-Mysik G. Clinical patterns of hypersensitivity to nonsteroidal anti-inflammatory drugs and their pathogenesis. J Allergy Clin Immunol 1977;60(5):276–84.

14. Mathison DA, Stevenson DD. Hypersensitivity to nonsteroidal antiinflammatory drugs: indications and methods for oral challenges. J Allergy Clin Immunol 1979;64(6 pt 2):669–74.

15. Mastalerz L, Setkowicz M, Szczeklik A. Mechanism of chronic urticaria exacerbation by aspirin. Curr Allergy Asthma Rep 2005;5(4):277–83.

16. Zembowicz A, Mastalerz L, Setkowicz M, et al. Safety of cyclooxygenase 2 inhibitors and increased leukotriene synthesis in chronic idiopathic urticaria with sensitivity to nonsteroidal anti-inflammatory drugs. Arch Dermatol 2003; 139(12):1577–82.

17. Asero R. Etoricoxib challenge in patients with chronic urticaria with NSAID intolerance. Clin Exp Dermatol 2007;32(6):661–3.

18. Setkowicz M, Mastalerz L, Podolec-Rubis M, et al. Clinical course and urinary eicosanoids in patients with aspirin-induced urticaria followed up for 4 years. J Allergy Clin Immunol 2009;123(1):174–8.

19. Nizankowska-Mogilnicka E, Bochenek G, Mastalerz L, et al. EAACI/GA2LEN guideline: aspirin provocation tests for diagnosis of aspirin hypersensitivity. Allergy 2007;62(10):1111–8.

20. Rajan JP, Simon RA, Bosso JV. Prevalence of sensitivity to food and drug additives in patients with chronic idiopathic urticaria. J Allergy Clin Immunol Pract 2014;2(2):168–71.

21. McMullan KL, Wedner HJ. Safety of aspirin desensitization in patients with reported aspirin allergy and cardiovascular disease. Clin Cardiol 2013;36(1): 25–30.

22. White AA, Stevenson DD, Woessner KM, et al. Approach to patients with aspirin hypersensitivity and acute cardiovascular emergencies. Allergy Asthma Proc 2013;34(2):138–42.

23. Simon RA. Prevention and treatment of reactions to NSAIDs. Clin Rev Allergy Immunol 2003;24(2):189–98.

24. Slowik SM, Slavin RG. Aspirin desensitization in a patient with aspirin sensitivity and chronic idiopathic urticaria. Ann Allergy Asthma Immunol 2009;102(2): 171–2.

25. Lee J. Aspirin desensitization as a treatment for aspirin-sensitive chronic spontaneous urticaria. Dermatol Ther 2015;28(1):4–6.

26. Leeyaphan C, Kulthanan K, Jongjarearnprasert K, et al. Drug-induced angioedema without urticaria: prevalence and clinical features. J Eur Acad Dermatol Venereol 2010;24(6):685–91.

27. Katz Y, Goldberg N, Kivity S. Localized periorbital edema induced by aspirin. Allergy 1993;48(5):366–9.

28. Quiralte J, Blanco C, Delgado J, et al. Challenge-based clinical patterns of 223 Spanish patients with nonsteroidal anti-inflammatory-drug-induced-reactions. J Investig Allergol Clin Immunol 2007;17(3):182–8.

29. Asero R. Intolerance to nonsteroidal anti-inflammatory drugs might precede by years the onset of chronic urticaria. J Allergy Clin Immunol 2003;111(5):1095–8.

30. Doña I, Blanca-López N, Torres MJ, et al. NSAID-induced urticaria/angioedema does not evolve into chronic urticaria: a 12-year follow-up study. Allergy 2014; 69(4):438–44.

31. Kowalski ML, Woessner K, Sanak M. Approaches to the diagnosis and management of patients with a history of nonsteroidal anti-inflammatory drug-related urticaria and angioedema. J Allergy Clin Immunol 2015;136(2):245–51.

32. Scott DR, White AA. Approach to desensitization in aspirin-exacerbated respiratory disease. Ann Allergy Asthma Immunol 2014;112(1):13–7.

33. Doña I, Barrionuevo E, Salas M, et al. Natural evolution in patients with nonsteroidal anti-inflammatory drug-induced urticaria/angioedema. Allergy 2017;72(9):1346–55.

34. Woessner KM, Simon RA. Cardiovascular prophylaxis and aspirin "allergy". Immunol Allergy Clin North Am 2013;33(2):263–74.

35. Dona I, Blanca-Lopez N, Cornejo-Garcia JA, et al. Characteristics of subjects experiencing hypersensitivity to non-steroidal anti-inflammatory drugs: patterns of response. Clin Exp Allergy 2011;41(1):86–95.

36. Kowalski ML, Bienkiewicz B, Woszczek G, et al. Diagnosis of pyrazolone drug sensitivity: clinical history versus skin testing and in vitro testing. Allergy Asthma Proc 1999;20(6):347–52.

37. van der Klauw MM, Wilson JH, Stricker BH. Drug-associated anaphylaxis: 20 years of reporting in The Netherlands (1974-1994) and review of the literature. Clin Exp Allergy 1996;26(12):1355–63.

38. Quiralte J, Blanco C, Castillo R, et al. Intolerance to nonsteroidal antiinflammatory drugs: results of controlled drug challenges in 98 patients. J Allergy Clin Immunol 1996;98(3):678–85.

39. Quiralte J, Blanco C, Castillo R, et al. Anaphylactoid reactions due to nonsteroidal antiinflammatory drugs: clinical and cross-reactivity studies. Ann Allergy Asthma Immunol 1997;78(3):293–6.

40. Chaudhry T, Hissaria P, Wiese M, et al. Oral drug challenges in non-steroidal anti-inflammatory drug-induced urticaria, angioedema and anaphylaxis. Intern Med J 2012;42(6):665–71.

41. Canto MG, Andreu I, Fernandez J, et al. Selective immediate hypersensitivity reactions to NSAIDs. Curr Opin Allergy Clin Immunol 2009;9(4):293–7.

42. Viola M, Rumi G, Valluzzi RL, et al. Assessing potential determinants of positive provocation tests in subjects with NSAID hypersensitivity. Clin Exp Allergy 2011; 41(1):96–103.

43. Rajan JP, Wineinger NE, Stevenson DD, et al. Prevalence of aspirin-exacerbated respiratory disease among asthmatic patients: a meta-analysis of the literature. J Allergy Clin Immunol 2015;135(3):676–81.e1.

44. Ta V, White AA. Survey-defined patient experiences with aspirin-exacerbated respiratory disease. J Allergy Clin Immunol Pract 2015;3(5):711–8.

45. Cardet JC, White AA, Barrett NA, et al. Alcohol-induced respiratory symptoms are common in patients with aspirin exacerbated respiratory disease. J Allergy Clin Immunol Pract 2014;2(2):208–13.

46. Kim JE, Kountakis SE. The prevalence of Samter's triad in patients undergoing functional endoscopic sinus surgery. Ear Nose Throat J 2007;86(7):396–9.

47. Lee JH, Haselkorn T, Borish L, et al. Risk factors associated with persistent airflow limitation in severe or difficult-to-treat asthma: insights from the TENOR study. Chest 2007;132(6):1882–9.

48. Mascia K, Haselkorn T, Deniz YM, et al. Aspirin sensitivity and severity of asthma: evidence for irreversible airway obstruction in patients with severe or difficult-to-treat asthma. J Allergy Clin Immunol 2005;116(5):970–5.

49. Koga T, Oshita Y, Kamimura T, et al. Characterisation of patients with frequent exacerbation of asthma. Respir Med 2006;100(2):273–8.

50. O'Byrne PM, Israel E, Drazen JM. Antileukotrienes in the treatment of asthma. Ann Intern Med 1997;127(6):472–80.

51. Stevenson DD, Zuraw BL. Pathogenesis of aspirin-exacerbated respiratory disease. Clin Rev Allergy Immunol 2003;24(2):169–88.

52. Yamashita T, Tsuji H, Maeda N, et al. Etiology of nasal polyps associated with aspirin-sensitive asthma. Rhinol Suppl 1989;8:15–24.

53. Ruhno J, Howie K, Anderson M, et al. The increased number of epithelial mast cells in nasal polyps and adjacent turbinates is not allergy-dependent. Allergy 1990;45(5):370–4.

54. Sladek K, Szczeklik A. Cysteinyl leukotrienes overproduction and mast cell activation in aspirin-provoked bronchospasm in asthma. Eur Respir J 1993;6(3): 391–9.

55. Bochenek G, Nagraba K, Nizankowska E, et al. A controlled study of 9 alpha,11 beta-PGF2 (a prostaglandin D-2 metabolite) in plasma and urine of patients with bronchial asthma and healthy controls after aspirin challenge. J Allergy Clin Immunol 2003;111(4):743–9.

56. Fischer AR, Rosenberg MA, Lilly CM, et al. Direct evidence for a role of the mast cell in the nasal response to aspirin in aspirin-sensitive asthma. J Allergy Clin Immunol 1994;94(6 Pt 1):1046–56.

57. Robuschi M, Gambaro G, Sestini P, et al. Attenuation of aspirin-induced bronchoconstriction by sodium cromoglycate and nedocromil sodium. Am J Respir Crit Care Med 1997;155(4):1461–4.

58. Yoshida S, Amayasu H, Sakamoto H, et al. Cromolyn sodium prevents bronchoconstriction and urinary LTE4 excretion in aspirin-induced asthma. Ann Allergy Asthma Immunol 1998;80(2):171–6.

59. Szczeklik A, Mastalerz L, Nizankowska E, et al. Protective and bronchodilator effects of prostaglandin E and salbutamol in aspirin-induced asthma. Am J Respir Crit Care Med 1996;153(2):567–71. Available at: http://onlinelibrary.wiley. com/o/cochrane/clcentral/articles/179/CN-00123179/frame.html.

60. Sestini P, Armetti L, Gambaro G, et al. Inhaled PGE2 prevents aspirin-induced bronchoconstriction and urinary LTE4 excretion in aspirin-sensitive asthma. Am J Respir Crit Care Med 1996;153(2):572–5.

61. Ferreri NR, Howland WC, Stevenson DD, et al. Release of leukotrienes, prostaglandins, and histamine into nasal secretions of aspirin-sensitive asthmatics during reaction to aspirin. Am Rev Respir Dis 1988;137(4):847–54.

62. Narayanankutty A, Resendiz-Hernandez JM, Falfan-Valencia R, et al. Biochemical pathogenesis of aspirin exacerbated respiratory disease (AERD). Clin Biochem 2013;46(7–8):566–78.

63. Moon TC, Campos-Alberto E, Yoshimura T, et al. Expression of DP2 (CRTh2), a prostaglandin D_2 receptor, in human mast cells. PLoS One 2014;9(9):e108595.

64. Cahill KN, Bensko JC, Boyce JA, et al. Prostaglandin D(2): a dominant mediator of aspirin-exacerbated respiratory disease. J Allergy Clin Immunol 2015;135(1): 245–52.

65. Takahashi G, Tanaka H, Higuchi N, et al. The potential role of prostaglandin D2 in nasal congestion observed in a guinea pig model of allergic rhinitis. Int Arch Allergy Immunol 2012;158(4):359–68.

66. Chang JE, Doherty TA, Baum R, et al. Prostaglandin D2 regulates human type 2 innate lymphoid cell chemotaxis. J Allergy Clin Immunol 2014;133(3): 899–901.e3.

67. Xue L, Salimi M, Panse I, et al. Prostaglandin D2 activates group 2 innate lymphoid cells through chemoattractant receptor-homologous molecule expressed on TH2 cells. J Allergy Clin Immunol 2014;133(4):1184–94.

68. Spik I, Brenuchon C, Angeli V, et al. Activation of the prostaglandin D2 receptor DP2/CRTH2 increases allergic inflammation in mouse. J Immunol 2005;174(6): 3703–8.

69. Di Lorenzo G, Drago A, Esposito Pellitteri M, et al. Measurement of inflammatory mediators of mast cells and eosinophils in native nasal lavage fluid in nasal polyposis. Int Arch Allergy Immunol 2001;125(2):164–75.

70. Landolina N, Gangwar RS, Levi-Schaffer F. Mast cells' integrated actions with eosinophils and fibroblasts in allergic inflammation: implications for therapy. Adv Immunol 2015;125:41–85.

71. Payne SC, Early SB, Huyett P, et al. Evidence for distinct histologic profile of nasal polyps with and without eosinophilia. Laryngoscope 2011;121(10): 2262–7.

72. Steinke JW, Negri J, Liu L, et al. Aspirin activation of eosinophils and mast cells: implications in the pathogenesis of aspirin-exacerbated respiratory disease. J Immunol 2014;193(1):41–7.

73. Cowburn AS, Sladek K, Soja J, et al. Overexpression of leukotriene C-4 synthase in bronchial biopsies from patients with aspirin-intolerant asthma. J Clin Invest 1998;101(4):834–46.

74. Laidlaw TM, Kidder MS, Bhattacharyya N, et al. Cysteinyl leukotriene overproduction in aspirin-exacerbated respiratory disease is driven by platelet-adherent leukocytes. Blood 2012;119(16):3790–8.

75. Laidlaw TM, Cutler AJ, Kidder MS, et al. Prostaglandin E2 resistance in granulocytes from patients with aspirin-exacerbated respiratory disease. J Allergy Clin Immunol 2014;133(6):1692–701.e3.

76. Dahlen B, Nizankowska E, Szczeklik A, et al. Benefits from adding the 5-lipoxygenase inhibitor zileuton to conventional therapy in aspirin-intolerant asthmatics. Am J Respir Crit Care Med 1998;157(4 Pt 1):1187–94.

77. Israel E, Fischer AR, Rosenberg MA, et al. The pivotal role of 5-lipoxygenase products in the reaction of aspirin-sensitive asthmatics to aspirin. Am Rev Respir Dis 1993;148(6 Pt 1):1447–51.

78. Cai Y, Bjermer L, Halstensen TS. Bronchial mast cells are the dominating LTC4S-expressing cells in aspirin-tolerant asthma. Am J Respir Cell Mol Biol 2003; 29(6):683–93.

79. Chen YS, Langhammer T, Westhofen M, et al. Relationship between matrix metalloproteinases MMP-2, MMP-9, tissue inhibitor of matrix metalloproteinases-1 and IL-5, IL-8 in nasal polyps. Allergy 2007;62(1):66–72.

80. Yeo NK, Eom DW, Oh MY, et al. Expression of matrix metalloproteinase 2 and 9 and tissue inhibitor of metalloproteinase 1 in nonrecurrent vs recurrent nasal polyps. Ann Allergy Asthma Immunol 2013;111(3):205–10.

81. Lee YM, Kim SS, Kim HA, et al. Eosinophil inflammation of nasal polyp tissue: relationships with matrix metalloproteinases, tissue inhibitor of metalloproteinase-1, and transforming growth factor-beta1. J Korean Med Sci 2003;18(1):97–102.

82. Coste A, Lefaucheur JP, Wang QP, et al. Expression of the transforming growth factor beta isoforms in inflammatory cells of nasal polyps. Arch Otolaryngol Head Neck Surg 1998;124(12):1361–6.

83. Pawankar R, Lee KH, Nonaka M, et al. Role of mast cells and basophils in chronic rhinosinusitis. Clin Allergy Immunol 2007;20:93–101.

84. Pawankar R. Mast cells in allergic airway disease and chronic rhinosinusitis. Chem Immunol Allergy 2005;87:111–29.

85. Cahill KN, Raby BA, Zhou X, et al. Impaired EP expression causes resistance to prostaglandin E in nasal polyp fibroblasts from subjects with AERD. Am J Respir Cell Mol Biol 2015;54(1):34–40.

86. Cahill KN, Laidlaw TM. Aspirin exacerbated respiratory disease: the search for a biomarker. Ann Allergy Asthma Immunol 2014;113(5):500–1.

87. Williams AN, Simon RA, Woessner KM, et al. The relationship between historical aspirin-induced asthma and severity of asthma induced during oral aspirin challenges. J Allergy Clin Immunol 2007;120(2):273–7.

88. Dahlen B, Zetterstrom O. Comparison of bronchial and per oral provocation with aspirin in aspirin-sensitive asthmatics. Eur Respir J 1990;3(5):527–34.

89. Nizankowska E, Bestyńska-Krypel A, Cmiel A, et al. Oral and bronchial provocation tests with aspirin for diagnosis of aspirin-induced asthma. Eur Respir J 2000;15(5):863–9. Available at: http://onlinelibrary.wiley.com/o/cochrane/clcentral/articles/431/CN-00297431/frame.html.

90. Celikel S, Stevenson D, Erkorkmaz U, et al. Use of nasal inspiratory flow rates in the measurement of aspirin-induced respiratory reactions. Ann Allergy Asthma Immunol 2013;111(4):252–5.

91. Chen JR, Buchmiller BL, Khan DA. An Hourly Dose-Escalation Desensitization Protocol for Aspirin-Exacerbated Respiratory Disease. J Allergy Clin Immunol Pract 2015;3(6):926–31.e1.

92. Lee RU, White AA, Ding D, et al. Use of intranasal ketorolac and modified oral aspirin challenge for desensitization of aspirin-exacerbated respiratory disease. Ann Allergy Asthma Immunol 2010;105(2):130–5.

93. Berges-Gimeno MP, Simon RA, Stevenson DD. The effect of leukotriene-modifier drugs on aspirin-induced asthma and rhinitis reactions. Clin Exp Allergy 2002; 32(10):1491–6.

94. White A, Ludington E, Mehra P, et al. Effect of leukotriene modifier drugs on the safety of oral aspirin challenges. Ann Allergy Asthma Immunol 2006;97(5): 688–93.

95. Cook K, Modena M, Wineinger N, et al. Use of a composite symptom score during challenge in patients with suspected aspirin-exacerbated respiratory disease. Ann Allergy Asthma Immunol 2017;118(5):597–602.

96. White AA, Stevenson DD, Simon RA. The blocking effect of essential controller medications during aspirin challenges in patients with aspirin-exacerbated respiratory disease. Ann Allergy Asthma Immunol 2005;95(4):330–5.

97. Stevenson DD, Simon RA. Lack of cross-reactivity between rofecoxib and aspirin in aspirin-sensitive patients with asthma. J Allergy Clin Immunol 2001; 108(1):47–51.

98. Gyllfors P, Bochenek G, Overholt J, et al. Biochemical and clinical evidence that aspirin-intolerant asthmatic subjects tolerate the cyclooxygenase 2-selective analgesic drug celecoxib. J Allergy Clin Immunol 2003;111(5):1116–21. Available at: http://onlinelibrary.wiley.com/o/cochrane/clcentral/articles/357/CN-00437357/frame.html.

99. Morales DR, Guthrie B, Lipworth BJ, et al. NSAID-exacerbated respiratory disease: a meta-analysis evaluating prevalence, mean provocative dose of aspirin and increased asthma morbidity. Allergy 2015;70(7):828–35.

100. Bobolea I, Cabañas R, Jurado-Palomo J, et al. Concurrent coxibs and antiplatelet therapy unmasks aspirin-exacerbated respiratory disease. Eur Respir J 2013;42(5):1418–20.

101. Daham K, Song WL, Lawson JA, et al. Effects of celecoxib on major prostaglandins in asthma. Clin Exp Allergy 2011;41(1):36–45.

102. Machado-Carvalho L, Martín M, Torres R, et al. Low E-prostanoid 2 receptor levels and deficient induction of the IL-1β/IL-1 type I receptor/COX-2 pathway: vicious circle in patients with aspirin-exacerbated respiratory disease. J Allergy Clin Immunol 2016;137(1):99–107.e7.

103. Senna GE, Andri G, Dama AR, et al. Tolerability of imidazole salicylate in aspirin-sensitive patients. Allergy Proc 1995;16(5):251–4.

104. Nizankowska E, Dworski R, Soja J, et al. Salicylate pre-treatment attenuates intensity of bronchial and nasal symptoms precipitated by aspirin in aspirin-intolerant patients. Clin Exp Allergy 1990;20(6):647–52.

105. Szczeklik A, Nizankowska E, Dworski R. Choline magnesium trisalicylate in patients with aspirin-induced asthma. Eur Respir J 1990;3(5):535–9. Available at: http://onlinelibrary.wiley.com/o/cochrane/clcentral/articles/194/CN-00069194/frame.html.

106. Tuttle KL, Schneider TR, Henrickson SE, et al. Aspirin-exacerbated respiratory disease: not always "adult-onset". J Allergy Clin Immunol Pract 2016;4(4):756–8.

107. Ertoy Karagol HI, Yilmaz O, Topal E, et al. Nonsteroidal anti-inflammatory drugs-exacerbated respiratory disease in adolescents. Int Forum Allergy Rhinol 2015;5(5):392–8.

108. Zambonino MA, Torres MJ, Muñoz C, et al. Drug provocation tests in the diagnosis of hypersensitivity reactions to non-steroidal anti-inflammatory drugs in children. Pediatr Allergy Immunol 2013;24(2):151–9.

109. Arikoglu T, Aslan G, Yildirim DD, et al. Discrepancies in the diagnosis and classification of nonsteroidal anti-inflammatory drug hypersensitivity reactions in children. Allergol Int 2016;66(3):418–24.

110. Topal E, Celiksoy MH, Catal F, et al. The value of the clinical history for the diagnosis of immediate nonsteroidal anti-inflammatory drug hypersensitivity and safe alternative drugs in children. Allergy Asthma Proc 2016;37(1):57–63.

111. Misirlioglu ED, Toyran M, Capanoglu M, et al. Negative predictive value of drug provocation tests in children. Pediatr Allergy Immunol 2014;25(7):685–90.

112. Cousin M, Chiriac A, Molinari N, et al. Phenotypical characterization of children with hypersensitivity reactions to NSAIDs. Pediatr Allergy Immunol 2016;27(7):743–8.

113. Cavkaytar O, Arik Yilmaz E, Karaatmaca B, et al. Different phenotypes of nonsteroidal anti-inflammatory drug hypersensitivity during childhood. Int Arch Allergy Immunol 2015;167(3):211–21.

114. Debley JS, Carter ER, Gibson RL, et al. The prevalence of ibuprofen-sensitive asthma in children: a randomized controlled bronchoprovocation challenge study. J Pediatr 2005;147(2):233–8.

115. Rachelefsky GS, Coulson A, Siegel SC, et al. Aspirin intolerance in chronic childhood asthma: detected by oral challenge. Pediatrics 1975;56(3):443–8. Available at: http://onlinelibrary.wiley.com/o/cochrane/clcentral/articles/131/CN-00704131/frame.html.

116. Hassani A, Ponvert C, Karila C, et al. Hypersensitivity to cyclooxygenase inhibitory drugs in children: a study of 164 cases. Eur J Dermatol 2008;18(5):561–5.

117. Sanchez-Borges M, Capriles-Behrens E, Caballero-Fonseca F. Hypersensitivity to non-steroidal anti-inflammatory drugs in childhood. Pediatr Allergy Immunol 2004;15(4):376–80.

118. Wong JT, Nagy CS, Krinzman SJ, et al. Rapid oral challenge-desensitization for patients with aspirin-related urticaria-angioedema. J Allergy Clin Immunol 2000; 105(5):997–1001.

119. Rossini R, Angiolillo DJ, Musumeci G, et al. Aspirin desensitization in patients undergoing percutaneous coronary interventions with stent implantation. Am J Cardiol 2008;101(6):786–9.

120. Silberman S, Neukirch-Stoop C, Steg PG. Rapid desensitization procedure for patients with aspirin hypersensitivity undergoing coronary stenting. Am J Cardiol 2005;95(4):509–10.

121. Rossini R, Iorio A, Pozzi R, et al. Aspirin desensitization in patients with coronary artery disease: results of the multicenter ADAPTED Registry (Aspirin Desensitization in Patients With Coronary Artery Disease). Circ Cardiovasc Interv 2017; 10(2) [pii:e004368].

122. Trautmann A, Anders D, Stoevesandt J. H1-antihistamine premedication in NSAID-associated urticaria. J Allergy Clin Immunol Pract 2016;4(6):1205–12.

Delayed Cutaneous Hypersensitivity Reactions to Antibiotics

Management with Desensitization

Caitlin M.G. McNulty, MD, Miguel A. Park, MD*

KEYWORDS

- Antibiotic allergy • Delayed cutaneous adverse reactions • Desensitization
- Management

KEY POINTS

- Mild to moderate delayed cutaneous adverse reactions to antibiotics can be successfully desensitized.
- Severe cutaneous adverse reaction to antibiotics is a contraindication to desensitization.
- Future research opportunities to the mechanism and protocol standardization for delayed cutaneous adverse reactions to antibiotics is needed.

INTRODUCTION

Drug reactions are a common event complicating patient care and can be immunologically mediated. Studies estimate that the incidence of drug reactions mediated by an immunologic mechanism is between 2.3 to 3.6 per 1000 patients, with almost all these reactions involving the skin and antibiotics being the most frequent precipitants of cutaneous reactions.[1–4] The incidence of delayed drug reactions is not well characterized because most epidemiologic studies of cutaneous drug reactions are retrospective and firm demonstration of causality is difficult. One study estimates that Gel-Coombs type IV reactions account for approximately 25% of hypersensitivity reactions and 5% of all adverse drug reactions; however, other studies estimate that 64% of drug reactions are delayed.[3,5] Management of patients with delayed cutaneous adverse reactions to antibiotics is mainly avoidance and use of alternative antibiotics. Alternatively, desensitization to an antibiotic that is suspected to have caused the delayed cutaneous adverse reactions has been described in the literature.

Disclosure Statement: None.
Division of Allergic Diseases, Mayo Clinic, 200 1st Street Southwest, Rochester, MN 55905, USA
* Corresponding author.
E-mail address: park.miguel@mayo.edu

This article explores the current literature of desensitization to delayed cutaneous adverse reactions to antibiotics.

PATHOPHYSIOLOGY

Given recent advancements in the understanding and management of drug allergy, a new classification system has been proposed by the recent PRACTALL guidelines to aid in the appropriate use of available testing and risk stratification.[6,7] This new classification system involves dividing drug reactions by phenotype and endotype, rather than using the traditional Gel-Coombs classification system, which is cumbersome in the face of recent understanding of the diverse mechanisms of drug allergy.[7] Here, phenotype refers to the timing of the drug reaction, with reactions occurring within 6 hours of administration as representative of immediate drug reactions, whereas reactions occurring in the days to weeks following administration are delayed.[7] Drug reactions are further classified by endotype, which describes the mechanism through which the reaction occurs. For example, immediate onset of urticaria following administration of penicillin would have been classified as a Gel-Coombs type 1 reaction, which now would be understood as an immediate, immunoglobulin (Ig)-E–mediated drug allergy, whereas the classic reaction to abacavir would be described as a delayed, human leukocyte antigen (HLA)-associated drug reaction (**Table 1**). This allows more precise labeling of drug allergy as understanding of drug-mediated reactions increases.

Delayed drug reactions have a variety of manifestations and the pathways by which they occur have not been fully elucidated. Drug reaction with eosinophilia and systemic symptoms (DRESS), as well as maculopapular exanthema with eosinophilia, are manifestations of an eosinophil-mediated endotype, whereas Stevens-Johnson syndrome (SJS) and toxic epidermal necrolysis (TEN) are secondary to a cytotoxic T-cell–mediated endotype. Agranulocytosis exanthematous pustulosis (AGEP) is characterized by the formation of sterile pustules by neutrophil recruitment. The effects of delayed drug reactions can affect the liver, kidneys, and lungs, in addition to hematopoiesis; however, skin reactions are the most common manifestation. This is thought to be due to the presence of high numbers of primed cells of both innate and adaptive immunity in the skin.[5] Due to the heterogeneous immune mechanisms that can precipitate a delayed adverse cutaneous drug eruption, there is diversity in the way drug reactions manifest in the skin. Maculopapular rashes are the most frequent, although life-threatening reactions are rare.[4] The mortality rate of these reactions is 1% to 5% in SJS and up to 25% to 35% in TEN.[8]

Outside of genetic tests for certain HLA haplotypes that are associated with severe adverse cutaneous reactions, there is no validated testing to determine if a patient is

Table 1
Phenotypes and endotypes of drug allergy to trimethoprim sulfamethoxazole

Reaction	Phenotype	Endotype
Anaphylaxis	Immediate	IgE-mediated
SJS	Delayed	Cytotoxic T cell
Maculopapular Rash	Delayed	Unknown
Serum Sickness	Delayed	Immune complex deposition
Aseptic Meningitis	Delayed	Possibly neutrophilic

Data from Refs.[25,26,30,32,33]

going to experience a delayed drug reaction affecting the skin. Although skin prick testing (SPT) and intradermal testing (IDT) are widely used in IgE-mediated hypersensitivity reactions, their specificity is limited in delayed drug reactions.[9] Patch testing has been proposed as a safe alternative to SPT or IDT; however, there is no positive control available and the negative predictive value is limited.[9] In one case series, patch testing for penicillin-containing antibiotics showed high reproducibility for patients who had experienced a delayed reaction; however, this has not been borne out in other series.[10–12]

MANAGEMENT

A desensitization procedure may be performed to induce tolerance to a culprit drug in a patient with a history of an immunologically mediated drug reaction. Desensitization has long been used to induce tolerance to life-saving antimicrobials but has increasingly been used in recent years for monoclonal antibodies and chemotherapeutic agents.[13–19] In general, starting concentrations range from about 1 per 10,000 to 1 per 100 depending on the severity of the initial reaction.[16,20] This dose is then often doubled over the course of minutes to several days. In immediate hypersensitivity reactions, it is thought that this induces a temporary state of tolerance in mast cells by binding to IgE at doses too low to trigger the activation threshold.[20] Most desensitization protocols have been published for immediate drug reactions; however, there is an increasing body of evidence that desensitization procedures can be applied in the context of delayed drug reactions.[13,21,22] However, the mechanism of tolerance induction in delayed hypersensitivity reactions remains elusive but likely involves changes in the basophil and T-cell response.[23]

There is a risk of inducing a hypersensitivity reaction when performing desensitization; therefore, appropriate patient selection is crucial. Desensitization is indicated when there is a lack of availability of therapeutic options of equivalent potency or efficacy. Desensitization is absolutely contraindicated in certain delayed reactions. These include vasculitis, hemolytic anemias, and DRESS, in addition to SJS or TEN, because there is a concern that even the small amounts of medication used in a desensitization protocol could possibly trigger one of these reactions and, unlike anaphylaxis, there is no known effective condition-specific treatment.[20] Desensitization is additionally relatively contraindicated in poorly controlled asthma.[20,24] Due to the risk of a hypersensitivity reaction, desensitization procedures should be carried out under the supervision of staff trained to recognize and treat life-threatening hypersensitivity reactions promptly. Importantly, it should be emphasized that desensitization procedures induce tolerance only for as long as the medication is given regularly. Lapses in regular administration of the drug can result in an allergic hypersensitivity reaction. Before proceeding with desensitization, it should be emphasized with the patient and referring physician that desensitization does not confer tolerance in the long term and that adherence is crucial.

Amoxicillin and trimethoprim-sulfamethoxazole are widely used and very efficacious antimicrobials that also, unfortunately, have the highest rates of inciting both immediate and delayed hypersensitivity reactions.[1,3,4] Indeed, one study found that trimethoprim-sulfamethoxazole was implicated in 66.6% of cutaneous drug reactions requiring hospitalization.[4] Delayed drug reactions to both amoxicillin and trimethoprim-sulfamethoxazole have diverse manifestations, reflecting a variety of endotypical mechanisms that are often poorly understood. Trimethoprim-sulfamethoxazole is most notorious for precipitating SJS or TEN, which is mediated by cytotoxic T-cell mechanisms as well as a delayed maculopapular rash, the mechanism of which is unknown.[25,26] Penicillin-containing antibiotics have also been reported to cause SJS or TEN, as well as AGEP and fixed-drug eruptions.[27–29] Serum sickness secondary to immune complex deposition has occurred in the context of trimethoprim-sulfamethoxazole and penicillins.[30,31] Aseptic meningitis has also been reported to trimethoprim-sulfamethoxazole, which is possibly mediated by a neutrophilic reaction.[32]

The literature is somewhat lacking regarding desensitization to nonimmediate reactions to antibiotics; however, in the case of trimethoprim-sulfamethoxazole, given its wide use and its predilection for causing cutaneous adverse drug reactions, numerous desensitization protocols have been published in both human immunodeficiency virus (HIV)-infected populations and non-HIV infected populations.[21,24,34–41] Many trimethoprim-sulfamethoxazole case reports and series, unfortunately, do not differentiate between immediate and delayed-type hypersensitivity reactions, though many of the published cases involve apparent delayed cutaneous drug reaction.

One of the first case reports detailing successful trimethoprim-sulfamethoxazole desensitization over 6 weeks involved a patient with fever, rash, and joint pain.[42] The clinical history presented in this case raises suspicion for serum sickness or other delayed reaction.[42] In a paper on desensitization-graded challenge by Demoly and colleagues,[43] 2 of the 44 initially desensitized subjects developed maculopapular rash and fever on day 10 of trimethoprim-sulfamethoxazole therapy, 1 of whom was successfully desensitized at a later date with a 10-day protocol (**Table 2**). In a case series by Caumes and colleagues,[35] at the initial adverse drug reaction, the median time of rash onset was 10 days after initiating therapy; 37 of the 48 subjects who underwent the 8-step, 2-day protocol were successfully desensitized.

There are 2 case series reported that detail convincing delayed-drug reaction histories with reports of successful desensitization to trimethoprim-sulfamethoxazole. Kalanadhabhatta and colleagues[38] included at least 3 subjects with delayed drug eruption in their 1996 trimethoprim-sulfamethoxazole desensitization case series

Table 2
One-day trimethoprim-sulfamethoxazole graded administration protocol: 12 steps

Step	Dose (mg)
1	0.001/0.0002
2	0.003/0.006
3	0.009/0.0018
4	0.03/0.006
5	0.09/0.018
6	0.3/0.06
7	1/0.2
8	3/0.6
9	9/1.8
10	30/6
11	90/18
12	300/60

Dosing interval is 30 minutes apart.
Adapted from Demoly P, Messaad D, Sahla H, et al. Six-hour trimethoprim-sulfamethoxazole-graded challenge in HIV-infected patients. J Allergy Clin Immunol 1998;102(6 Pt 1):1034; with permission.

(**Table 3**). Three of the subjects profiled in that study had onset of maculopapular rash 7 to 14 days after initiation of trimethoprim-sulfamethoxazole; all 3 of these subjects were successfully desensitized using a 3-phase, 36-step regimen.[38]

Pyle and colleagues[21] presented the largest case series of trimethoprim-sulfamethoxazole desensitization in subjects without HIV. Most of these subjects had nonurticarial rashes reported as their primary adverse drug reaction.[21] Three desensitization protocols were studied, including 2 1-day protocols. One of these was a 6-step protocol starting at 0.004 mg of trimethoprim and 0.02 of sulfamethoxazole and using flexible intervals from 15 to 60 minutes based a previously published protocol by Gluckstein and Ruskin.[21,37] The other 1-day protocol, modified from the Kalanadhabhatta and

Table 3		
One-day trimethoprim-sulfamethoxazole graded administration Protocol: 3 Phase, Multi-Step		
Phase	**Step**	**Dose (mg/mL)**
Phase 1: 15-min dosing interval	1	0.000004/0.00002
	2	0.000008/0.00004
	3	0.000016/0.00008
	4	0.000032/0.00016
	5	0.00004/0.0002
	6	0.00008/0.0004
	7	0.00016/0.0008
	8	0.00032/0.0016
	9	0.0004/0.002
	10	0.0008/0.004
	11	0.0016/0.008
	12	0.0032/0.016
	13	0.004/0.02
	14	0.008/0.04
	15	0.016/0.08
	16	0.032/0.16
	17	0.04/0.2
	18	0.08/0.4
	19	0.16/0.8
	20	0.32/1.6
	21	0.4/2
	22	0.8/4
	23	1.6/8
	24	3.2/16
	25	4/20
Phase 2: 30-min dosing interval	1	8/40
	2	16/80
Phase 3: 2-h dosing interval	1	16/80
	2	16/80
	3	16/80
	4	16/80
	5	24/120
	6	40/200
	7	64/320
	8	80/400
	9	80/400
	10	80/400

Adapted from Kalanadhabhatta V, Muppidi D, Sahni H, et al. Successful oral desensitization to trimethoprim-sulfamethoxazole in acquired immune deficiency syndrome. Ann Allergy Asthma Immunol 1996;77(5):397; with permission.

colleagues 1996 protocol,[39] involved a 14-step, 4 hour desensitization starting a dose of 0.08 mg of trimethoprim and 0.016 mg of sulfamethoxazole.[22] These studies offer the most convincing evidence of the success of desensitization in a delayed reaction to trimethoprim-sulfamethoxazole.

Unfortunately, there are no published case series on successful desensitization to amoxicillin after a delayed drug reaction, though successful desensitization has been reported for several other antibiotics. Most of the literature available on desensitization in the setting of penicillin hypersensitivity involves immediate reactions to penicillin.[44–49] However, there have been 2 case series from the cystic fibrosis literature that offer evidence of successful desensitization in the case of delayed drug eruption secondary to antibiotics. In 2011, Whitaker and colleagues[50] published a retrospective review of 275 desensitizations in a population of 42 adult subjects with cystic fibrosis. In this population, repeat desensitizations to different antimicrobials are needed due to frequent infections from resistant organisms. Subjects were included if they experienced a drug reaction without typical IgE-mediated features that occurred greater than 24 hours after the antibiotic was initiated.[50] These subjects reported reactions to tazocin, ceftazidime, meropenem, aztreonam, tobramycin, and colomycin.[50] Multiple desensitizations were performed on the same subjects.[50] Using a 7-step, 2-hour and 20-minute procedure that involved 10-fold increases with each step, a 91% success rate was achieved, with success defined as successful completion of the antibiotic course.[50] In another retrospective study of 19 subjects with cystic fibrosis, 71 desensitization procedures were performed.[51] The classes to which these desensitizations were performed included penicillins, cephalosporins, carbapenems, monobactams, vancomycin, sulfonamides, chloramphenicol, quinolones, and colomycins.[51] This case series included 18 cases of delayed reaction. Of the 71 desensitization procedures that were performed, 76% were successful, though it is unclear how many of these successful desensitizations involved delayed reactions. These studies, particularly Whitaker and colleagues,[50] offer the most convincing evidence of the successful use of rapid desensitization protocols in the setting of delayed drug reactions.

Given the prevalence of delayed reactions to antimicrobials, as well as the potential life-saving value of successful desensitization to these essential medications, it is encouraging that rapid desensitization protocols have shown success in allowing subjects to tolerate various classes of antimicrobials that previously incited delayed reactions.[21,35,38,50,51] In the study by Pyle and colleagues,[21] the short-term and long-term (defined as a mean follow-up time of 11 months) success rates of both the 14-step and the 6-step protocols exhibited a success rate of 98%, whereas the short-term and long-term success rates of the 10-day protocol were 93% and 81%, respectively. The rate of adverse reactions was greater in the multiday protocol, and only one short protocol desensitization needed to be stopped secondary to an adverse event that consisted of a rash and lip swelling.[21] Similarly, Whitaker and colleagues[50] using their 7-step, 2-hour and 20-minute protocol were able to achieve a 91% successful desensitization rate, with these subjects able to tolerate the antibiotic for the duration of its course. The reactions that lead to failure of desensitization were all reported as mild; many of these patients were able to tolerate desensitization to another antimicrobial.[50] These studies show that rapid desensitizations to antimicrobials lasting between 2 and 4 hours result in desensitizations that are not only safe and durable, but also more convenient for the patient.

The authors offer a basic outline of a rapid desensitization protocol to be used for various classes of antimicrobials, based on the work of Pyle and colleagues,[21] Whitaker and colleagues,[50] and the 12-step to 16-step protocol for desensitization

Step	Dose (mg)
Table 4 **One-day trimethoprim-sulfamethoxazole graded administration protocol: 14 steps**	
1	0.08/0.016
2	0.16/0.032
3	0.32/0.064
4	0.64/0.128
5	1.28/0.256
6	2.5/0.512
7	5/1
8	10/2
9	20/4
10	40/8
11	80/16
12	160/32
13	320/64
14	440/88

Dosing interval is 15 minutes apart.

Data from Pyle RC, Butterfield JH, Volcheck GW, et al. Successful outpatient graded administration of trimethoprim-sulfamethoxazole in patients without HIV and with a history of sulfonamide adverse drug reaction. J Allergy Clin Immunol Pract 2014;2(1):52–8.

pioneered by Dr. Castells' group,[13,16,24] the general principles of desensitization outlined in the position paper on desensitization by Cernadas and colleagues,[20] and the position paper by Scherer and colleagues.[52] With the success of short protocols, the authors propose a 14-step protocol with 15 minutes between each dosing interval (the safety and efficacy of rapid protocol is previously delineated).[21,50] The initial concentration of antibiotic should be 1/1000 to 1/10,000 of the full-strength dose (**Table 4**).[16,20,21] Doses should be doubled at 15-minute intervals because this dosing strategy has been proposed to trigger inhibitory mechanisms in immediate hypersensitivity reactions and are, perhaps, associated with less side effects than 10-fold increases.[20,23] If this strategy fails, it may be prudent to proceed with a multiday desensitization approach, such as the 10-day protocol outlined by Pyle and colleagues[21] and inspired by the 1994 protocol by Absar and colleagues,[34] which involves daily dose doubling. Although there is uncertainty as to how desensitization in the context of delayed drug reactions works, these studies provide evidence that temporary induction of tolerance is indeed possible.

As previously detailed, absolute contraindications to this protocol and all desensitizations include a history of severe exfoliative dermatosis, including SJS or TEN, as well as vasculitis, autoimmune cytopenias, and DRESS. Desensitization should only be performed with on-site staff that is trained in the management of acute hypersensitivity reactions.

SUMMARY

These cases illustrate that desensitization in patients with a history of delayed drug reaction is possible, though the mechanism remains unclear. The existing evidence is limited by underreporting of unsuccessful desensitizations; additionally, true sensitization is unconfirmed in most case series. Further prospective studies are needed to further establish the role of desensitization in cases of delayed cutaneous drug reactions.

REFERENCES

1. Bigby M, Jick S, Jick H, et al. Drug-induced cutaneous reactions. A report from the Boston Collaborative Drug Surveillance Program on 15,438 consecutive inpatients, 1975 to 1982. JAMA 1986;256(24):3358–63.
2. Fiszenson-Albala F, Auzerie V, Mahe E, et al. A 6-month prospective survey of cutaneous drug reactions in a hospital setting. Br J Dermatol 2003;149(5): 1018–22.
3. Thong BY-H, Leong K-P, Tang C-Y, et al. Drug allergy in a general hospital: results of a novel prospective inpatient reporting system. Ann Allergy Asthma Immunol 2003;90(3):342–7.
4. Hernandez-Salazar A, de Leon-Rosales SP, Rangel-Frausto S, et al. Epidemiology of adverse cutaneous drug reactions. A prospective study in hospitalized patients. Arch Med Res 2006;37(7):899–902.
5. Böhm R, Cascorbi I. Pharmacogenetics and predictive testing of drug hypersensitivity reactions. Front Pharmacol 2016;7:1–11.
6. Castells MC. Drug allergy: phenotypes, endotypes, and biomarkers. J Allergy Clin Immunol Pract 2017;5(3):626–7.
7. Muraro A, Lemanske RF Jr, Castells M, et al. Precision medicine in allergic disease-food allergy, drug allergy, and anaphylaxis-PRACTALL document of the European Academy of Allergy and Clinical Immunology and the American Academy of Allergy, Asthma and Immunology. Allergy 2017;72:1006–21.
8. Hoetzenecker W, Nägeli M, Mehra ET, et al. Adverse cutaneous drug eruptions: current understanding. Semin Immunopathol 2016;38(1):75–86.
9. Konvinse K, Phillips E, White K, et al. Old dog begging for new tricks – Current practices and future directions in the diagnosis of delayed antimicrobial hypersensitivity HHS public access. Curr Opin Infect Dis 2016;29(6):561–76.
10. Pinho A, Marta A, Coutinho I, et al. Long-term reproducibility of positive patch test reactions in patients with non-immediate cutaneous adverse drug reactions to antibiotics. Contact Dermatitis 2017;76(4):204–9.
11. Gompels MM, Simpson N, Snow M, et al. Desensitization to co-trimoxazole (trimethoprim-sulphamethoxazole) in HIV-infected patients: is patch testing a useful predictor of reaction? J Infect 1999;38(2):111–5.
12. Problems C, Sensitivity P. Leaving high speed overturning. 2017;(c).
13. Bavbek S, Ataman Ş, Akinci A, et al. Rapid subcutaneous desensitization for the management of local and systemic hypersensitivity reactions to etanercept and adalimumab in 12 patients. J Allergy Clin Immunol Pract 2015;3(4):629–32.
14. Brennan PJ, Bouza TR, Hsu FI, et al. Hypersensitivity reactions to mAbs: 105 desensitizations in 23 patients, from evaluation to treatment. J Allergy Clin Immunol 2009;124(6):1259–66.
15. Castells MC, Tennant NM, Sloane DE, et al. Hypersensitivity reactions to chemotherapy: outcomes and safety of rapid desensitization in 413 cases. J Allergy Clin Immunol 2008;122(3):574–80.
16. Castells M. Rapid desensitization for hypersensitivity reactions to medications. Immunol Allergy Clin North Am 2009;29:585–606.
17. Feldweg AM, Lee CW, Matulonis UA, et al. Rapid desensitization for hypersensitivity reactions to paclitaxel and docetaxel: a new standard protocol used in 77 successful treatments. Gynecol Oncol 2005;96(3):824–9.

18. Lee CW, Matulonis UA, Castells MC. Carboplatin hypersensitivity: a 6-h 12-step protocol effective in 35 desensitizations in patients with gynecological malignancies and mast cell/IgE-mediated reactions. Gynecol Oncol 2004;95(2):370–6.

19. Lee CW, Matulonis UA, Castells MC. Rapid inpatient/outpatient desensitization for chemotherapy hypersensitivity: standard protocol effective in 57 patients for 255 courses. Gynecol Oncol 2005;99(2):393–9.

20. Cernadas JR, Brockow K, Romano A, et al. General considerations on rapid desensitization for drug hypersensitivity - A consensus statement. Allergy 2010; 65(11):1357–66.

21. Pyle RC, Butterfield JH, Volcheck GW, et al. Successful outpatient graded administration of trimethoprim-sulfamethoxazole in patients without HIV and with a history of sulfonamide adverse drug reaction. J Allergy Clin Immunol Pract 2014; 2(1):52–8.

22. Di Paolo C, Minetti S, Mineni M, et al. Desensitization to febuxostat: report of two cases. J Allergy Clin Immunol Pract 2015;3(4):633–6.

23. Castells MC. A new era for drug desensitizations. J Allergy Clin Immunol Pract 2015;3(4):639–40.

24. Legere HJ, Palis R, Rodriguez Bouza T, et al. A safe protocol for rapid desensitization in patients with cystic fibrosis and antibiotic hypersensitivity. J Cyst Fibros 2009;8(6):418–24.

25. Hemstreet BA, Page RL 2nd. Sulfonamide allergies and outcomes related to use of potentially cross-reactive drugs in hospitalized patients. Pharmacotherapy 2006;26(4):551–7.

26. Jick H. Adverse reactions to trimethoprim-sulfamethoxazole in hospitalized patients. Rev Infect Dis 1982;4(2):426–8.

27. Ferrandiz-pulido C, Garcia-patos V. A review of causes of Stevens-Johnson syndrome and toxic epidermal necrolysis in children. Arch Dis Child 2013;98: 998–1003.

28. Talati S, Lala M, Kapupara H. Acute generalized exanthematous pustulosis: a rare clinical entity with use of piperacillin/tazobactam. Am J Ther 2009;592:591–2.

29. Vanessa L, Guevara P, Yges EL, et al. Fixed drug eruption due to amoxicillin and quinolones. Ann Allergy Asthma Immunol 2013;110(1):61–2.

30. Heckbert SR, Stryker WS, Coltin KL, et al. Serum sickness in children after antibiotic exposure: estimates of occurrence and morbidity in a health maintenance organization population. Am J Epidemiol 1990;132(2):336–42.

31. Tatum AJ, Ditto AM, Patterson R. Severe serum sickness-like reaction to oral penicillin drugs: three case reports. Ann Allergy Asthma Immunol 2001;86(3):330–4.

32. Bruner KE, Coop CA, White KM. Trimethoprim-sulfamethoxazole-induced aseptic meningitis-not just another sulfa allergy. Ann Allergy Asthma Immunol 2014; 113(5):520–6.

33. Harle DG, Baldo BA, Wells JV. Drugs as allergens: detection and combining site specificities of IgE antibodies to sulfamethoxazole. Mol Immunol 1988;25(12): 1347–54.

34. Absar N, Daneshvar H, Beall G. Desensitization to trimethoprim/sulfamethoxazole in HIV-infected patients. J Allergy Clin Immunol 1993;93(6):1001–5.

35. Caumes E, Guermonprez G, Lecomte C, et al. Efficacy and safety of desensitization with sulfamethoxazole and trimethoprim in 48 previously hypersensitive patients infected with human immunodeficiency virus. Arch Dermatol 1997;133(4): 465–9.

36. Fegueux S, De Truchis P, Balloul H, et al. Sulphadiazine desensitization in AIDS patients. AIDS 1991;5(10):1275–6.

37. Gluckstein D, Ruskin J. Rapid oral desensitization to trimethoprim-sulfamethoxazole (TMP-SMZ): use in prophylaxis for pneumocystis carinii pneumonia in patients with aids who were previously intolerant to TMP-SMZ. Clin Infect Dis 1995;20(4):849–53. Available at: http://www.jstor.org/stable/4458447.
38. Kalanadhabhatta V, Muppidi D, Sahni H, et al. Successful oral desensitization to trimethoprim- sulfamethoxazole in acquired immune deficiency syndrome. Ann Allergy Asthma Immunol 1996;77:394–400.
39. Leoung GS, Stanford JF, Giordano MF, et al. Trimethoprim-Sulfamethoxazole (TMP-SMZ) Dose Escalation versus Direct Rechallenge from Pneumocystis Carinii Pneumonia Prophylaxis in Human Immunodeficiency Virus-Infected Patients with Previous Adverse Reaction to TMP-SMZ. J Infect Dis 2001;184:992–7.
40. Nguyen M-T, Weiss PJ, Wallace MR. Two-day oral desensitization to trimethoprim-sulfamethoxazole in HIV-infected patients. AIDS 1995;9:573–5.
41. Nucera E, Schiavino D, Buonomo A, et al. Tolerance induction to cotrimoxazole. Allergy 2000;55:681–2.
42. Park R, Brit M. Sulphonamide Allergy: Persistence of Desensitization. Br Med J 1944;2(816):51.
43. Demoly P, Messaad D, Sahla H, et al. Six-hour trimethoprim-sulfamethoxazole-graded challenge in HIV-infected patients. J Allergy Clin Immunol 1998;102:1033–6.
44. Peck SM, Siegal S, Glick AW, et al. Clinical problems in penicillin sensitivity. JAMA 1947;138(9):631–40.
45. Reisman RE, Rosc NR, Witebsky E, et al. Penicillin allergy and desensitization. J Allergy 1962;33(2):180–6.
46. Stark BJ, Earl HS, Gross GN, et al. Acute and chronic desensitization of penicillin-allergic patients using oral penicillin. J Allergy Clin Immunol 1987;79(3):523–32.
47. Sullivan TJ. Antigen-specific desensitization of patients allergic to penicillin. J Allergy Clin Immunol 1982;69(6):500–8.
48. Sullivan TJ, Yecies LD, Shatz GS, et al. Desensitization of patients allergic to penicillin using orally administered beta-lactam antibiotics. J Allergy Clin Immunol 1982;69(3):275–82.
49. Wendel GD, Stark BJ, Jamison RB, et al. Penicillin allergy and desensitization in serious infectious during pregnancy. N Engl J Med 1985;312(19):1229–32.
50. Whitaker P, Shaw N, Gooi J, et al. Rapid desensitization for non-immediate reactions in patients with cystic fibrosis. J Cyst Fibros 2011;10(4):282–5.
51. Burrows JA, Toon M, Bell SC. Antibiotic desensitization in adults with cystic fibrosis. Respirology 2003;8:359–64.
52. Scherer K, Brockow K, Aberer W, et al. Desensitization in delayed drug hypersensitivity reactions - An EAACI position paper of the Drug Allergy Interest Group. Allergy Eur J Allergy Clin Immunol 2013;68(7):844–52.

Subcutaneous Injectable Drugs Hypersensitivity and Desensitization

Insulin and Monoclonal Antibodies

Sevim Bavbek, MD[a],*, Min Jung Lee, MD[b]

KEYWORDS

- Adalimumab • Etanercept • Omalizumab • Insulin • Injection site reactions
- Systemic hypersensitivity reactions • MoAbs • TNF-α inhibitors

KEY POINTS

- Etanercept and adalimumab are valid alternatives in the treatment of refractory inflammatory and autoimmune diseases, but local and systemic hypersensitivity reactions (HSRs) may prevent their use in sensitized patients.
- Rapid subcutaneous desensitization in patients with local and systemic HSRs to anti-tumor necrosis factor-α seems to be an effective treatment strategy.
- Rare incidences of systemic HSRs to insulin may be managed through desensitization.
- The mechanism of HSRs to omalizumab is not well-understood and desensitization has an unclear role for this agent.

TUMOR NECROSIS FACTOR-α INHIBITORS

Tumor necrosis factor-α (TNF-α) is one of the central mediators of inflammation, and TNF-α inhibitors are useful in certain "refractory" cases of inflammatory and autoimmune disorders in which TNF-α plays a major role in pathogenesis.[1] Today, 5 registered TNF-α antagonists—namely, infliximab, etanercept, adalimumab, certolizumab, and golimumab—are available on the market.[2] These agents are generally well-tolerated and safe, but they can induce a wide variety of adverse reactions. Among TNF-α inhibitor–induced adverse reactions, hypersensitivity reactions (HSRs), local

The authors do not have any commercial or financial conflict of interest and any funding sources relevant to this article.

[a] Division of Immunology and Allergy, Department of Chest Diseases, Ankara University School of Medicine, Mamak Street, Ankara 06100, Turkey; [b] Division of Allergy and Immunology, The University of Texas Southwestern Medical Center, 5323 Harry Hines Boulevard, Dallas, TX 75390, USA
* Corresponding author.
E-mail address: bavbek@medicine.ankara.edu.tr

or systemic, are infrequent; although the true incidence is unknown.[3] We limit our discussion to 2 injectable TNF-α antagonists, etanercept and adalimumab.

Etanercept

Etanercept is a fusion protein that binds irreversibly and competitively to membrane and circulant TNF-α molecule, and prevents them from binding to their receptors on immune effector cells. Etanercept is used in the treatment of multiple rheumatologic conditions such as rheumatoid arthritis, ankylosing spondylitis, psoriatic arthritis, and juvenile idiopathic arthritis; however, it may cause local and less commonly systemic HSR, limiting its use in sensitized patients.[4,5]

Adalimumab

Adalimumab is a recombinant, fully human IgG1 monoclonal antibody against TNF-α and is also indicated for the treatment of several chronic inflammatory diseases.[6] Adalimumab, as a fully humanized anti–TNF-α inhibitor, has not been expected to cause immune-mediated reactions, but has been infrequently associated with HSR.[7,8]

Clinical Presentations of Hypersensitivity Reactions to Etanercept and Adalimumab

Although generally well-tolerated and safe, a variety of adverse effects including HSR are increasingly being recognized in the setting of TNF-α inhibitors. The most common reactions with etanercept and adalimumab are local infusion and injection reactions, which are induced by subcutaneous biologic agents, are called injection site reactions (ISR), and are characterized by erythema, swelling, itching, or infiltrated plaques[7,9,10] (**Fig. 1**A, B). In clinical trials, ISRs have been found in up to 37% of etanercept-treated patients compared with 10% of the placebo-treated patients.[11,12] Like etanercept, in placebo-controlled clinical trials, an ISR was reported in between 3.2% to 20% of the adalimumab-treated patients compared with 1.8% to 14% of the placebo-treated patients.[13] These reactions may occur within a few minutes (immediate reactions) or later (delayed reactions) and generally were mild to moderate in severity, lasted 1 to 5 days, and occurred during the first month of treatment.[14,15]

In contrast, both immediate and delayed types, local and systemic immune-mediated HSR have been described with etanercept and adalimumab.[7,9,16] Both etanercept and adalimumab-induced immediate systemic HSR such as pruritus, urticaria, angioedema, and anaphylaxis have been reported rarely in the medical literature.[10,17–20]

In addition, delayed-type HSRs, thromboembolic events, serum sickness–like reactions, and cutaneous reactions, including maculopapular rash, leukocytoclastic vasculitis, erythema multiforme, Stevens-Johnson syndrome, and toxic epidermal necrolysis, have also described with the use of etanercept and adalimumab. In cases with severe skin reactions, the majority of the affected subjects were female and were being treated for rheumatoid arthritis.[12,21]

Underlying Mechanisms and Diagnostic Approach to Local and Systemic Hypersensitivity Reactions to Etanercept and Adalimumab

The mechanisms underlying HSR to etanercept and adalimumab have not been extensively studied. However, immediate HSRs to biologic agents have been closely related to the development of antidrug antibodies, both IgE and non-IgE isotypes.[6,22] Prick and intradermal skin tests with early readings have been used to detect the presence and biological activity of serum IgE to relevant biologic agents. In this regard, a few attempts have been done with skin testings to etanercept and adalimumab. Prick testing have been performed using commercially available etanercept and

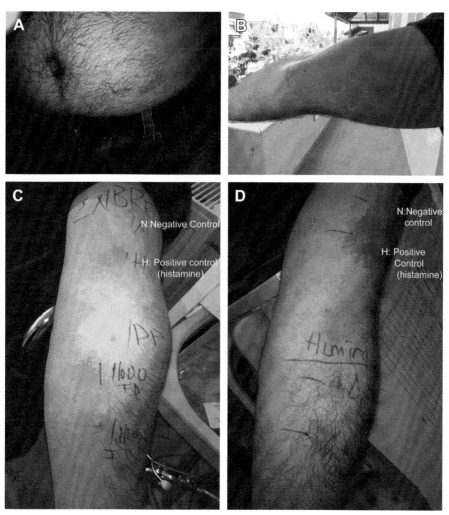

Fig. 1. Injection site reactions to (*A*) etanercept and (*B*) adalimumab. Skin test positivity to (*C*) etanercept and (*D*) adalimumab. H, positive control (histamine); N, negative control.

adalimumab with concentrations up to 25 to 50 mg/mL and 50 mg/mL, respectively. For prick and intradermal tests, the drugs have been diluted up to 1:10 with 0.9% NaCl.[10] In our series, we had a patient who had reacted to fifth dose of etanercept with severe systemic reaction requiring epinephrine. He showed strong positive reaction at 1:100 dilution of the prick and intradermal test to the drug.[10] This result is suggestive of an immediate-type allergic reaction, possibly an IgE-mediated mechanism. In previous reports describing 4 cases with anaphylaxis to etanercept, the diagnosis has been based on history and clinical alone. By history, anaphylaxis had occurred within hours after injection after several months of etanercept treatment and no recurrence of anaphylaxis after etanercept discontinuation.[17,18] A skin prick test with adalimumab (50 mg/mL) has elicited a positive response in a patient who developed nasal obstruction, generalized itching, and urticaria within a few minutes of a sixth injection of adalimumab.[23]

Although ISRs are the most common adverse reactions, studies about mechanisms are scarce. ISRs may be irritative or immune mediated.[9,15] Most ISRs might be an example of a T lymphocyte–mediated delayed-type HSR[9]; however, another study presented an unusual case with eosinophilic cellulitis-like reaction in biopsy specimen from the etanercept injection site.[16] These were the first data suggesting that the underlying immune mechanism may be a T_H2-mediated reaction in some patients with an ISR to etanercept. Two years later, supporting the data, early reading of prick and intradermal tests with the drug have been found positive in 2 patients with ISRs, which occurred within 6 hours after etanercept injection.[7] In our hands, prick tests with etanercept were negative but prick and intradermal tests were positive at a 1:100 and 1:10 dilutions in patients with ISR to etanercept[10] (see **Fig. 1**C).

Similarly, few reports have assessed the immunologic mechanism of ISRs to adalimumab.[7,8,10] In one of them, prick and intradermal tests with adalimumab were only positive at late reading, with a negative reaction in the prick test suggesting a cell-mediated reaction in 2 cases of ISRs to adalimumab.[7] In contrast, the other study, for the first time, suggested an IgE-mediated immediate-type hypersensitivity by demonstrating positivity on skin prick, an early reading intradermal test, and histamine release assay in 2 patients with progressively worsening ISRs to adalimumab.[8] In our experience, the prick test result with 40 mg/mL of adalimumab was positive in 4 cases and positive by prick and intradermal tests at a concentration of 1:1000 in all patients in 4 patients with ISR and one with urticaria[10] (see **Fig. 1**D).

The pathogenesis of delayed cutaneous reactions, even if they remain resolved, are most probably sustained by the activation of cellular immune mechanisms. However, the role of the patch test or late reading prick and intradermal tests have never been defined in the diagnosis of delayed cutaneous reactions to TNF-α inhibitors.[14]

Management of Hypersensitivity Reactions to Tumor Necrosis Factor-α Inhibitors with Desensitization

The simplest and most practical approach is to use other anti–TNF-α drugs in case of HSR to relevant drug. However, desensitization is a promising method for the delivery of monoclonal antibodies after a moderate or severe immediate type HSR in which there is no suitable alternative.[24] There are only 2 case ports of desensitization to adalimumab after a systemic reaction, such as generalized urticaria, rhinitis, and anaphylaxis.[17,23] Quercia and colleagues[17] describe a patient with anaphylaxis (at the 10th exposure to adalimumab, a rush desensitization protocol [2 hours in duration]) has been applied and the patient has been receiving full adalimumab doses for the past 2 years. In another case report, Rodriguez and colleagues[23] report another patient with generalized urticaria and rhinitis after adalimumab injection who was treated via desensitization. The protocol starts with an initial subcutaneous dose of 0.5 mg (1/100) that is increased to a cumulative dose of 44.25 mg with 60-minute intervals in the patient who reacted to adalimumab with generalized urticaria and rhinitis.

Beside desensitization protocols for immediate systemic HSRs to subcutaneous TNF-α inhibitors, there was no protocol for desensitization for immediate ISR induced by subcutaneous TNF-α inhibitors, although they are more common. Our group recently reported 2 successful desensitization protocols for patients with ISR to etanercept and adalimumab.[25,26] The first case was a patient with ankylosing spondylitis who became sensitized to both adalimumab and etanercept. The patient had developed local swelling, diffuse pruritus, and shortness of breath after his 26th adalimumab injection and was then switched to etanercept. He had an ISR followed by a disseminated urticarial rash after his 22nd etanercept injection. The patient was positive on prick and intradermal tests to 1/100 dilution of etanercept compared with 2 negative controls and then desensitized after a 3-day protocol that consisted of 6 injections on each day spaced by 30 to 90 minutes starting at 1/100 dilution of the final dose and doubling the dose with each step. Oral diphenhydramine (Benadryl) 25 mg, and famotidine 20 mg, aspirin 325 mg, and Montelukast 10 mg were given 1 hour before desensitization. The patient achieved the target dose and was subsequently maintained on etanercept twice weekly as a single injections with only small (<3 cm in diameter) local ISRs.[25] The second case was a 26-year-old woman with rheumatoid arthritis and progressive ISR (4 × 4 cm in diameter at the site of injection within 1 hour of the 11th injection, followed pruritus, redness, and swelling 8 × 8 cm and 8 × 10 in diameter, respectively, at the site of injection at second and third injection) to adalimumab who had a positive skin test both at direct prick and at prick and intradermal tests to 1/1000 dilution of the final dose of adalimumab. Oral diphenhydramine 25 mg, and famotidine 20 mg, were given 30 minutes before desensitization. The patient received initially doubling doses starting at 1 mg of adalimumab and ending at 24 mg of the drug; the cumulative dose for the desensitization was 55 mg. Subsequently, the patient received 40 mg at each treatment, which is the recommended therapeutic dose. The patient was maintained on weekly adalimumab self-injection for 3 months with diphenhydramine 25 mg and twice daily cetirizine. Because she experienced no reactions for the first 3 months, the adalimumab injections were spaced out to every other week.[26] However, desensitization protocols have not been standardized for the treatment of ISRs and systemic reactions after subcutaneous medication injections. On the basis of our experience with previously reported cases, we standardized the protocols for subcutaneous administration in patients sensitized to etanercept and adalimumab. Desensitization protocols for 50 mg of weekly etanercept and 40 mg of adalimumab were generated as shown in **Tables 1** and **2**. Using this protocol, successfully subcutaneous recommended daily dosages

Table 1
Subcutaneous desensitization protocol with etanercept (for 50 mg/mL, weekly injection)

Time (min)	Dose (mg)	Dilution (Concentration)	Volume Administered (mL)
Days 1, 2 (Monday, Wednesday)			
0	0.50	1:100, (0.5 mg/mL)	1
30	1.0	1:10, (5 mg/mL)	0.2
60	2	1:10, (5 mg/mL)	0.4
90	4	1:10,(5 mg/mL)	0.8
120	8	1:1, (50 mg/mL)	0.16
150	9	1:1, (50 mg/mL)	0.18
Total dose	24.5		
Day 3 (Monday)			
0	0.50	1:100, (0.5 mg/mL)	1.0
30	1.00	1:10, (5 mg/mL)	0.2
60	2.00	1:10, (5 mg/mL)	0.4
90	4.00	1:10, (5 mg/mL)	0.8
120	8.00	1:1, (50 mg/mL)	0.16
150	16.00	1:1, (50 mg/mL)	0.32
180	18.5	1:1, (50 mg/mL)	0.37
Total dose	50		

Table 2
Subcutaneous desensitization protocol with adalimumab (for 50 mg/mL, weekly injection)

Time (min)	Dilution Concentration (50 mg/mL)	Volume (mL)	Dose (mg)	Cumulative Dose (mg)
0	1:100 (0.5 mg/mL)	1.00	0.50	0.50
30	1:10 (5 mg/mL)	0.15	0.75	1.25
60	1:10 (5 mg/mL)	0.25	1.25	2.50
90	1:1 (5 mg/mL)	0.50	2.50	5.00
120	1:1 (50 mg/mL)	0.10	5.00	10.00
150	1:1 (50 mg/mL)	0.20	10.00	20.00
180	1:1 (50 mg/mL)	0.40	20.00	40.00

were reported in 7 patients who experienced adverse reactions to etanercept (6 ISRs and 1 systemic reaction), and 5 patients with reactions to adalimumab (4 ISR and 1 urticaria). All patients have been able to continue with etanercept, with minor local erythema resolving within 1 to 2 hours. Similarly, all patients were successfully desensitized and maintained on weekly adalimumab for 3 months with premedication. Adalimumab injections were then spaced to every other week without further problems.[10] Recently, a shorter protocol was reported by de la Varga Martínez et al.[27] In this report, 2 patients with psoriatic arthritis developed ISR followed by generalized urticaria without angioedema in 1 patient. Patients have been found negative at prick and intradermal tests, but positive on basophil activation test. After premedication with dexamethasone (20 mg orally) and dexchlorpheniramine (5 mg intramuscular) 1 hour before the first desensitization, patients have been desensitized protocol that is consisted of subcutaneous administration of 8 doses every 15 minutes until reaching a cumulative therapeutic dose of 50 mg.

INSULIN

Insulin is a key component in the management of type I and type II diabetes mellitus. With the transition from animal-sourced insulin to human-derived insulin in the 1980s, the reports of HSRs have decreased significantly.[28] Currently, the most widely used insulin types are human insulin (NPH, regular insulin) and insulin analogues (ie, Aspart, Lispro, Detemir, Glargine). Here, we focus mainly on immediate-type HSRs related to insulin with brief discussion of ISRs.

Clinical Presentations of Hypersensitivity Reactions to Insulin

Both immediate and delayed reactions to insulin have been reported in the literature. Immediate reactions usually occur within 1 hour of administration and can be broadly categorized as ISR (usually limited to local or limited skin involvement) or HSR (usually systemic), extending beyond the areas of injection that can be IgE mediated with or without a complement-mediated mechanism. Delayed reactions to insulin usually occur hours after exposure and likely involve types III or IV reactions.[28–31]

Given that ISRs are more commonly reported, it would be prudent for the treating physician to be aware of the signs and symptoms of HSRs associated with insulin. Foremost, injection site technique including the preparation of the injection site should be noted and excluded as a possible cause for local site reaction. ISRs are usually localized to the site of injection, occurring in varying onset after injection, and may spontaneously resolve rather than worsening over time.[30] In contrast, the signs of

HSR have the following characteristics: rapid, extensive involvement, and/or worsening nature of the symptoms over time. The symptoms of HSRs to insulin can include pruritus, hives, angioedema, shortness of breath, and other symptoms of anaphylaxis.[29,30] Rarely, fatal reports have been described, with some related to insulin itself or its constituents such as protamine.[32,33]

Diagnostic Approach to Hypersensitivity Reactions to Insulin

Once the history suggests immediate systemic reactions or HSRs, the skin testing evaluation of the reactions should include the insulin itself, additives in the preparation (protamine and cresol), and/or latex.[29] Protamine is used in human insulin to prolong the activity of insulin and is also used for heparin reversal during cardiac intervention. Cresol is a preservative present in all currently available human insulin and insulin analogues. Although skin testing has been done to show sensitization in patients with HSRs, the sensitivity has not been established given limited number of patients involved. False-positive results to insulin skin testing have been reported in patients with diabetes mellitus without history of HSRs.[34] With that in mind, skin prick testing has been done with 50 to 100 U/mL and intradermal concentration further diluted 10- to 100-fold. With the same precaution, protamine skin prick testing has been done at 350 μg/mL and intradermal concentration further diluted 10- to 100-fold. Cresol also has been used for skin prick testing at 1.5 to 3 mg/mL.[34,35] If there is a suspicion for latex sensitivity, latex-specific IgE and/or skin prick testing can be done, which may be limited based on availability.[36] The usefulness of late reading (24–48 hours) after skin testing and/or patch testing to insulin and its constituents has not been validated and may have limited clinical value.

Management of Hypersensitivity Reactions to Insulin with Desensitization

Immediate systemic reactions to insulin that are persistent despite change in the insulin preparation may need desensitization for further administration. Coordination with an endocrinology team would be essential to monitor for glucose on a regular interval during the procedure. Multiple desensitization protocols have been reported with varying starting concentration (1,000,000-fold to 1000-fold diluted from 100 IU/mL), which can be increased either 10-fold or 2-fold to reach a goal dose every 15 to 30 minutes[37] (**Table 3**). Other routes, such as continuous

Table 3
Example of subcutaneous desensitization protocol with insulin (goal: 10 U/mL, injection)

Steps	Dose (IU)
1	0.001[a]
2[b]	0.01
3[b]	0.1
4[b]	1
5	2
6	4
7	10

Starting at 10^{-6} or 10^{-3} IU.

[a] Starting dose may be more dilute depending on the severity of initial reaction. Increase 10-fold every 15 to 30 minutes until reaching 1 IU. After 1 IU is reached, increase about 2-fold (or double) every 15 to 30 minutes until reaching the goal dose.

[b] Monitor glucose level at each step or at least 30- to 60-minute intervals.

subcutaneous insulin infusion and intravenous methods, have also been used with successful outcomes.[38,39] In a few rare reports, concomitant use of omalizumab or immunosuppression during insulin desensitization has been described for difficult cases.[40]

OMALIZUMAB

Omalizumab is a humanized monoclonal antibody directed against the Fcε portion of IgE. It has been approved for moderate to severe persistent, allergic asthma in patients age 6 and older as well as chronic idiopathic urticaria in age 12 and older (package insert). In addition, there are ongoing investigational uses of omalizumab in conjunction with food or allergen and venom immunotherapy.

Clinical Presentations of Hypersensitivity Reactions to Omalizumab

HSRs to omalizumab can be either immediate or delayed and the mechanism is largely unknown. Although most common reactions to omalizumab are ISRs in up to 45% of treated patients, anaphylaxis has been rarely reported with symptoms including bronchospasm, hypotension, syncope, urticarial, and/or angioedema in the first 3 doses or after many doses.[41] In 2007, the Omalizumab Joint Task Force reviewed the clinical trials and postmarketing data since its approval in 2003 and identified rate of anaphylaxis as 0.09% in 39,510 patients who were treated between June 1, 2001, and December 31, 2005. There were no reports of death or respiratory distress requiring intubation. The task force has recommended the following advisories, which include 2-hour observation periods for the first 3 initial injections and 30-minute observation times for subsequent injections.[42] Then again in 2011, the Joint Task Force has upheld its previous recommendations, which would recognize 77% of reactions in the medical settings. Interestingly, all patients with anaphylaxis had asthma, and tryptase that was checked in few occasions were not elevated.[43] In contrast, there are also reports of serum sickness–like reactions (such as arthralgia) noted in both package inserts and in a few case reports.[44,45]

The mechanism behind omalizumab-associated HSRs is not well-understood. The interesting and unusual characteristics of omalizumab reactions are that up to 77% of HSRs can occur immediately (within hours), but the rest of the reactions can occur delayed fashion (>12 hours or even days after administration).[42,43] These findings suggest that omalizumab is unlikely to follow our typical understanding of immediate HSRs, which usually includes sensitization (omalizumab reactions can occur after first injection) and immediate occurrence (omalizumab reactions can occur in hours to days). These clinical findings suggest that the pathogenesis of anaphylaxis to omalizumab is unclear and may or may not involve an IgE-mediated mechanism against the small murine component of omalizumab or its excipients, such as polysorbate.[46]

Diagnostic Approach to Hypersensitivity Reactions to Omalizumab

Skin testing to omalizumab has yielded variable reports and a nonirritating concentration for skin testing has not been established. One study suggests the nonirritating concentration for intradermal testing is 1:100,000 or 1.25 μg/mL diluted in saline[47]; however, this has not been validated.

Management of Hypersensitivity Reactions to Omalizumab with Desensitization

There are few case reports of desensitizations to omalizumab with variable outcomes. The first case reported was of a woman with uncontrolled asthma and chronic urticaria who developed mild symptoms (diffuse erythema with pruritus) to omalizumab. She was desensitized starting 7.5 mg, doubling every 30 minutes for a total goal dose of 150 mg. However, she continued to develop similar initial symptoms and later developed fever and petechiae that were suggestive of serum sickness–like reaction, leading to discontinuation.[44] Next, a case series of 3 patients with HSRs consisting of cough, urticaria, and angioedema were desensitized starting with 0.0625 mg, doubling every 30 minutes to a total cumulative dose of 113 to 190 mg. These patients tolerated subsequent doses with 2 of them receiving it weekly.[48] In contrast, Paranjpe and colleagues[49] reported a case of failed desensitization in a patient with moderate to severe symptoms consisting of dyspnea, nausea, and hypotension that were initially treated with 2 epinephrine injections. After negative skin prick testing, the patient was started on 0.125 mg, increasing every 30 minutes until a 31.25 mg dose, when she reported cough, chest tightness, dyspnea with an $FEV_1\%$ of 30% predicted from baseline of 65%, which was treated with epinephrine injection and albuterol nebulizer. The lack of understanding of the pathogenesis as well as experience with this drug would require careful consideration in the evaluation and management of patients with omalizumab-associated HSRs.

REFERENCES

1. Murdaca G, Colombo BM, Puppo F. Anti-TNF-alpha inhibitors: a new therapeutic approach for inflammatory immune-mediated diseases: an update upon efficacy and adverse events. Int J Immunopathol Pharmacol 2009;22(3):557–65.
2. Tracey D, Klareskog L, Sasso EH, et al. Tumor necrosis factor antagonist mechanisms of action: a comprehensive review. Pharmacol Ther 2008;117:244–79.
3. Corominas M, Gastaminza G, Lobera T. Hypersensitivity reactions to biological drugs. J Investig Allergol Clin Immunol 2014;24:212e25.
4. Culy CR, Keating GM. Etanercept: an updated review of its use in rheumatoid arthritis, psoriatic arthritis and juvenile rheumatoid arthritis. Drugs 2002;62: 2493–537.
5. Fleischmann R, Baumgartner SW, Weisman MH, et al. Long term safety of etanercept in elderly subjects with rheumatic diseases. Ann Rheum Dis 2006;65: 379–84.
6. Voulgari PV, Kaltsonoudis E, Papagoras C, et al. Adalimumab in the treatment of rheumatoid arthritis. Expert Opin Biol Ther 2012;12(12):1679–86.
7. Benucci M, Manfredi M, Demoly P, et al. Injection site reactions to TNF-α blocking agents with positive skin tests. Allergy 2008;63:138–9.
8. Paltiel M, Gober LM, Deng A, et al. Immediate type I hypersensitivity response implicated in worsening injection site reactions to adalimumab. Arch Dermatol 2008;144(9):1190–4.
9. Zeltser R, Valle L, Tanck C, et al. Clinical, histological, and immunophenotypic characteristics of injection site reactions associated with etanercept: a recombinant tumor necrosis factor alpha-receptor: Fc fusion protein. Arch Dermatol 2001; 137(7):893–9.
10. Bavbek S, Ataman Ş, Akıncı A, et al. Rapid subcutaneous desensitization for the management of local and systemic hypersensitivity reactions to etanercept and adalimumab in 12 patients. J Allergy Clin Immunol Pract 2015;3:629e32.
11. Dore RK, Mathews S, Schechtman J, et al. The immunogenicity, safety, and efficacy of etanercept liquid administered once weekly in patients with rheumatoid arthritis. Clin Exp Rheumatol 2007;25:40–6.
12. Borrás-Blasco J, Navarro-Ruiz A, Borrás C, et al. Adverse cutaneous reactions induced by TNF-α antagonist therapy. South Med J 2009;102(11):1133–9.

13. Humira (adalimumab) Prescribing Information [package insert]. Abbott Park, IL: Abbott Laboratories; 2008.

14. Vultaggio A, Matucci A, Nencini F, et al. Hypersensitivity reactions to biologicals: true allergy? Curr Treat Options Allergy 2016;3:147–57.

15. Batycka-Baran A, Flaig M, Molin S, et al. Etanercept-induced injection site reactions: potential pathomechanisms and clinical assessment. Expert Opin Drug Saf 2012;11(6):911–21.

16. Winfield H, Lain E, Horn T, et al. Eosinophilic cellulites like reaction to subcutaneous etanercept injection. Arch Dermatol 2006;142:218–20.

17. Quercia O, Emiliani F, Foschi FG, et al. Adalimumab desensitization after anaphylactic reaction. Ann Allergy Asthma Immunol 2011;106:547–8.

18. Crayne CB, Gerhold K, Cron RQ. Anaphylaxis to etanercept in two children with juvenile idiopathic arthritis. J Clin Rheumatol 2013;19:129–31.

19. Quismorio A, Brahmbhatt B, Houng M, et al. Etanercept allergy and anaphylaxis. J Rheumatol 2012;39:11.

20. George SJ, Anderson HL, Hsu S. Adalimumab-induced urticaria. Dermatol Online J 2006;12:4.

21. Masson PL. Thromboembolic events and anti-tumor necrosis factor therapies. Int Immunopharmacol 2012;14(4):444–5.

22. Matucci A, Pratesi S, Petroni G, et al. Allergological in vitro and in vivo evaluation of patients with hypersensitivity reactions to infliximab. Clin Exp Allergy 2013; 43(6):659–64.

23. Rodríguez-Jiménez B, Dominquez-Ortega J. Successful adalimumab desensitization after generalized urticaria and rhinitis. J Investig Allergol Clin Immunol 2009;19:246–7.

24. Brennan PJ, Rodriguez Bouza T, Hsu FI, et al. Hypersensitivity reactions to mAbs: 105 desensitizations in 23 patients, from evaluation to treatment. J Allergy Clin Immunol 2009;124(6):1259–66.

25. Bavbek S, Aydın O, Ataman S, et al. Injection-site reaction to etanercept: role of skin test in the diagnosis of such reaction and successful desensitization. Allergy 2011;66(9):1256–7.

26. Bavbek S, Ataman Ş, Bankova L, et al. Injection site reaction to adalimumab: positive skin test and successful rapid desensitization. Allergol Immunopathol 2012; 41(3):204–6.

27. de la Varga Martínez R, Gutierrez Fernandez D, Foncubierta Fernandez A, et al. Rapid subcutaneous desensitization for treatment of hypersensitivity reactions to etanercept in two patients with positive basophil activation test. Allergol Int 2017; 66(2):357–9.

28. Schernthaner G. Immunogenicity and allergic potential of animal and human insulins. Diabetes Care 1993;16(Suppl 3):155–65.

29. Ghazavi ML, Johnston GA. Insulin allergy. Clin Dermatol 2011;29:300–5.

30. Heinzerling L, Raile K, Rochlitz H, et al. Insulin allergy: clinical manifestations and management strategies. Allergy 2008;63:148–55.

31. Rojas J, Villalobos M, Sofia Martinez M, et al. Successful management of insulin allergy and autoimmune polyendocrine syndrome type 4 with desensitization therapy and glucocorticoid treatment: a case report and review of literature. Case Reports Immunol 2014;2014:394754.

32. Chu YQ, Cai LJ, Jiang DC, et al. Allergic shock and death associated with protamine administration in a diabetic patient. Clin Ther 2010;32:1729.

33. Kaya A, Gungor K, Karakose S. Severe anaphylactic reaction to human insulin in a diabetic patient. J Diabet Complications 2007;21:124.

34. Lee AY, Chey WY, Choi J, et al. Insulin induced drug eruptions and reliability of skin tests. Acta Derm Venereol 2002;82:114–7.
35. Botger U, Wittrup M. A rational clinical approach to suspected insulin allergy: status after five years and 22 cases. Diabet Med 2005;22:102–6.
36. Roest MA, Shaw S, Orton DI. Insulin-injection-site reactions associated with type I latex allergy. N Engl J Med 2003;348(3):265–6.
37. Hoffman AG, Schram SE, Ercan-Fang NG, et al. Type I allergy to insulin: case report and review of localized and systemic reactions to insulin. Dermatitis 2008;19(1):52–8.
38. Fujikawa T, Imbe H, Date M, et al. Severe insulin allergy successfully treated with continuous subcutaneous insulin infusion. Diabetes Res Clin Pract 2012;97:e31.
39. Asai M, Yoshida M, Miura Y. Immunologic tolerance to intravenously injected insulin. N Engl J Med 2006;354:307.
40. Yong PF, Malik R, Arif S, et al. Rituximab and omalizumab in severe, refractory insulin allergy. N Engl J Med 2009;360:1045.
41. XOLAIR (omalizumab) [package insert]. San Francisco, CA: Genentech, Inc; 2016.
42. Cox L, Platts-Mills TA, Finegold I, et al. American Academy of Allergy, Asthma &Immunology/American College of Allergy, Asthma and Immunology Joint Task force-Report on omalizumab-associated anaphylaxis. J Allergy Clin Immunol 2007;120:1373–7.
43. Cox L, Lieberman P, Wallace D, et al. American Academy of Allergy, Asthma &Immunology/American College of Allergy, Asthma and Immunology Omalizumab-Associated anaphylaxis Joint Task Force follow-up Report on omalizumab-associated anaphylaxis. J Allergy Clin Immunol 2011;128:210–2.
44. Dreyfus DH, Randolph CC. Characterization of an anaphylactoid reaction to omalizumab. Ann Allergy Asthma Immunol 2006;96(4):624–7.
45. Pilette C, Coppens N, Houssiau FA, et al. Severe serum sickness-like syndrome after omalizumab therapy for asthma. J Allergy Clin Immunol 2007;124(4):972–3.
46. Lieberman P. The unusual suspects: a surprise regarding reactions to omalizumab. Allergy Asthma Proc 2007;28:259–61.
47. Liebermen P, Rahmaoui A, Wong DA. The safety and interpretability of skin tests with omalizumab. Ann Allergy Asthma Immunol 2010;1105:493–5.
48. Owens G, Petro A. Successful desensitization of three patients with hypersensitivity reactions to omalizumab. Curr Drug Saf 2011;6(5):339–42.
49. Paranjpe P, Hilton K, Khan DA. Failure of omalizumab desensitization resulting in anaphylaxis in a patient with severe asthma. Ann Allergy Asthma Immunol 2009; 103(5):A124.

Progestogen Hypersensitivity

An Evidence-Based Approach to Diagnosis and Management in Clinical Practice

Dinah Foer, MD[a],*, Kathleen M. Buchheit, MD[a,b]

KEYWORDS

- Progesterone • Progestin • Progestogen hypersensitivity
- Autoimmune progesterone dermatitis • Desensitization • In vitro fertilization

KEY POINTS

- Progestogen hypersensitivity (PH) may be triggered by endogenous progesterone or exogenous progestin exposure.
- The heterogeneity of progestogen exposures and PH symptoms underscore the importance of a systematic and thorough history and physical during the patient encounter.
- Current skin-testing methods for PH yield equivocal results and is an active area of research.
- Patient-specific symptom profiles and patient goals should guide treatment.
- Desensitization to progestogens has been demonstrated as a safe, reproducible option for women pursuing pregnancy through in vitro fertilization as well as for refractory symptoms.

INTRODUCTION

Although the term progestogen hypersensitivity (PH) is a relatively new addition to the allergy/immunologist lexicon,[1] progesterone hypersensitivity syndromes were first described more than 50 years ago.[2] In the intervening years, the term autoimmune progesterone dermatitis was a common reference to a heterogeneous collection of symptoms. However, as recent studies have demonstrated, there is little evidence

Disclosure: The authors have no relevant commercial or financial conflicts of interests to disclose.
[a] Department of Medicine, Division of Rheumatology, Immunology and Allergy, Brigham and Women's Hospital, Harvard Medical School, Boston, MA, USA; [b] Department of Medicine, Division of Rheumatology, Immunology and Allergy, Brigham and Women's Hospital, Harvard Medical School, 60 Fenwood Road, Boston, MA 02115, USA
* Corresponding author. Brigham and Women's Hospital, 75 Francis Street, Boston, MA 02445.
E-mail address: dfoer@bwh.harvard.edu

Immunol Allergy Clin N Am 37 (2017) 773–784
http://dx.doi.org/10.1016/j.iac.2017.07.006   immunology.theclinics.com
0889-8561/17/© 2017 Elsevier Inc. All rights reserved.

supporting an autoimmune pathophysiology, and the range of PH symptoms include both immediate and delayed-type hypersensitivity. This article reviews a systematic approach to patient diagnosis, centered on a triad of history, physical examination, and testing. This approach will then form the basis for a discussion of current evidence on treatment strategies, including desensitization and longitudinal symptom management.

DEFINITIONS

Progestogen describes a group of steroid hormones that includes both progesterone and progestins.

Progesterone is an endogenously synthesized hormone derived from cholesterol. The roles of progesterone in obstetrics and gynecology has been well defined, particularly in its role as a mediator of the menstrual cycle. Levels rise in the luteal phase, and fall in the follicular phase, leading to menstruation.[3,4] In pregnancy, progesterone is produced by the corpus luteum and then the placenta.[5,6] Progesterone has also been implicated in endocrine signaling to a variety of other organs including the brain and lungs.[7] Investigating progesterone's role in sex differences in common diseases, such as asthma, is an active area of research without conclusive evidence to whether it mitigates or facilitates respiratory inflammation.[8,9]

Progestins are synthetically derived by editing side chains on a different group of hormones, primarily 19-nortestosterone, 17 α-hydroxyprogesterone or acetoxyprogestin.[10] Therefore, oral and implantable contraceptives and intrauterine devices (IUDs) are composed of a distinctly different chemical structure than endogenous progesterone, yet still fall under the rubric of progestogens.

EPIDEMIOLOGY

Despite its description more than 50 years ago, the prevalence of PH remains unknown. Women between menarche and menopause can be affected, with the average age of onset to be in the third decade of life, with a mean age of 27.3 years (range 12–47) and 29.7 years (range 13–48) in 2 different studies.[1,11] A single case report of hypersensitivity to progestin has been reported in a man, who reacted to megestrol acetate and confirmed by positive skin testing to progesterone acetate.[12]

THE CLINICAL ENCOUNTER

The history and physical is an essential starting point for the diagnosis of PH, as outlined in **Table 1**.

History

The heterogeneity of progestogen exposures and PH symptoms underscores the importance of a systematic and thorough history and physical during the patient encounter. A classification schema for PH presentation has been previously proposed (**Table 2**).

Progestogen hypersensitivity from endogenous progesterone exposure generally correlates with monthly symptoms that occur 3 to 10 days before the onset of menses (**Fig. 1**). However, as in the general population, some women with PH may have metrorrhagia and experience PH at other intervals. These symptoms may remiss at menopause or may persist.[13,14] Keeping a menstrual diary of symptoms may help identify symptoms correlating with each period, albeit irregular in timing. The pattern of PH in pregnancy and its natural history is not well documented, as intrapartum

Table 1		
Key elements of the history and physical examination for PH diagnosis		
Clinical Encounter	**Area of Focus**	**Key Findings**
History	Symptom timing	• Cyclical pattern
	OB-GYN history	• Menses
		• Pregnancies and terminations
		• Assisted fertility
	Medication use	• Progestogens
		• NSAIDs
Physical	Dermatologic	• Rash
		• Urticaria
		• Angioedema
	Pulmonary	• Wheezes
	Pelvic	• Pruritus
		• Labial swelling

Abbreviations: NSAIDs, nonsteroidal anti-inflammatory drugs; OB-GYN, obstetrics-gynecology; PH, progestogen hypersensitivity.

improvement has been reported.[15] In other case reports, patients have developed symptoms during pregnancy and postpartum.[16–22] Patients may have previously tolerated menses but develop cyclical symptoms later in life following endogenous (ie, pregnancy) or exogenous progestogen exposure. Nguyen and Razzaque Ahmed[11] found that 40 (44.94%) of the 89 cases they reviewed had known prior exposure to exogenous progestogen. Of note, family history of PH is not thought to be a risk factor, but there is one case report of 3 sisters with PH.[23]

Exogenous sources of progestogens are an important and growing consideration in PH diagnosis and successful management. Sources include progestins in oral contraceptive pills (OCPs),[14,20,24] long-acting depot preparations such as

Table 2		
Classification of progestogen hypersensitivity presentation		
Exposure Classification	**Trigger**	**Timing**
Endogenous		
Primary	Menses	Perimenstrual symptoms
	Pregnancy	Monthly symptoms after completion of non–in vitro fertilization pregnancy
Exogenous		
Secondary	Supplemental progestogen[a]	Symptoms only during supplemental progestogen administration
Mixed[b]	Supplemental progestogen[a]	Took supplemental progestogen, then develops perimenstrual symptoms

[a] Includes synthetic progesterone and progestins.
[b] Defined as initial reaction due to exogenous exposure, with subsequent reactions to both exogenous and endogenous sources of progestogen.

Adapted from Foer D, Buchheit KM, Gargiulo AR, et al. Progestogen hypersensitivity in 24 cases: diagnosis, management, and proposed renaming and classification. J Allergy Clin Immunol Pract 2016;4(4):725; with permission.

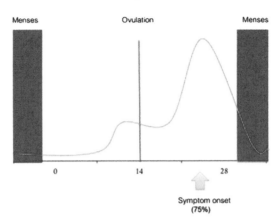

Fig. 1. Progesterone levels during the menstrual cycle. (*From* Foer D, Buchheit KM, Gargiulo AR, et al. Progestogen hypersensitivity in 24 cases: diagnosis, management, and proposed renaming and classification. J Allergy Clin Immunol Pract 2016;4(4):726; with permission.)

medroxyprogesterone acetate,[3,22,25] vaginal rings,[26] emergency contraception, and IUDs.[1] The rise of in vitro fertilization (IVF) and use of high-dose progesterone is now well documented as an emerging source of PH and a further barrier to achieving pregnancy using assisted reproductive technologies.[20] Of note, there are no published cases of PH secondary to hormone replacement therapy, although the diagnosis

> Therefore, on history, 2 questions can help guide diagnosis of PH: What is the presumed progestogen exposure, and what is the timing of patient symptoms? Taken together, these can help the clinician avoid common diagnostic delays.[3,24]

should be considered in the differential with a suggestive history and physical.

Physical

Patients may present with active physical manifestations of PH, photos of past flares, or asymptomatically based on symptom timing. Dermatologic findings are most common and include a broad range of pathology, including urticaria with or without angioedema,[3,21,27–30] eczematous dermatitis,[20,31] maculopapular rash, vesiculobullous and vesiculopustular lesions,[2,15,24] petechiae and purpura,[32,33] fixed drug eruption,[34,35] stomatitis,[36,37] and erythema multiforme.[19,38] Some of these findings may be localized to the pelvic area, including vulvovaginal pruritus,[39] and labial swelling.[40] Respiratory symptoms, such as asthma, have been reported and there are also reports of anaphylaxis[14,21,25,34,41]; in some patients both dermatologic and nondermatologic manifestations have been described.[14,34,38,42]

Following the clinical encounter, the differential diagnosis for PH includes other steroid-based syndromes, medication triggers other than progestogens, and a variety of primary dermatologic pathologies (**Table 3**). Of note, eliciting a thorough medication history is important in differentiating PH from other immediate or delayed-type hypersensitivity syndromes.

Table 3
Differential diagnosis for progestogen hypersensitivity

Medications	Particularly nonsteroidal anti-inflammatory drugs, commonly used in premenstrual period[26]
Primary dermatologic pathology	Chronic idiopathic urticaria, atopic dermatitis, allergic contact dermatitis
Steroid hypersensitivity syndromes	
Catamenial anaphylaxis	Symptoms correlate with ONSET of menstrual cycle[43]
Estrogen hypersensitivity	Exogenous or endogenous estrogen leads to premenstrual urticaria or delayed-type dermatitis with positive estrogen skin test[43–47]
Lactation anaphylaxis	Clinical correlation with breastfeeding or manual expression of breast milk[48–53]

DIAGNOSTIC TESTING OPTIONS

Common diagnostic modalities in clinical practice include progesterone skin testing and challenge.[29,30,54] However, the equivocal results from current skin-testing methodologies discussed as follows highlight the importance of a convincing clinical history in making the diagnosis of PH.

Skin Testing

Skin prick testing is conducted with progesterone (50 mg/mL) in serial dilutions. Diluents can be ethanol or oil based. False-positive reactions caused benzyl alcohol or oil-based diluents have been described.[1] Wheal and flare are compared with diluent (either oil or ethanol) and positive histamine controls.[1,29,55] Testing with water-soluble progestins has been proposed as an alternative to progesterone skin testing. However, similar limitations exist given additives to progestins such as polyethylene glycol, which can also cause irritant reactions.[54,56] Under study by our group is the possible use of water-soluble depo-progestins, which would eliminate the irritant effects in current skin-testing methods.[1] In a recent study of 24 patients with clinical history consistent with PH, only 50% of patients had positive progestogen skin testing. This included patients with observed respiratory symptoms during skin testing, but negative skin test results. Therefore, the positive predictive value and negative predictive value of skin testing is unknown and cannot alone rule in or rule out PH.

Progesterone Challenge

The utility of progesterone challenge is limited in the diagnosis of PH. A clear history of symptoms following exogenous progestogen exposure may obviate the need for further progesterone challenge. Risks of challenge include symptom exacerbation.[2,19] Rather than challenge, empiric treatment focused on patient symptoms or desensitization may be an appropriate next step (**Fig. 2**).

Patch Testing

Attempts at progesterone patch testing have not been shown to be a more useful diagnostic tool than existing modalities.[55] This is a potential area for further investigation, as patch testing is an attractive method for testing for delayed-type hypersensitivity reactions.

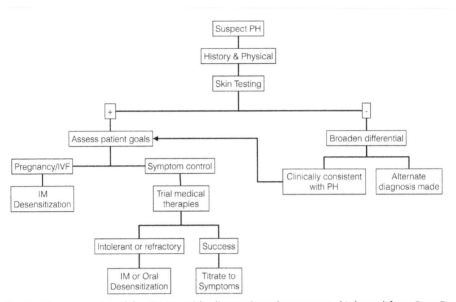

Fig. 2. Management tool for PH to guide diagnosis and treatment. (*Adapted from* Foer D, Buchheit KM, Gargiulo AR, et al. Progestogen hypersensitivity in 24 cases: diagnosis, management, and proposed renaming and classification. J Allergy Clin Immunol Pract 2016;4(4):727; with permission.)

Precision diagnostic testing is an active area of research, as discussed later in this article.

MANAGEMENT

Management of PH is directed by the severity of patient symptoms and patient goals, as outlined in **Fig. 2**. Interestingly, the specific progestogen trigger does not seem to matter in terms of responsiveness to medical management and treatment with desensitization.[2,13,17]

Table 4 outlines current treatment options for PH. Medical management with antihistamines or topical or oral corticosteroids can be initially trialed for patients desiring symptom control.[21,41,42,57] Tolerance of these therapies is variable, and often limited by adverse side effects for long-term use. Three months has been suggested as a reasonable trial period for medication management, although this may be at the discretion of the patient and clinician. Patients who do not respond to symptom management may require suppression of ovulation or desensitization as described in the following paragraph.

Suppression of ovulation with OCPs can control symptoms in many patients. However, some patients cannot tolerate the low-dose progestin in OCPs and instead require treatments with other medications that suppress ovulation, such as gonadotropin-releasing hormone (GnRH) agonists,[3,14,22,41,58,59] alkylated androgens,[50,59] and tamoxifen.[4,19,37] However, symptoms of hypoestrogenemia with GnRH agonists and tamoxifen, and androgen-induced side effects with the 17-α-alkylated steroids severely limit their use. Oophorectomy remains a definitive, curative option for PH of endogenous or mixed etiology, although should be considered only in refractory cases or based on patient preference.[2,36,60,61]

Table 4
Treatment options in progestogen hypersensitivity

Treatment Category	Drug Class	Potential Benefits	Potential Limitations
Symptomatic relief	Oral antihistamines	Acute relief of itching, swelling	Incomplete efficacy
	Topical glucocorticoids	Acute relief of itching, swelling	Incomplete efficacy, long-term side effects
	Systemic glucocorticoids	Acute relief of itching, swelling, wheezing	Incomplete efficacy, long-term side effects
Ovulation suppression	Combined oral contraceptive pills	Readily available	Possible hypersensitivity reaction to low-dose progestin[a]
	GnRH agonists	Alternative if unable to tolerate OCPs	Estrogen withdrawal symptoms including bone loss, hot flashes, urogenital atrophy
	Selective estrogen-receptor modulators	Alternative if unable to tolerate OCPs	Estrogen withdrawal symptoms including bone loss, hot flashes, urogenital atrophy
	17-α-alkylated steroids	Alternative if unable to tolerate OCPs	Hirsutism, mood changes, LFT abnormalities
	Oophorectomy	Definitive symptoms relief in cases of endogenous PH	Premature menopause, permanent loss of fertility
Desensitization	Rapid desensitization to IM or intravaginal progestogens	Can be precisely timed to IVF needs; enables successful pregnancy	Resource intensive, risk of hypersensitivity reactions during desensitization
	Rapid or slow desensitization to oral progestins	Can be tailored to goal dose of progestin; long-term symptom control	Risk of hypersensitivity reactions during desensitization; long-term cycling on hormones to avoid resensitization

Abbreviations: GnRH, gonadotropin-releasing hormone; IM, intramuscular; IVF, invitro fertilization; LFT, liver function tests; OCPs, oral contraceptive pills; PH, progestogen hypersensitivity.
[a] Desensitization to OCPs is an option for managing this side effect.[1]

For patients undergoing fertility treatment/IVF requiring high-dose progesterone, symptom management described previously is not an option. In these cases, progesterone desensitization has been shown to be a successful, reproducible modality for treatment, allowing patients to tolerate high-dose progesterone required to maintain pregnancy. Although intramuscular (IM) and vaginal protocols appear to have equal efficacy, IM has been recommended as the easiest modality for rapid desensitization.[2,12,13] The timing of desensitization relative to embryo transfer is determined in collaboration with a reproductive endocrinologist.

The success and safety of desensitization to date positions it as an option to more readily consider in cases outside the IVF realm. Indications include severe symptoms not optimally controlled with symptom-focused medications.[2,36,60,61] In these cases, a rapid or slow oral desensitization protocol may be used. The protocols have been detailed elsewhere in the literature.[2,13] Following desensitization, patients must continually cycle on the OCP to maintain a steady state of progesterone to avoid resensitization.

ACTIVE AREAS OF RESEARCH
Pathomechanisms of Progestogen Hypersensitivity

The underlying cause of PH in unknown. It has been theorized that patients with PH are sensitized via exposure to exogenous progesterone and progestins used for either contraception or fertility treatments.[62] However, as described previously, only half of patients with PH have history of prior exposure to progestogens.[11] An alternative mechanism by which patients may become sensitized to progestogens is cross-sensitization to related corticosteroids.[63] Regardless of the cause of PH, it appears that multiple mechanisms may be at play given the wide variety of clinical manifestations that can occur in PH. Proposed mechanisms include mast-cell activation[64] and immune complex deposition.[19,65]

Advances in Diagnostic Testing

Given the problems with progestogen skin testing described previously, development of more accurate in vitro tests would greatly assist the allergist in diagnosing PH. Several experimental tests have been used to diagnose PH. A direct leukocyte histamine release assay and a progesterone-specific immunoglobulin (Ig)E enzyme-linked immunosorbent assay have been used by Bernstein and colleagues.[14] An assay to detect interferon-gamma release also has been proposed.[66]

Potential Treatment Options

Omalizumab, a monoclonal antibody directed against IgE, was used to treat a patient with cyclic episodes of anaphylaxis, not responsive to antihistamines and oral corticosteroids, and positive skin testing to progesterone. Resolution of the recurrent episodes of anaphylaxis occurred quickly and the patient tolerated the treatment well.[40] Omalizumab may represent an excellent choice for patients with PH who develop urticaria and anaphylaxis. It is not clear that this treatment will be helpful to patients with more delayed-type reactions and is an area for further study.

SUMMARY

PH manifests as a wide variety of hypersensitivity reactions and can occur with endogenous or exogenous progestogen exposure. The allergist/immunologist is uniquely suited to diagnose and treat PH. A careful clinical history and identification of progestogen as a trigger is paramount to the diagnosis of PH. Patient-specific symptom profiles and patient goals should guide treatment.

REFERENCES

1. Foer D, Buchheit KM, Gargiulo AR, et al. Progestogen hypersensitivity in 24 cases: diagnosis, management, and proposed renaming and classification. J Allergy Clin Immunol Pract 2016;4(4):723–9.
2. Shelley WB, Preucel RW, Spoont SS. Autoimmune progesterone dermatitis. Cure by oophorectomy. JAMA 1964;190:35–8.
3. Baptist AP, Baldwin JL. Autoimmune progesterone dermatitis in a patient with endometriosis: case report and review of the literature. Clin Mol Allergy 2004; 2(1):10.
4. Cocuroccia B, Gisondi P, Gubinelli E, et al. Autoimmune progesterone dermatitis. Gynecol Endocrinol 2006;22(1):54–6.
5. Bierman SM. Autoimmune progesterone dermatitis of pregnancy. Arch Dermatol 1973;107(6):896–901.
6. Georgouras K. Autoimmune progesterone dermatitis. Australas J Dermatol 1981; 22(3):109–12.
7. Bosse Y. Endocrine regulation of airway contractility is overlooked. J Endocrinol 2014;222(2):R61–73.
8. Newcomb DC, Cephus JY, Boswell MG, et al. Estrogen and progesterone decrease let-7f microRNA expression and increase IL-23/IL-23 receptor signaling and IL-17A production in patients with severe asthma. J Allergy Clin Immunol 2015;136(4):1025–34.e11.
9. Nwaru BI, Sheikh A. Hormonal contraceptives and asthma in women of reproductive age: analysis of data from serial national Scottish Health Surveys. J R Soc Med 2015;108(9):358–71.
10. Taraborrelli S. Physiology, production and action of progesterone. Acta Obstet Gynecol Scand 2015;94(Suppl 161):8–16.
11. Nguyen T, Razzaque Ahmed A. Autoimmune progesterone dermatitis: update and insights. Autoimmun Rev 2016;15(2):191–7.
12. Fisher DA. Drug-induced progesterone dermatitis. J Am Acad Dermatol 1996; 34(5 Pt 1):863–4.
13. Lee MK, Lee WY, Yong SJ, et al. A case of autoimmune progesterone dermatitis misdiagnosed as allergic contact dermatitis. Allergy Asthma Immunol Res 2011; 3(2):141–4.
14. Bernstein IL, Bernstein DI, Lummus ZL, et al. A case of progesterone-induced anaphylaxis, cyclic urticaria/angioedema, and autoimmune dermatitis. J Womens Health (Larchmt) 2011;20(4):643–8.
15. Herzberg AJ, Strohmeyer CR, Cirillo-Hyland VA. Autoimmune progesterone dermatitis. J Am Acad Dermatol 1995;32(2 Pt 2):333–8.
16. Brestel EP, Thrush LB. The treatment of glucocorticosteroid-dependent chronic urticaria with stanozolol. J Allergy Clin Immunol 1988;82(2):265–9.
17. Medeiros S, Rodrigues-Alves R, Costa M, et al. Autoimmune progesterone dermatitis: treatment with oophorectomy. Clin Exp Dermatol 2010;35(3):e12–3.
18. Teelucksingh S, Edwards CR. Autoimmune progesterone dermatitis. J Intern Med 1990;227(2):143–4.
19. Wojnarowska F, Greaves MW, Peachey RD, et al. Progesterone-induced erythema multiforme. J R Soc Med 1985;78(5):407–8.

20. Jenkins J, Geng A, Robinson-Bostom L. Autoimmune progesterone dermatitis associated with infertility treatment. J Am Acad Dermatol 2008;58(2):353–5.
21. Poole JA, Rosenwasser LJ. Chronic idiopathic urticaria exacerbated with progesterone therapy treated with novel desensitization protocol. J Allergy Clin Immunol 2004;114(2):456–7.
22. Toms-Whittle LM, John LH, Griffiths DJ, et al. Autoimmune progesterone dermatitis: a diagnosis easily missed. Clin Exp Dermatol 2011;36(4):378–80.
23. Chawla SV, Quirk C, Sondheimer SJ, et al. Autoimmune progesterone dermatitis. Arch Dermatol 2009;145(3):341–2.
24. Hart R. Autoimmune progesterone dermatitis. Arch Dermatol 1977;113(4):426–30.
25. Snyder JL, Krishnaswamy G. Autoimmune progesterone dermatitis and its manifestation as anaphylaxis: a case report and literature review. Ann Allergy Asthma Immunol 2003;90(5):469–77 [quiz: 477, 571].
26. Camoes S, Sampaio J, Rocha J, et al. Autoimmune progesterone dermatitis: case report of an unexpected treatment reaction. S Afr Med J 2016;106(4):48–50.
27. Prieto-Garcia A, Sloane DE, Gargiulo AR, et al. Autoimmune progesterone dermatitis: clinical presentation and management with progesterone desensitization for successful in vitro fertilization. Fertil Steril 2011;95(3):1121.e9-13.
28. Farah FS, Shbaklu Z. Autoimmune progesterone urticaria. J Allergy Clin Immunol 1971;48(5):257–61.
29. Hill JL, Carr TF. Iatrogenic autoimmune progesterone dermatitis treated with a novel intramuscular progesterone desensitization protocol. J Allergy Clin Immunol Pract 2013;1(5):537–8.
30. Vasconcelos C, Xavier P, Vieira AP, et al. Autoimmune progesterone urticaria. Gynecol Endocrinol 2000;14(4):245–7.
31. Jones WN, Gordon VH. Auto-immune progesterone eczema. An endogenous progesterone hypersensitivity. Arch Dermatol 1969;99(1):57–9.
32. Wintzen M, Goor-van Egmond MB, Noz KC. Autoimmune progesterone dermatitis presenting with purpura and petechiae. Clin Exp Dermatol 2004;29(3):316.
33. Mbonile L. Autoimmune progesterone dermatitis: case report with history of urticaria, petechiae and palpable pinpoint purpura triggered by medical abortion. S Afr Med J 2016;106(4):48–50.
34. Honda T, Kabashima K, Fujii Y, et al. Autoimmune progesterone dermatitis that changed its clinical manifestation from anaphylaxis to fixed drug eruption-like erythema. J Dermatol 2014;41(5):447–8.
35. Asai J, Katoh N, Nakano M, et al. Case of autoimmune progesterone dermatitis presenting as fixed drug eruption. J Dermatol 2009;36(12):643–5.
36. Berger H. Progesterone. Arch Dermatol 1969;100(1):117.
37. Moghadam BK, Hersini S, Barker BF. Autoimmune progesterone dermatitis and stomatitis. Oral Surg Oral Med Oral Pathol Oral Radiol 1998;85(5):537–41.
38. Maguire T. Autoimmune progesterone dermatitis. Dermatol Nurs 2009;21(4):190–2.
39. Banerjee AK, de Chazal R. Chronic vulvovaginal pruritus treated successfully with GnRH analogue. Postgrad Med J 2006;82(970):e22.
40. Heffler E, Fichera S, Nicolosi G, et al. Anaphylaxis due to progesterone hypersensitivity successfully treated with omalizumab. J Allergy Clin Immunol Pract 2017;5(3):852–4.
41. Meggs WJ, Pescovitz OH, Metcalfe D, et al. Progesterone sensitivity as a cause of recurrent anaphylaxis. N Engl J Med 1984;311(19):1236–8.

42. Walling HW, Scupham RK. Autoimmune progesterone dermatitis. Case report with histologic overlap of erythema multiforme and urticaria. Int J Dermatol 2008;47(4):380–2.

43. Shelley WB, Shelley ED, Talanin NY, et al. Estrogen dermatitis. J Am Acad Dermatol 1995;32(1):25–31.

44. Leylek OA, Unlu S, Ozturkcan S, et al. Estrogen dermatitis. Eur J Obstet Gynecol Reprod Biol 1997;72(1):97–103.

45. Mayou SC, Charles-Holmes R, Kenney A, et al. A premenstrual urticarial eruption treated with bilateral oophorectomy and hysterectomy. Clin Exp Dermatol 1988; 13(2):114–6.

46. Yotsumoto S, Shimomai K, Hashiguchi T, et al. Estrogen dermatitis: a dendritic-cell-mediated allergic condition. Dermatology 2003;207(3):265–8.

47. Randall K, Steele R. Estrogen dermatitis: treatment with progestin-only pill. Arch Dermatol 2005;141(6):792–3.

48. McKinney KK, Scranton SE. A case report of breastfeeding anaphylaxis: successful prophylaxis with oral antihistamines. Allergy 2011;66(3):435–6.

49. Durgakeri P, Jones B. A rare case of lactation anaphylaxis. Australas Med J 2015; 8(3):103–5.

50. Shank JJ, Olney SC, Lin FL, et al. Recurrent postpartum anaphylaxis with breast-feeding. Obstet Gynecol 2009;114(2 Pt 2):415–6.

51. Villalta D, Martelli P. A case of breastfeeding anaphylaxis. Eur Ann Allergy Clin Immunol 2007;39(1):26–7.

52. MacDonell JW, Ito S. Breastfeeding anaphylaxis case study. J Hum Lact 1998; 14(3):243–4.

53. Mullins RJ, Russell A, McGrath GJ, et al. Breastfeeding anaphylaxis. Lancet 1991;338(8777):1279–80.

54. Garcia-Ortega P, Scorza E. Progesterone autoimmune dermatitis with positive autologous serum skin test result. Obstet Gynecol 2011;117(2 Pt 2):495–8.

55. Stranahan D, Rausch D, Deng A, et al. The role of intradermal skin testing and patch testing in the diagnosis of autoimmune progesterone dermatitis. Dermatitis 2006;17(1):39–42.

56. Bauer CS, Kampitak T, Messieh ML, et al. Heterogeneity in presentation and treatment of catamenial anaphylaxis. Ann Allergy Asthma Immunol 2013;111(2): 107–11.

57. Shahar E, Bergman R, Pollack S. Autoimmune progesterone dermatitis: effective prophylactic treatment with danazol. Int J Dermatol 1997;36(9):708–11.

58. Yee KC, Cunliffe WJ. Progesterone-induced urticaria: response to buserelin. Br J Dermatol 1994;130(1):121–3.

59. Slater JE, Raphael G, Cutler GB Jr, et al. Recurrent anaphylaxis in menstruating women: treatment with a luteinizing hormone-releasing hormone agonist–a preliminary report. Obstet Gynecol 1987;70(4):542–6.

60. Moody BR, Schatten S. Autoimmune progesterone dermatitis: onset in a women without previous exogenous progesterone exposure. South Med J 1997;90(8): 845–6.

61. Rodenas JM, Herranz MT, Tercedor J. Autoimmune progesterone dermatitis: treatment with oophorectomy. Br J Dermatol 1998;139(3):508–11.

62. Meltzer L. Hypersensitivity to gonadal hormones. South Med J 1963;56:538–42.

63. Schoenmakers A, Vermorken A, Degreef H, et al. Corticosteroid or steroid allergy? Contact Dermatitis 1992;26(3):159–62.

64. Slater JE, Kaliner M. Effects of sex hormones on basophil histamine release in recurrent idiopathic anaphylaxis. J Allergy Clin Immunol 1987;80(3 Pt 1):285–90.

65. Cheesman KL, Gaynor LV, Chatterton RT Jr, et al. Identification of a 17-hydroxy-progesterone-binding immunoglobulin in the serum of a woman with periodic rashes. J Clin Endocrinol Metab 1982;55(3):597–9.

66. Halevy S, Cohen AD, Lunenfeld E, et al. Autoimmune progesterone dermatitis manifested as erythema annulare centrifugum: confirmation of progesterone sensitivity by in vitro interferon-gamma release. J Am Acad Dermatol 2002; 47(2):311–3.

Severe Delayed Drug Reactions

Role of Genetics and Viral Infections

Rebecca Pavlos, PhD[a,1], Katie D. White, MD, PhD[b,1],
Celestine Wanjalla, MD, PhD[b], Simon A. Mallal, MBBS[a,b,c],
Elizabeth J. Phillips, MD[a,b,c,d],*

KEYWORDS

- Human leukocyte antigen • T-cell receptor • Adverse drug reaction
- Pharmacogenomics • Human herpes virus
- Drug reaction with eosinophilia and systemic symptoms • Steven Johnson syndrome
- Toxic epidermal necrolysis

KEY POINTS

- Severe delayed drug reactions are typically off-target reactions that are immunologically mediated and associated with long-lasting immunologic memory.
- There are many strong associations between these immunologically mediated adverse drug reactions (IM-ADR) and the major histocompatibility complex.
- Despite this, the minority of these have been implemented into clinical practice as cost-effective pretreatment screening tests.
- A heterologous immune model of delayed drug hypersensitivity may explain why, for most drugs, less than 5% of those carrying an HLA risk allele will develop an IM-ADR.
- It is proposed that pathogen-specific T-cell responses generate either migratory or resident memory T-cells which cross-react with drug-modified self-peptide epitopes when the risk drug is introduced later in life.

INTRODUCTION

Adverse drug reactions (ADRs) account for a significant source of patient morbidity and mortality and represent a major burden to the health care and drug development systems. It is estimated that up to 50% of such reactions are preventable.[1–8] Although

[a] Institute for Immunology and Infectious Diseases, Murdoch University, 6150 Murdoch, Western Australia, Australia; [b] Department of Medicine, Vanderbilt University Medical Center, Nashville, TN, USA; [c] Department of Pathology, Microbiology and Immunology, Vanderbilt University Medical Center, Nashville, TN, USA; [d] Department of Pharmacology, Vanderbilt University Medical Center, Nashville, TN, USA
[1] Co-first authors.
* Corresponding author. 1161 21st Avenue South, A-2200 Medical Center North, Nashville, TN 37232-2582.
E-mail address: elizabeth.j.phillips@vanderbilt.edu

Immunol Allergy Clin N Am 37 (2017) 785–815
http://dx.doi.org/10.1016/j.iac.2017.07.007
0889-8561/17/© 2017 Elsevier Inc. All rights reserved.
immunology.theclinics.com

many ADRs can be predicted based on the on-target pharmacologic activity of the drug (**Fig. 1**),[1–3,6,8–10] ADRs arising from drug interactions with off-target receptors are now more commonly recognized. Off-target ADRs include the immune-mediated ADRs (IM-ADRs) as well as pharmacologic drug effects such as those associated with non–IgE-mediated mast cell activation (see **Fig. 1**).[11] In this review, we discuss what is known about the immunogenetics and pathogenesis of IM-ADRs and the hypothesized role of preexisting pathogen exposure as a predisposing factor for the development of an IM-ADR.

CLINICAL PHENOTYPES OF IMMUNE-MEDIATED ADVERSE DRUG REACTIONS

IM-ADRs encompass a number of phenotypically distinct clinical diagnoses that include both B-cell (antibody-mediated, Gell Coombs types I–III) and purely T-cell–mediated reactions (Gell-Coombs type IV). T-cell–mediated IM-ADRs have been classified into delayed exanthema without systemic symptoms (ie, maculopapular eruption), contact dermatitis, drug-induced hypersensitivity syndrome, drug reaction with eosinophilia and systemic symptoms (DRESS), hypersensitivity syndrome, Stevens-Johnson syndrome (SJS), toxic epidermal necrolysis (TEN), acute generalized exanthematous pustulosis, fixed drug eruption, single organ involvement pathologies such as drug-induced liver injury, and the abacavir hypersensitivity syndrome.[12,13]

Drug Reaction with Eosinophilia and Systemic Symptoms

The clinical presentation of DRESS is characterized by a generalized rash of varying severity without skin separation, fever, internal organ involvement (usually hepatitis), and hematologic abnormalities (often atypical lymphocytes and/or eosinophilia). Clinical features of this syndrome are variable, but may also include diffuse lymphadenopathy, pneumonitis, encephalitis, myocarditis, and nephritis. Onset of symptoms typically occurs 2 to 8 weeks after initiation of the inciting drug and the patient may have a protracted clinical course. Prolonged or recurrent symptoms, sometimes weeks after cessation of the offending drug and often related to discontinuation of systemic corticosteroids, is frequently observed and late onset autoimmune diseases including thyroiditis, systemic lupus, and type I diabetes are well-described long-term sequelae that can occur at least up to 4 years after the resolution of acute disease.[14–22]

Stevens–Johnson Syndrome and Toxic Epidermal Necrolysis

SJS and TEN are the most severe cutaneous hypersensitivity syndromes and are thought to represent a spectrum of disease defined by the percentage of total body surface area (TBSA) involvement. Characteristic features include epidermal necrosis leading to the formation of fluid-filled blisters and epidermal sloughing, fever, mucosal and eye involvement, internal organ involvement, and secondary complications such as sepsis. Generally, SJS is diagnosed in cases where less than 10% of TBSA has blistering and epidermal detachment, whereas TEN is diagnosed in instances where more than 30% of the TBSA is affected. SJS/TEN describes the overlap in this spectrum in which 10% to 30% of TBSA is affected. However, patients with severe epidermal detachment and skin necrosis are classified as TEN regardless of the percentage of TBSA involved. These syndromes are often associated with significant mortality as well as short- and long-term morbidity, including respiratory, gastrointestinal, and genitourinary complications, as well as permanent corneal scarring and vision loss.[7,12] The mortality associated with TEN is higher with aging and comorbidities and may reach 30% to 50%.[12,13,23,24]

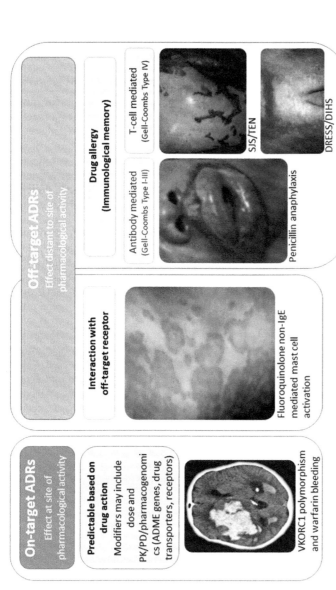

Fig. 1. Classification of adverse drug reactions (ADRs). ADRs may result from either on-target or off-target interactions between the drug and cellular proteins. On-target ADRs account for 80% or more of ADRs and are generally predictable based on the drug pharmacology. Variation in the cellular processes that modulate drug absorption, distribution, metabolism, and excretion (ADME), drug transporters, target receptor expression, and drug dosing or administration errors contribute to ADRs that are primarily mediated by pharmacologic mechanisms. Off-target adverse effects account for a smaller proportion of total ADRs (≤20%) and include both immune-mediated and non–immune-mediated syndromes. The non-IgE mediated mast cell activation syndrome, which phenotypically resembles anaphylaxis, has recently been shown in a murine model to result from off-target binding of drug to G-protein–coupled receptors without involvement of the adaptive immune system.[11] The IM-ADRs include both B-cell–mediated and T-cell–mediated reactions (types I–IV reactions according to the Gell-Coombs schema) and are associated with immunologic memory. DRESS/DIHS, drug reaction with eosinophilia and systemic symptoms/drug-induced hypersensitivity syndrome; SJS/TENS, Stevens–Johns syndrome/toxic epidermal necrolysis; PD, pharmacodynamic; PK, pharmacokinetic. (*Adapted from* Peter JG, Lehloenya R, Dlamini S, et al. Severe Delayed Cutaneous and Systemic Reactions to Drugs: A Global Perspective on the Science and Art of Current Practice. J Allergy Clin Immunol Pract 2017;5(3):549; with permission.)

The Abacavir Hypersensitivity Syndrome

Abacavir is a guanosine analogue that is used for the treatment of infection with human immunodeficiency virus type 1 (HIV-1). In the premarketing phase of drug development, a hypersensitivity syndrome characterized by fever, malaise, gastrointestinal, respiratory symptoms, and/or generalized rash was reported in approximately 5% to 8% of patients within the first 6 weeks after initiation of abacavir. The immunologic basis for the abacavir hypersensitivity syndrome has been well-described and is discussed in subsequent sections of this review.

Emerging Immune-mediated Adverse Drug Reactions: Immune Checkpoint Inhibitors

Novel monoclonal antibodies that target surface proteins that suppress T-cell cytotoxic function have shown significant efficacy as cancer therapeutics. The immune checkpoint inhibitors ipilimumab (targeting anti-cytotoxic T-lymphocyte antigen 4 [CTLA-4]) and nivolumab or pembrolizumab (targeting the anti–programmed death receptor-1 [PD-1]), used alone or in combination, and are now first line therapies for the treatment of metastatic melanoma. The checkpoint inhibitors and are also licensed for treatment of selected types of skin cancer, head and neck cancer, lung cancer, bladder cancer, lymphoma, and kidney cancer (available at: https://medi-paper.com/approved-immunotherapies/). Immune checkpoint inhibitors have been associated with an increasing range of organ specific IM-ADRs, also called immune-related adverse events (irAEs), including rash (rarely, SJS/TEN), gastrointestinal syndromes, hepatitis, endocrine syndromes (thyroiditis, pancreatitis, hypophysitis), hematologic syndromes (red cell aplasia), neurologic (Guillain–Barre syndrome, aseptic meningitis), myocarditis, and rheumatologic syndromes (systemic lupus erythematosus, polyarthritis). Onset of irAEs most commonly occur 3 to 6 months after initiation of immune checkpoint inhibitor therapy and usually manifest as mild syndromes that are not treatment limiting and often steroid responsive. However, an increasing number of severe reactions with high morbidity and mortality have been recently described, particularly with the use of combination CTLA-4 and PD-1 blockade.[25–27] Recent studies showing superior tumor response to checkpoint inhibitor therapy in patients who develop irAEs support the hypothesis that these irAEs are mediated by a cross-reactive memory T-cell response between the tumor and a self or pathogen epitope.[26] Further, a report of 2 cases of fatal myocarditis after combination PD-1 and CTLA-4 inhibitor therapy for the treatment of metastatic melanoma demonstrated that an identical dominant T-cell clonotype and overall repertoire was present in posttherapy tumor tissue and myocardium.[28] The relative risk of T-cell–mediated ADRs in the presence of immune checkpoint inhibitor is unknown and is a focus of ongoing research.

Clinical Mimics of Stevens–Johnson Syndrome and Toxic Epidermal Necrolysis

Bullous erythema multiforme is a severe acute bullous disorder characterized by raised typical or atypical target lesions affecting less than 10% of the TBSA.[29] Unlike SJS, erythema multiforme is most commonly associated with infectious diseases including herpes simplex virus (HSV)[30–35] and *Mycoplasma pneumoniae*.[36,37] Although SJS/TEN is most often associated with drug exposure, there are many reported cases of SJS/TEN for which there is no causative drug implicated. In such cases, a coincident viral infection similar to those seen with erythema multiforme may explain the observed clinical features. In 1922, M. Stevens and F. C. Johnson described the first 2 cases of SJS, neither of which were associated with antecedent medication exposure. One of these cases had a concurrent pneumonia, a presentation that is consistent with what is now known as *M pneumoniae*–induced rash and mucositis.[38,39] Studies have reported that 14% to 63% of children with clinical SJS/TEN have detectable *M pneumoniae* serum antibodies[40,41] and *M pneumoniae* is recognized as a major trigger for recurrent SJS episodes, particularly in children and adolescents.[40,42] SJS/TEN with eye involvement is more common in children with concurrent *M pneumoniae* (26.7%) or HSV (15.6%) infections.[31]

There are reports of atypical hand, foot, and mouth disease caused by coxsackievirus A6 that share features of drug-induced eruptions. Patients exhibit widespread blistering mucocutaneous reactions with inflammatory infiltration of cytotoxic T cells and granulysin producing natural killer cells.[43] Intact coxsackievirus A6 virus particles have been detected in the blister fluids and skin lesions of these patients.[44]

GENETIC ASSOCIATIONS OF IMMUNE-MEDIATED ADVERSE DRUG REACTIONS
Human Leukocyte Antigen

Many strong associations have been described between human leukocyte antigen (HLA) alleles and drug-specific IM-ADRs such as DRESS/drug-induced hypersensitivity syndrome, SJS/TEN, and drug-induced liver injury. The T-cell receptors (TCRs) on the surface of a T cell recognize peptides that are bound and displayed by surface HLA molecules expressed on various cells of the immune system. Class I major histocompatibility complex (MHC) molecules (HLA-A, -B, and -C) are expressed on all nucleated cells and are responsible for activating $CD8^+$ cytotoxic T lymphocytes, whereas class II MHC molecules (HLA-DP, HLA-DQ, and HLA-DR) are expressed only on professional antigen presenting cells (B cells, macrophages, and dendritic cells) and activate $CD4^+$ helper T lymphocytes. In an era when HLA typing was performed by serology, weak 2-digit associations were described for allopurinol (B58) and sulfa antimicrobial hypersensitivity.[45–47] The strong association between HLA-B*57:01 and the abacavir hypersensitivity syndrome was identified in 2002 and marked the advent of a new era of discovery made possible by high-resolution HLA typing in patients with specifically phenotyped drug hypersensitivity syndromes.[48,49] This discovery was followed by the reported associations between carbamazepine SJS/TEN and HLA-B*15:02 and allopurinol DRESS/SJS/TEN and HLA-B*58:01[48,50–52] (**Table 1**). Investigations of these 3 well-characterized drug related syndromes have since suggested new models for the immunopathogenesis of T-cell–mediated IM-ADRs.

The crystal structure(s) of abacavir noncovalently bound to the floor of the peptide binding groove of HLA-B*57:01 demonstrated how the drug is able to affect the peptide binding properties of the HLA molecule.[53,54] It is as yet unclear whether the same mechanism will generalize to other HLA-associated IM-ADRs. Abacavir hypersensitivity syndrome only occurs in individuals with HLA-B*57:01, and 55% of those with HLA-B*57:01 exposed to the drug will develop hypersensitivity. This 100% negative predictive value combined with this unusually high positive predictive value (PPV) facilitated successful implementation of allele screening before the initiation of abacavir therapy.[55] Other HLA-associated IM-ADRs have much lower PPVs (<3%) for the development of hypersensitivity. Although HLA risk alleles are necessary but not sufficient for IM-ADRs, identifying other genetic or ecological factors that account for the "*PPV gap*" will be necessary to enhance current mechanistic models of the pathogenesis of these syndromes.

Carbamazepine is an aromatic amine anticonvulsant known to cause a spectrum of IM-ADRs, including maculopapular exanthema, DRESS, and SJS/TEN. The original association between HLA-B*15:02 and the development of SJS/TEN was reported

Table 1
Pharmacogenomics of off-target reactions associated with immunologic memory

Drug	DHR	Alleles[c]	PPV	NPV	NNT	Populations	LOE[a]
Abacavir	HSS, DIHS	B*57:01[48,49,55,136]	55%	100%	13	European, African	1a
Carbamazepine	SJS, TEN	B*15:02[50,52,57,62,137-141]	3%	100% in Han Chinese	1000	Han Chinese, Thai, Malaysian, Indian	1a
		B*15:11[60,142]				Korean, Japanese	3
		B*15:18, B*59:01 and C*07:04[143]				Japanese	3
		A*31:01[65-67,142]				Japanese, northern European, Korean	2b
	HSS, DIHS, DRESS	A*11:01[68]				Spanish	
		8.1 AH (HLA A*01:01, Cw*07:01, B*08:01, DRB1*03:01, DQA1*05:01, DQB1*02:01)[144]				Caucasians	3
		A*31:01[145]	0.89%	99.98%	3334	Europeans	1a
		A*31:01[145]	0.59%	99.97%	5000	Chinese	1a
		A*31:01[65-68,142]				Northern Europeans, Japanese, and Korean, Spanish	1a
	MPE	A*11 and B*51 (weak)[66]				Japanese	3
		A*31:01[52]	34.9%	96.7%	91		1a
Allopurinol	SJS, TEN, DIHS, DRESS	B*58:01 (or B*58 haplotype)[45,51,71,146-150]	3%	100% in Han Chinese	250	Han Chinese, Thai, European, Italian, Korean	1a
Oxcarbazepine	SJS, TEN	B*15:02 and B*15:18[63,64,151,152]				Han Chinese, Taiwanese	2b
Lamotrigine	SJS, TEN	B*15:02 (positive)[63]				Han Chinese	3
		B*38:01[68]				Spanish	3
		B*15:02 (no association)[153,154]				Han Chinese	3
	DRESS	A*24:02[68]				Spanish	3
	SCAR	A*31:01[155]				Korean	3

Drug	Reaction	Association			Population	Evidence
Phenytoin	SJS, TEN	B*15:02 (weak), Cw*08:01 and DRB1*16:02[62,63,78,138]			Han Chinese	3
		B*13:01, B*56:02/04, CYP2C19*3[79,80]			Thailand	3
		CYP2C9*3[78]				
		A*02:01/Cw15:02[68]			Spanish	3
	DRESS, MPE	B*13:01(weak), B*5101 (weak)[78]			Han Chinese	3
		CYP2C9*3[78]				1a
Phenobarbital	SCAR, MP rash	A*01:01 and B*13:01, CYP2C19*2[156,157]			Thailand	3
		B*15:02 and −B*15:11[158]			Chinese	3
Nevirapine	SJS, TEN	C*04:01[88]			Malawian	3
	HSS, DIHS, DRESS	DRB1*01:01 and DRB1*01:01 (hepatitis and low CD4+)[85,86]	18%	96%	Australian, European and South African	1b
		DRB1*01:02				1b
		Cw*8 or Cw*8-B*14 haplotype[84,159]			Italian and Japanese	2b
		Cw*4[85,160]			Blacks, Asians, Whites	2b
					Han Chinese	1b
		B*35[104]	16%	97%	Asian	1b
		B*35:01[83]				1b
		B*35:05[87]				2b
	Delayed rash	DRB1*01[161]			French	3
		Cw*04[85,162]			African, Asian, European, and Thai	
		B*35:05, rs1576*G CCHCR1 status[87,163]			Thai	2b

(continued on next page)

Table 1
(continued)

Drug	DHR	Alleles[c]	PPV	NPV	NNT	Populations	LOE[a]
Dapsone	HSS	B*13:01[164]	7.8%	99.8%	84		1b
		B*13:01[132]				Chinese	1b
Co-trimoxazole	SJS, TEN	B*15:02, C*06:02, and C*08:01[165]				Thailand	3
Piperacillin, tazobactam	DRESS	B*62[166]				UK	3
Strontium ranelate	SJS, TEN	A*33:03, B*58:01[167]				Han Chinese	3
Efavirenz	Delayed rash	DRB1*01[161]				French	3
Sulfamethoxazole	SJS, TEN	B*38[148]				European	3
Amoxicillin-clavulanate	DILI	DRB1*15:01				European	1b
		A*02:01					1b
		DRB1*07 and HLA-A1 (protective)					3
		DQB1*06:02					1b
		And rs3135388, a tag SNP of DRB1*15:01-DQB1*06:02[168–170]					1b
Lumiracoxib	DILI	DRB1*15:01-DQB1*06:02-DRB5*01:01-DQA1*01:02 haplotype[171]				International, multicenter	3
Ximelagatran	DILI	DRB1*07 and DQA1*02[172]				Swedish	2b
Diclofenac	DILI	B11, C-24T, UGT2B7*2, IL-4 C-590-A[173–175]				European	3
Flucloxacillin	DILI	B*57:01 DRB1*01:07-DQB1*01:03[174,176]	0.12%	99.99%	13,819	European	1b

Drug	Reaction	Genetic marker			Population	Level
Lapatinib	DILI	DRB1*07:01-DQA2*02:01-DQB1*02:02/02:02[177]			International, multicenter	1b
Minocycline	DILI	B*35:02[178]			Caucasian	3
Asparaginase	Anaphylaxis	DRB1*07:01[131]			European	2b
Penicillin[b]	IgE- mediated allergy	IL-4Ralpha Q576R[179]			Chinese	3
		STAT6 in 2SNP3[180]			Spanish	3
		DRA rs7192 and rs8084, ZNF300 rs4958427[181]				
	Urticaria	IL-4Ralpha I75V[179]			Chinese	3
Methimazole, carbimazole	Agranulocytosis	B*38:02[182,183]	7%	99.9%	Southeast Asian	1b
Antithyroid drugs		B*27:05[184] (3 SNPs)	30%	>99%	European	1b
Statin	Myopathy	DRB1*04:06[185]			Japanese	3
Raltegravir	DRESS	B*53-C*04 haplotype[186]			African	4

Abbreviations: DHR, Drug hypersensitivity reaction; DIHS, drug-induced hypersensitivity syndrome; DILI, drug-induced liver injury; DRESS, drug reaction with eosinophilia and systemic symptoms; HSS, hypersensitivity syndrome; LOE, levels of evidence; MP rash, maculopapular rash; MPE, maculopapular eruption; NNT, number needed to treat; NPV, negative predictive value; PPV, positive predictive value; SCAR, severe cutaneous adverse reactions; SJS, Stevens-Johnson syndrome; SNP, single nucleotide polymorphism; TEN, toxic epidermal necrolysis.

[a] Levels of evidence (PharmGKB [102]): Level 1a, Annotation for a variant–drug combination in a Clinical Pharmacogenetics Implementation Consortium (CPIC) or medical society-endorsed pharmacogenomics guideline, or implemented at a Pharmacogenomics Research Network (PGRN) site, or in another major health system; Level 1b, Annotation for a variant–drug combination in which the preponderance of evidence shows an association. This association must be replicated in more than one cohort with significant P-values and preferably with a strong effect size; Level 2a, Annotation for a variant–drug combination that qualifies for level 2b, in which the variant is within a Very Important Pharmacogene (VIP) as defined by PharmGKB where their functional significance is more likely known; Level 2b, Annotation for a variant–drug combination with moderate evidence of an association. This association must be replicated, but there may be some studies that do not show statistical significance, and/or the effect size may be small; Level 3, Annotation for a variant–drug combination based on a single significant (not yet replicated) study or annotation for a variant–drug combination evaluated in multiple studies but lacking clear evidence of an association; Level 4, Annotation based on a case report, nonsignificant study, *in vitro*, molecular or functional assay evidence only.

[b] Associated with immunologic memory but responses are not maintained over time (loss of skin test reactivity).

[c] HLA alleles.

in the Han Chinese, and other South-East Asian populations where the frequency of HLA-B*15:02 carriage is relatively high.[52,56–58] This association is specific to the carbamazepine–SJS/TEN phenotype and HLA-B*15:02 has not been reported with DRESS or maculopapular eruption.[59] However, HLA molecules of the same B75 serotype (HLA-B*15:08, -B*15:11, and –B*15:21) with similar peptide binding properties have also been implicated in carbamazepine-induced SJS/TEN.[56,60,61] In addition, IM-ADR secondary to other aromatic amine anticonvulsants, including oxcarbazepine, phenytoin, and lamotrigine, are also associated with HLA-B*15:02, suggesting a potential shared interaction between the HLA allele and the drugs.[62–64] Overall, the carbamazepine example highlights that structural interactions between the drug and specific HLA alleles as well as risk allele carriage frequency in different populations are likely to affect the likelihood of identifying genetic associations. For many of the HLA alleles that are associated with IM-ADRs, the risk allele is present on a conserved haplotype that has been maintained at high frequency in particular populations, whereas haplotypes with nonrisk HLA alleles dominate in other ethnic groups.

In South-East Asian populations, carbamazepine–SJS/TEN is most often associated with HLA-B*15:02 and less commonly associated with other HLA-B75 serotype alleles. In European and Japanese populations, however, where HLA-B*15:02 and other B75 serotype HLA carriage is less than 1%, carbamazepine–DRESS, maculopapular exanthema, and SJS/TEN have been associated with the carriage of HLA-A*31:01.[65–67] Similarly, in South and Southeast Asians, the risk for HLA-B*15:02-associated IM-ADRs secondary to other aromatic amine anticonvulsants such as phenytoin and lamotrigine is lower than for carbamazepine and oxcarbazepine and HLA associations are unique in Europeans (see **Table 1**).[68]

Drug Metabolism and Transport

In contrast with the HLA allele-specific phenotype associations observed for carbamazepine IM-ADRs, HLA-B*58:01 is a genetic marker for both SJS/TEN and DRESS induced by allopurinol, a xanthine oxidase inhibitor used in the treatment of hyperuricemia and gout.[51] First described in the Han Chinese, the association of HLA-B*58:01 with severe cutaneous adverse reactions (SCAR) is also reported in Japanese and European populations.[51,69–72] Oxypurinol is the main metabolite of allopurinol produced via aldehyde oxidoreductase and is cleared almost entirely by urinary excretion. In keeping with this, renal impairment, increased plasma levels, and delayed clearance of oxypurinol correlate with an increased risk and mortality from allopurinol SCAR.[73] Several studies have examined genetic variability in genes of allopurinol metabolism and clearance relative to allopurinol response and prescribed dose. For example, the single nucleotide polymorphism Hist1270Arg in aldehyde oxidase is significantly associated with therapeutic allopurinol dose and other studies have shown enhanced conversion of some substrates by aldehyde oxidase with this single nucleotide polymorphism and other genetic variants.[74,75] In addition, adenosine triphosphate–binding cassette subfamily G member 2 (ABCG2) is as an allopurinol transporter[76] and an ABCG2 missense allele (rs2231142) is associated with a reduced response to allopurinol.[77] As yet, these and similar candidate genes in allopurinol metabolism and clearance have not been examined specifically in relation to the development allopurinol induced IM-ADRs and are good candidates for further study.

The cytochrome P450 (CYP) group of enzymes metabolize thousands of endogenous and exogenous chemicals and are the major enzymes in drug metabolism. A combination of metabolic and immunologic factors is associated with predisposition for some drugs associated with IM-ADRs, such as phenytoin-associated SCARs, including maculopapular exanthema, DRESS, and SJS/TEN. A recent genome-wide association study across mixed ethnic populations, including individuals from Taiwan, Japan, and Malaysia, identified a missense variant of the CYP2C9 gene, whose protein product is responsible for metabolizing phenytoin in the liver. The variant identified as CYP2C9*3 was strongly associated with development of SCARs and reduced phenytoin clearance.[78,79] However, delayed clearance was also observed in individuals without this variant allele, suggesting other contributing factors such as hepatic or renal insufficiency or a drug–drug interaction. This study, which mainly consisted of Southeast Asians (Taiwanese and Malaysians) and a smaller population of Japanese participants, also demonstrated weaker genetic associations with HLA-B alleles, including HLA-B*13:01, HLA-B*15:02, and HLA-B*51:01, respectively.[79–82] Therefore, a combination of both pharmacologic and immunologic mechanisms contributes to the development of phenytoin-related SCAR.

The nonnucleoside reverse transcriptase inhibitor nevirapine, used to treat HIV-1 infection, is associated with both cutaneous and hepatitis hypersensitivity variants that have class I and II MHC associations. Nevirapine is associated with a spectrum of cutaneous adverse reactions ranging from mild rash to the severe SJS/TEN and DRESS.[83] HLA alleles associated with specific nevirapine phenotypes include HLA-B*35 and HLA-C*04 with cutaneous reactions, HLA-DRB1*01 with hepatic symptoms, and the HLA-B*14-C*08 haplotype with eosinophilia.[83–88] In addition, CYP2B6 516G > T and 983T > C are associated with reduced clearance of the drug and cutaneous adverse reactions, with the strongest effect in African populations, where this variant is present in 20% of the population.[85,89,90]

IMMUNE MECHANISMS OF IMMUNE-MEDIATED ADVERSE DRUG REACTIONS

As described, many type IV IM-ADRs are strongly associated with allelic variation in the class I and class II HLA genes, which encode the restricting elements for CD8$^+$ and CD4$^+$ T cells, respectively (see **Table 1**). Currently, 3 models have been proposed to describe how a drug might interact with immune proteins to elicit a T-cell response. These include the hapten/prohapten model, the pharmacologic interaction model, and the altered peptide repertoire model (**Fig. 2**).

In the hapten/prohapten model, the drug or drug metabolite covalently binds to an endogenous (self) protein that then undergoes intracellular processing to generate a pool of chemically modified peptides referred to as neoepitopes. When presented in the context of HLA proteins, these modified peptides will be recognized as "foreign" by T cells and elicit an immune response.[91,92] The pharmacologic interaction model postulates that the offending drug interacts in a noncovalent manner with either the TCR or HLA protein in a peptide-independent manner to directly activate T cells. This model has been hypothesized to explain in vitro T-cell reactivity that is labile (ie, reactivity is abrogated by washing drug from the surface of antigen-presenting cells) and/or is observed within seconds of drug exposure, a time course too short to require intracellular antigen processing.[93,94] The altered peptide repertoire model was defined through structural and peptide elution studies demonstrating the interactions of the antiretroviral drug abacavir and the HLA-B*57:01 protein. These studies demonstrated that abacavir binds to the HLA-B*57:01 peptide binding groove, thereby changing the chemistry of the binding cleft and resulting in presentation of a pool of peptides that are not normally bound to HLA-B*57:01 in the absence of drug. It is proposed that peptides presented in this context are recognized as "foreign" by the immune system and therefore elicit a T-cell response.[53,54]

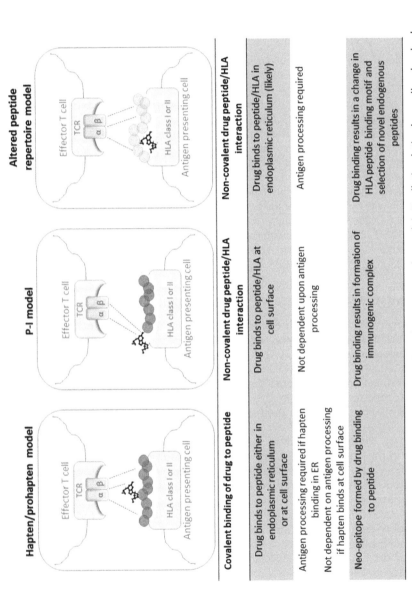

	Hapten/prohapten model	P-I model	Altered peptide repertoire model
	Covalent binding of drug to peptide	Non-covalent drug peptide/HLA interaction	Non-covalent drug peptide/HLA interaction
	Drug binds to peptide either in endoplasmic reticulum or at cell surface	Drug binds to peptide/HLA at cell surface	Drug binds to peptide/HLA in endoplasmic reticulum (likely)
	Antigen processing required if hapten binding in ER Not dependent on antigen processing if hapten binds at cell surface	Not dependent upon antigen processing	Antigen processing required
	Neo-epitope formed by drug binding to peptide	Drug binding results in formation of immunogenic complex	Drug binding results in a change in HLA peptide binding motif and selection of novel endogenous peptides

Fig. 2. Models of T-cell activation by small molecules. Three models have been proposed to explain T-cell stimulation by small molecule pharmaceuticals. The hapten/prohapten model postulates that the drug binds covalently to peptide (either in the intracellular environment before peptide processing and presentation or at the cell surface) to generate a neoantigen that stimulates a T-cell response. The P-I model proposes that a small molecule may bind to HLA in a noncovalent manner to directly stimulate T cells. The altered peptide model postulates that a small molecule can bind noncovalently to the major histocompatibility complex binding cleft to alter the specificity of peptide binding. This results in the presentation of novel peptide ligands to elicit an immune response. ER, endoplasmic reticulum; TCR, T-cell receptor. (*Adapted from* White KD, Chung WH, Hung SI, et al. Evolving models of the immunopathogenesis of T cell–mediated drug allergy: The role of host, pathogens, and drug response. J Allergy Clin Immunol 2015;136(2):223; [quiz: 235]; with permission.)

Stevens–Johnson Syndrome and Toxic Epidermal Necrolysis

The strong association between carriage of specific class I HLA alleles and risk of drug-induced SJS/TEN has been well-established (see **Table 1**) and is consistent with evidence suggesting that cytotoxic CD8$^+$ T cells, natural killer cells, and CD3$^+$CD56$^+$ natural killer T cells mediate epidermal cell death in SJS/TEN through the production of soluble cytotoxic factors, such as granulysin.[95–98] Granulysin is a cytolytic peptide that is present in high concentrations in blister fluid and serum levels of granulysin have been shown to correlate with the severity of acute SJS/TEN and predict mortality.[73,99]

Mutagenesis studies suggest that carbamazepine likely binds to B pocket of the HLA-B*15:02 peptide binding groove and that the B pocket residues Arg62, Asn63, Ile95, and Leu156 contribute to drug–HLA interactions. Experiments using next generation TCR sequencing of circulating and blister fluid–derived T cells from patients with HLA-B*15:02–associated carbamazepine SJS/TEN have identified a shared CD8$^+$ T-cell clonotype bearing a common CDR3 sequence that is not found in the peripheral blood of drug tolerant controls or in blister fluid from patients with SJS/TEN secondary to another drug.[100,101] This finding suggests that the pathogenesis of HLA-B*15:02 associated carbamazepine-SJS/TEN depends on the concomitant involvement of both a specific HLA allotype and a specific TCR clonotype.

As mentioned, the pathogenesis of HLA-B*58:01–associated allopurinol IM-ADRs is mediated by oxypurinol, the active metabolite of allopurinol. Mutagenesis and in silico modeling studies suggest that oxypurinol binds the HLA-B*58:01 peptide binding groove and this interaction depends on contact with the Arg97 residue of HLA-B*58:01.[102] Cell culture experiments have shown that T cells isolated from patients with allopurinol-associated IM-ADRs expand and acquire effector functions after stimulation with allopurinol or oxypurinol but that high concentrations of oxypurinol (up to 100 µg/mL, 10 times that expected with a therapeutic dose) is the primary driver of T-cell reactivity.[73,103] As seen for HLA-B*15:02–associated carbamazepine SJS/TEN, CD8$^+$ T cells are known mediators of pathogenesis in allopurinol SJS/TEN. However, 1 study using bulk next-generation TCR sequencing examined the CD8$^+$ T-cell repertoire among blister fluid and peripheral blood cells from multiple patients with allopurinol-associated SJS/TEN demonstrated some degree of clonotypic restriction for some, but not all, patients with no evidence of a shared clonotype as seen for carbamazepine-associated SJS/TEN.[103] The role of these clonotypes in the pathogenesis is under investigation.

Drug Reaction with Eosinophilia and Systemic Symptoms

DRESS is characterized by the expansion of circulating and dermal-infiltrating effector T cells and CD4$^+$FoxP3$^+$ regulatory T cells.[104,105] Skin homing CD4$^+$FoxP3$^+$ T cells are hypothesized to limit the severity of acute disease by suppressing effector T-cell responses.[106] Reactivation of human herpesviruses (HHV), including HHV-6, Epstein–Barr virus, HHV-7, and cytomegalovirus is often observed during acute and recovery phase DRESS (**Table 2**). HHV-6 and Epstein–Barr virus reactivation is observed as early as 2 to 3 weeks after onset of rash and antiviral CD8$^+$ effector T cells are concurrently expanded during acute disease. How viral reactivation and antiviral T-cell responses contribute to pathology in DRESS is currently under investigation. It is not clear whether viral replication contributes to the events inciting DRESS or is instead the result of general immune dysfunction, such as breakdown of regulatory T cells suppressor function or the upregulation of the HHV-6 receptor, CD134, on CD4$^+$ T cells.[105–108] Nevertheless, viral replication and virus-specific T-cell responses

Table 2
Viral reactivation reported during DRESS/DIHS

Drug	Virus	Reference
Allopurinol	HSV-2, HHV-6, HHV-7, CMV, EBV	108,114,187–190
Amoxicillin	HHV-6	191
Aspirin	HHV-6	192
Carbamazepine	HHV-6, HHV-7, CMV, EBV, Parvoviridae	82,108,109,187,193–200
Cold and flu tablets[a,b]	HHV-6	201,202
Ibuprofen	HHV-6	194
Isoniazid, rifampin, ethambutol, and pyrazinamide	HHV-7	203
Lamotrigine and valproic acid	HHV-6	204
Mexiletine	HHV-6, EBV, CMV	109,187
Minocycline	HHV-6	114
Phneobarbital, phenobarbital-zonisamide	HHV-6, HHV-7, CMV, EBV	109,187,188,205
Strontium ranelate	HHV-7	206
Sulfasalazine-salazosulfapyridine	HHV-6	187,194,207,208
Sulfamethoxazole	HHV-6, HHV-7, EBV	108
Trimethoprim-sulfamethoxazole	HHV-6	209,210
Vancomycin-teicoplanin	HHV-6	211
Zonisamide	HHV-6, HHV-7, CMV	187,188
Drug not specified for each case	HHV-6, HHV-7, EBV, CMV	212–215

Abbreviations: CMV, cytomegalovirus; DIHS, drug-induced hypersensitivity syndrome; DRESS, drug reaction with eosinophilia and systemic symptoms; EBV, Epstein–Barr virus; HHV, human herpes virus; HSV, herpes simples virus.
[a] Acetaminophen, clemastine fumarate, dihydrocodeine phosphate, noscapine, dl-methyl ephedrine hydrochloride, potassium guaiacolsulfonate, anhydrous caffeine, benfotiamine and lysozyme hydrochloride.
[b] Acetaminophen, isopropylantipyrine, and/or allylisopropyl-acetylurea.

likely contribute to the clinical features of DRESS including prolonged and relapsing disease and multiorgan involvement. Although there are more complex individual host factors involved, autoimmune diseases including thyroiditis, graft-versus-host disease–like lesions, autoimmune polyglandular syndrome, systemic lupus, fulminant type I diabetes, and hemophagocytic syndrome after resolution of acute DRESS are hypothesized to occur in the setting of viral reactivation.[17,109,110] These autoimmune diseases may occur as either subclinical or clinical later complications of DRESS. The most common long-term complication of DRESS is autoimmune thyroid disease.[111–114] Recent studies have shown an association between autoimmune thyroid disease and HHV-6 infection and in vitro HHV-6 virus modulation of micro-RNA expression in thyrocytes and T-cell lines.[115–118]

The Heterologous Immunity Hypothesis as a Model for the Pathogenesis and Risk of Immune-Mediated Adverse Drug Reactions

The adaptive immune system has evolved to contend with antigenic diversity through the generation of polyspecific TCRs that are capable of recognizing multiple epitopes thereby enhancing our ability to defend against the wide microbial universe. This concept is termed heterologous immunity, and there exist numerous examples of clinical and experimental observations to support this paradigm.[119,120] In the setting of organ transplantation, virus-specific memory T cells that are cross-reactive with allogenic HLA have been implicated in allograft rejection. Recently, it has been recognized that these virus-specific memory T cells may be cross-reactive, sometimes mediated by a public TCR shared by unrelated individuals.[121]

Several observations regarding the clinical presentation and epidemiology of severe delayed IM-ADRs suggest that factors in addition to carriage of specific HLA alleles confer risk for the development of these reactions.

- *The "PPV gap."* As noted, delayed IM-ADRs are characterized by a high negative predictive value for HLA association (approaching 100% in many cases) but a low PPV and, thus, only a minority of patients carrying an HLA risk allele will develop a hypersensitivity reaction (see **Table 1**). What are the genetic or ecologic factors that differ among those individuals who develop hypersensitivity and those who carry the risk HLA allele but tolerate the drug?

- *Diverse clinical phenotypes.* Delayed IM-ADRs are characterized by variable clinical phenotypes and specific phenotypes have been associated with carriage of different HLA alleles. What explains the phenotypic variation seen among these HLA-restricted IM-ADRs?

- *Latency period for clinical disease.* The time from first drug administration to the onset of clinical disease is widely variable across the delayed IM-ADR syndromes. For example, immunologically mediated abacavir hypersensitivity, defined as patch test–positive, HLA-B*57:01–positive abacavir reactivity, occurs in a narrow time window of less than 2 days to 3 weeks from first exposure to drug. SJS/TEN has a shorter latency period than DRESS and typically occurs 4 to 28 days after first drug exposure. Factors contributing to the variable timing of these syndromes are currently unclear.

- *Immunologic memory.* In some cases, immunologically mediated drug-specific recall reactions have been demonstrated several years after drug exposure and withdrawal. For example, abacavir- and carbamazepine-specific in vivo (skin patch test) and ex vivo (ELISpot) responses may remain positive many years after clinical IM-ADR in the absence of subsequent reexposure to a drug. Factors that lead to the maintenance of these long-lasting memory T-cell responses in some but not all T-cell–mediated ADRs are not known.

In the context of IM-ADRs, the requirement for preexisting virus-specific memory T cells that recognize drug-modified antigen could explain many clinical and immunologic features of IM-ADRs as well as the low PPV for HLA allele carriage as a sole predictor of IM-ADR risk[122,123] (**Fig. 3**A). Of the pathogens that might prime such cross-reactive T cells, the HHV stand out as likely candidates. HHV are ubiquitous pathogens that establish lifelong infection and cellular latency and include HSV-1 and HSV-2, varicella zoster virus, Epstein–Barr virus, and cytomegalovirus. HHV are known to prime heterologous immune responses and act as likely sources of persistent antigen for the generation of long-lasting cross-reactive memory T cells. The heterologous immunity hypothesis for IM-ADR predicts that polyspecific T cells that are primed and maintained by HHV antigen cross-react with drug-modified peptide epitopes to elicit memory T-cell responses that result in the clinical IM-ADR syndromes (see **Fig. 3**A, B). This is one model by which the risk of IM-ADR might be predicted based on both genetics (HLA genotype) and ecologic factors such as past pathogen exposure that shape the repertoire of the memory T-cell pool. Future work to precisely

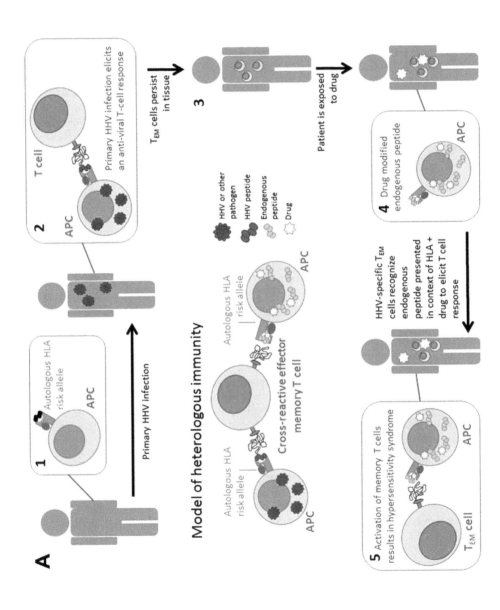

Model of heterologous immunity

A

1 Autologous HLA risk allele — APC

Primary HHV infection

2 T cell · APC — Primary HHV infection elicits an anti-viral T-cell response

3 T_EM cells persist in tissue

Patient is exposed to drug

4 Drug modified endogenous peptide — APC

HHV-specific T_EM cells recognize endogenous peptide presented in context of HLA + drug to elicit T cell response

5 Activation of memory T cells results in hypersensitivity syndrome — APC · T_EM cell

Autologous HLA risk allele — APC
Cross-reactive effector memory T cell
Autologous HLA risk allele — APC

HHV or other pathogen
HHV peptide
Endogenous peptide
Drug

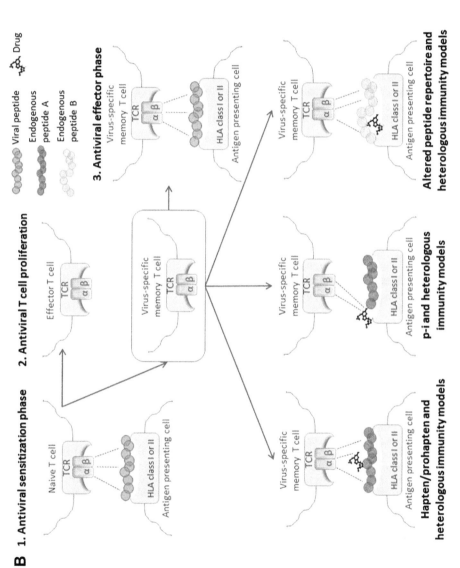

Fig. 3. (continued).

identify the T-cell subsets that participate in clinical IM-ADR is needed to define the pathogenesis of these ADRs.

OPPORTUNITIES FOR TRANSLATION INTO THE CLINICAL SETTING

The development of pharmacogenetic and immunologic assays to identify patients at risk for an IM-ADR before drug administration is a translational research priority given the substantial morbidity, mortality, and cost associated with these reactions. A few key examples demonstrate how basic science discoveries in this field have been translated into clinical practice to improve drug safety. After the PREDICT-1 and SHAPE trials in 2008, HLA-B*57:01 screening before abacavir prescription became part of international HIV treatment guidelines and has been incorporated into routine HIV clinical practice across the developed world.[124–128] In 2007, the US Food and Drug Administration recommended HLA-B*15:02 screening in persons of Southeast Asian ancestry, where carriage of this allele is prevalent, before carbamazepine prescription and avoidance of carbamazepine therapy in all HLA-B*15:02 carriers, regardless of ethnicity, unless the benefits of treatment clearly outweigh the risk of ADR.[129,130] In Taiwan, HLA-B*15:02 screening and restriction of off-label use of carbamazepine have resulted in dramatic decreases in the incidence of carbamazepine-associated IM-ADRs since these measures were implemented in 2010. Similar programs have been successfully implemented and shown to be cost effective in other parts of Southeast Asia. Screening for HLA-B*58:01 before the initiation of allopurinol has been recommended by the American College of Rheumatology for those with advanced renal failure and/or from high-risk populations such as persons of Southeast Asian ancestry.[131] Similar conclusions are observed for HLA-B*13:01 screening before the use of dapsone among high-risk populations and where the mortality from dapsone hypersensitivity syndrome has been shown to be significant.[132] For HLA screening to be safe and cost effective, it must be quality assured and used in the way intended to show "real world cost-effectiveness."[133] A Hong

---

Fig. 3. Generation of heterologous immune responses that may contribute to the pathogenesis of severe delayed adverse drug reaction (ADRs). (*A*) According to the heterologous immunity model, the pathogenesis of a T-cell–mediated ADR, considered over the course of an affected individual's lifetime, can be summarized as follows. (1) A prerequisite feature of each T-cell–mediated ADR is carriage of the HLA risk allele; this is necessary but not sufficient for the reaction. (2) Infection by human herpes virus (HHV; or other pathogen) elicits a polyclonal T-cell response that contains viral infection. HHV establishes latency in the host. (3) Virus-specific memory T cells persist in the host. (4) At a subsequent time point, the subject is exposed to the offending drug. Drug endogenous peptide HLA epitopes are formed as described by 1 of 3 models outlined in **Figs. 2** and **3**B. (5) Virus-specific memory T cells are cross-reactive with drug endogenous peptide-HLA epitopes and acquire cytotoxic function directed against cells displaying drug-modified epitopes. This results in clinical immune-mediated (IM)-ADR. (*B*) Integration of the models of T-cell activation by small molecules and heterologous immunity. In the heterologous immunity model, memory T cells are generated after pathogen exposure and reside at specific anatomic sites. These memory T cells may cross-react with (1) haptenated endogenous peptides presented in the context of the HLA risk allele, (2) drugs that bind the T-cell receptor (TCR) and/or major histocompatibility complex (MHC) in a noncovalent manner under the P-I model, or (3) an altered repertoire of endogenous peptides after drug binding to the MHC. APC, antigen-presenting cell. (*Adapted from* White KD, Chung WH, Hung SI, et al. Evolving models of the immunopathogenesis of T cell-mediated drug allergy: the role of host, pathogens, and drug response. J Allergy Clin Immunol 2015;136(2):226; [quiz: 235]; with permission.)

Kong trial showed that in the initial phase of mandatory HLA-B*15:02 screening the use of carbamazepine was displaced with use of phenytoin in HLA-B*15:02-negative individuals and the incidence of SJS/TEN overall remained unchanged.[134,135]

SUMMARY AND FUTURE DIRECTIONS

Key attributes that have contributed to the translation of some HLA–drug–IM-ADR associations into routine clinical screening include the 100% negative predictive value for lack of IM-ADR in the absence of HLA allele carriage in the target population, the prevalence of the IM-ADR, the low number needed to test to prevent one case, and the paucity of safe, efficacious, and effective therapeutic alternatives. For IM-ADR with known HLA associations that do not meet these criteria, such as seen with the antibiotic flucloxacillin, HLA genotyping is neither cost effective nor feasible. In the case of flucloxacillin, approximately 14,000 patients would need to be screened to prevent 1 case of flucloxacillin-associated drug induced liver injury, and this feature makes flucloxacillin a poor target for preprescription screening at present. All delayed IM-ADRs with a known HLA association aside from HLA-B*57:01–restricted abacavir hypersensitivity (PPV 55%) defined to date are associated with a low PPV (<1%–5%) for risk as determined by HLA genotype alone. As a result, screening strategies that focus solely on HLA genotyping will inevitably lead to the denial of therapy to a large number of carriers of HLA risk alleles who would ultimately tolerate the drug in question without complication. Elucidation of factors in addition to or outside of the MHC that predict risk for development of an IM-ADR will provide further insights into the immunopathogenesis of IM-ADRs and to capabilities for both preclinical (drug development and design) and clinical prevention of these reactions.

REFERENCES

1. Bates DW, Spell N, Cullen DJ, et al. The costs of adverse drug events in hospitalized patients. Adverse Drug Events Prevention Study Group. JAMA 1997; 277(4):307–11.
2. Classen DC, Pestotnik SL, Evans RS, et al. Adverse drug events in hospitalized patients. Excess length of stay, extra costs, and attributable mortality. JAMA 1997;277(4):301–6.
3. Hakkarainen KM, Hedna K, Petzold M, et al. Percentage of patients with preventable adverse drug reactions and preventability of adverse drug reactions–a meta-analysis. PLoS One 2012;7(3):e33236.
4. Kongkaew C, Noyce PR, Ashcroft DM. Hospital admissions associated with adverse drug reactions: a systematic review of prospective observational studies. Ann Pharmacother 2008;42(7):1017–25.
5. Lazarou J, Pomeranz BH, Corey PN. Incidence of adverse drug reactions in hospitalized patients: a meta-analysis of prospective studies. JAMA 1998; 279(15):1200–5.
6. Pirmohamed M, James S, Meakin S, et al. Adverse drug reactions as cause of admission to hospital: prospective analysis of 18 820 patients. BMJ 2004; 329(7456):15–9.
7. Roujeau JC, Stern RS. Severe adverse cutaneous reactions to drugs. N Engl J Med 1994;331(19):1272–85.
8. Suh DC, Woodall BS, Shin SK, et al. Clinical and economic impact of adverse drug reactions in hospitalized patients. Ann Pharmacother 2000;34(12):1373–9.
9. Edwards IR, Aronson JK. Adverse drug reactions: definitions, diagnosis, and management. Lancet 2000;356(9237):1255–9.

10. Rawlings MD, Thompson LW. Pathogenesis of adverse drug reactions. In: Davies DM, editor. Textbook of adverse drug reactions. London: Oxford University Press; 1977. p. 44.

11. McNeil BD, Pundir P, Meeker S, et al. Identification of a mast-cell-specific receptor crucial for pseudo-allergic drug reactions. Nature 2015;519(7542):237–41.

12. Pirmohamed M, Aithal GP, Behr E, et al. The phenotype standardization project: improving pharmacogenetic studies of serious adverse drug reactions. Clin Pharmacol Ther 2011;89(6):784–5.

13. Pirmohamed M, Friedmann PS, Molokhia M, et al. Phenotype standardization for immune-mediated drug-induced skin injury. Clin Pharmacol Ther 2011;89(6): 896–901.

14. Shiohara T, Kano Y, Takahashi R, et al. Drug-induced hypersensitivity syndrome: recent advances in the diagnosis, pathogenesis and management. Chem Immunol Allergy 2012;97:122–38.

15. Kano Y, Sakuma K, Shiohara T. Sclerodermoid graft-versus-host disease-like lesions occurring after drug-induced hypersensitivity syndrome. Br J Dermatol 2007;156(5):1061–3.

16. Kano Y, Tohyama M, Aihara M, et al. Sequelae in 145 patients with drug-induced hypersensitivity syndrome/drug reaction with eosinophilia and systemic symptoms: survey conducted by the Asian Research Committee on Severe Cutaneous Adverse Reactions (ASCAR). J Dermatol 2015;42(3):276–82.

17. Minegaki Y, Higashida Y, Ogawa M, et al. Drug-induced hypersensitivity syndrome complicated with concurrent fulminant type 1 diabetes mellitus and Hashimoto's thyroiditis. Int J Dermatol 2013;52(3):355–7.

18. Chiou CC, Chung WH, Hung SI, et al. Fulminant type 1 diabetes mellitus caused by drug hypersensitivity syndrome with human herpesvirus 6 infection. J Am Acad Dermatol 2006;54(2 Suppl):S14–7.

19. Chen YC, Chang CY, Cho YT, et al. Long-term sequelae of drug reaction with eosinophilia and systemic symptoms: a retrospective cohort study from Taiwan. J Am Acad Dermatol 2013;68(3):459–65.

20. Sekine N, Motokura T, Oki T, et al. Rapid loss of insulin secretion in a patient with fulminant type 1 diabetes mellitus and carbamazepine hypersensitivity syndrome. JAMA 2001;285(9):1153–4.

21. Sommers LM, Schoene RB. Allopurinol hypersensitivity syndrome associated with pancreatic exocrine abnormalities and new-onset diabetes mellitus. Arch Intern Med 2002;162(10):1190–2.

22. Onuma H, Tohyama M, Imagawa A, et al. High frequency of HLA B62 in fulminant type 1 diabetes with the drug-induced hypersensitivity syndrome. J Clin Endocrinol Metab 2012;97(12):E2277–81.

23. Mockenhaupt M. Stevens-Johnson syndrome and toxic epidermal necrolysis: clinical patterns, diagnostic considerations, etiology, and therapeutic management. Semin Cutan Med Surg 2014;33(1):10–6.

24. Zimmermann S, Sekula P, Venhoff M, et al. Systemic immunomodulating therapies for Stevens-Johnson syndrome and toxic epidermal necrolysis: a systematic review and meta-analysis. JAMA Dermatol 2017;153(6):514–22.

25. Camacho LH. CTLA-4 blockade with ipilimumab: biology, safety, efficacy, and future considerations. Cancer Med 2015;4(5):661–72.

26. Michot JM, Bigenwald C, Champiat S, et al. Immune-related adverse events with immune checkpoint blockade: a comprehensive review. Eur J Cancer 2016;54: 139–48.

27. Sibaud V, Meyer N, Lamant L, et al. Dermatologic complications of anti-PD-1/PD-L1 immune checkpoint antibodies. Curr Opin Oncol 2016;28(4):254–63.

28. Johnson DB, Balko JM, Compton ML, et al. Fulminant myocarditis with combination immune checkpoint blockade. N Engl J Med 2016;375(18):1749–55.

29. Bastuji-Garin S, Rzany B, Stern RS, et al. Clinical classification of cases of toxic epidermal necrolysis, Stevens-Johnson syndrome, and erythema multiforme. Arch Dermatol 1993;129(1):92–6.

30. Aurelian L, Ono F, Burnett J. Herpes simplex virus (HSV)-associated erythema multiforme (HAEM): a viral disease with an autoimmune component. Dermatol Online J 2003;9(1):1.

31. Moreau JF, Watson RS, Hartman ME, et al. Epidemiology of ophthalmologic disease associated with erythema multiforme, Stevens-Johnson syndrome, and toxic epidermal necrolysis in hospitalized children in the United States. Pediatr Dermatol 2014;31(2):163–8.

32. Brice SL, Leahy MA, Ong L, et al. Examination of non-involved skin, previously involved skin, and peripheral blood for herpes simplex virus DNA in patients with recurrent herpes-associated erythema multiforme. J Cutan Pathol 1994; 21(5):408–12.

33. Ng PP, Sun YJ, Tan HH, et al. Detection of herpes simplex virus genomic DNA in various subsets of Erythema multiforme by polymerase chain reaction. Dermatology 2003;207(4):349–53.

34. Biazar T, Shokri M, Hosseinnia H, et al. Erythema multiforme as a result of Orf disease; a case report. Emerg (Tehran) 2016;4(3):163–5.

35. Assier H, Bastuji-Garin S, Revuz J, et al. Erythema multiforme with mucous membrane involvement and Stevens-Johnson syndrome are clinically different disorders with distinct causes. Arch Dermatol 1995;131(5):539–43.

36. Schalock PC, Dinulos JG, Pace N, et al. Erythema multiforme due to Mycoplasma pneumoniae infection in two children. Pediatr Dermatol 2006;23(6): 546–55.

37. Sokumbi O, Wetter DA. Clinical features, diagnosis, and treatment of erythema multiforme: a review for the practicing dermatologist. Int J Dermatol 2012;51(8): 889–902.

38. Stevens AM, Johnson FC. A new eruptive fever associated with stomatitis and ophthalmia. Am J Dis Child 1922;24(6):526–33.

39. Callahan S, Oza V. Stevens-Johnson syndrome—a look back. JAMA Dermatol 2017;153(2):240.

40. Finkelstein Y, Soon GS, Acuna P, et al. Recurrence and outcomes of Stevens-Johnson syndrome and toxic epidermal necrolysis in children. Pediatrics 2011;128(4):723–8.

41. Olson D, Watkins LK, Demirjian A, et al. Outbreak of mycoplasma pneumoniae-associated Stevens-Johnson syndrome. Pediatrics 2015;136(2):e386–394.

42. Olson D, Abbott J, Lin C, et al. Characterization of children with recurrent episodes of Stevens Johnson syndrome. J Pediatric Infect Dis Soc 2017. [Epub ahead of print].

43. Second J, Velter C, Cales S, et al. Clinicopathologic analysis of atypical hand, foot, and mouth disease in adult patients. J Am Acad Dermatol 2017;76(4): 722–9.

44. Chung WH, Shih SR, Chang CF, et al. Clinicopathologic analysis of coxsackievirus a6 new variant induced widespread mucocutaneous bullous reactions mimicking severe cutaneous adverse reactions. J Infect Dis 2013;208(12): 1968–78.

45. Chan SH, Tan T. HLA and allopurinol drug eruption. Dermatologica 1989;179(1): 32–3.

46. Roujeau JC, Bracq C, Huyn NT, et al. HLA phenotypes and bullous cutaneous reactions to drugs. Tissue Antigens 1986;28(4):251–4.

47. Fischer PR, Shigeoka AO. Familial occurrence of Stevens-Johnson syndrome. Am J Dis Child 1983;137(9):914–6.

48. Mallal S, Nolan D, Witt C, et al. Association between presence of HLA-B*5701, HLA-DR7, and HLA-DQ3 and hypersensitivity to HIV-1 reverse-transcriptase inhibitor abacavir. Lancet 2002;359(9308):727–32.

49. Hetherington S, Hughes AR, Mosteller M, et al. Genetic variations in HLA-B region and hypersensitivity reactions to abacavir. Lancet 2002;359(9312):1121–2.

50. Chung WH, Hung SI, Hong HS, et al. Medical genetics: a marker for Stevens-Johnson syndrome. Nature 2004;428(6982):486.

51. Hung SI, Chung WH, Liou LB, et al. HLA-B*5801 allele as a genetic marker for severe cutaneous adverse reactions caused by allopurinol. Proc Natl Acad Sci U S A 2005;102(11):4134–9.

52. Hung SI, Chung WH, Jee SH, et al. Genetic susceptibility to carbamazepine-induced cutaneous adverse drug reactions. Pharmacogenet Genomics 2006; 16(4):297–306.

53. Ostrov DA, Grant BJ, Pompeu YA, et al. Drug hypersensitivity caused by alteration of the MHC-presented self-peptide repertoire. Proc Natl Acad Sci U S A 2012;109(25):9959–64.

54. Illing PT, Vivian JP, Dudek NL, et al. Immune self-reactivity triggered by drug-modified HLA-peptide repertoire. Nature 2012;486(7404):554–8.

55. Mallal S, Phillips E, Carosi G, et al. HLA-B*5701 screening for hypersensitivity to abacavir. N Engl J Med 2008;358(6):568–79.

56. Tassaneeyakul W, Tiamkao S, Jantararoungtong T, et al. Association between HLA-B*1502 and carbamazepine-induced severe cutaneous adverse drug reactions in a Thai population. Epilepsia 2010;51(5):926–30.

57. Then SM, Rani ZZ, Raymond AA, et al. Frequency of the HLA-B*1502 allele contributing to carbamazepine-induced hypersensitivity reactions in a cohort of Malaysian epilepsy patients. Asian Pac J Allergy Immunol 2011;29(3):290–3.

58. Wu XT, Hu FY, An DM, et al. Association between carbamazepine-induced cutaneous adverse drug reactions and the HLA-B*1502 allele among patients in central China. Epilepsy Behav 2010;19(3):405–8.

59. Phillips EJ, Chung WH, Mockenhaupt M, et al. Drug hypersensitivity: pharmacogenetics and clinical syndromes. J Allergy Clin Immunol 2011;127(3 Suppl): S60–6.

60. Kaniwa N, Saito Y, Aihara M, et al. HLA-B*1511 is a risk factor for carbamazepine-induced Stevens-Johnson syndrome and toxic epidermal necrolysis in Japanese patients. Epilepsia 2010;51(12):2461–5.

61. Mehta TY, Prajapati LM, Mittal B, et al. Association of HLA-B*1502 allele and carbamazepine-induced Stevens-Johnson syndrome among Indians. Indian J Dermatol Venereol Leprol 2009;75(6):579–82.

62. Locharernkul C, Loplumlert J, Limotai C, et al. Carbamazepine and phenytoin induced Stevens-Johnson syndrome is associated with HLA-B*1502 allele in Thai population. Epilepsia 2008;49(12):2087–91.

63. Hung SI, Chung WH, Liu ZS, et al. Common risk allele in aromatic antiepileptic-drug induced Stevens-Johnson syndrome and toxic epidermal necrolysis in Han Chinese. Pharmacogenomics 2010;11(3):349–56.

64. Chen CB, Hsiao YH, Wu T, et al. Risk and association of HLA with oxcarbazepine-induced cutaneous adverse reactions in Asians. Neurology 2017;88(1):78–86.

65. McCormack M, Alfirevic A, Bourgeois S, et al. HLA-A*3101 and carbamazepine-induced hypersensitivity reactions in Europeans. N Engl J Med 2011;364(12): 1134–43.

66. Niihara H, Kakamu T, Fujita Y, et al. HLA-A31 strongly associates with carbamazepine-induced adverse drug reactions but not with carbamazepine-induced lymphocyte proliferation in a Japanese population. J Dermatol 2011; 39(7):594–601.

67. Ozeki T, Mushiroda T, Yowang A, et al. Genome-wide association study identifies HLA-A*3101 allele as a genetic risk factor for carbamazepine-induced cutaneous adverse drug reactions in Japanese population. Hum Mol Genet 2011;20(5):1034–41.

68. Ramirez E, Bellon T, Tong HY, et al. Significant HLA class I type associations with aromatic antiepileptic drug (AED)-induced SJS/TEN are different from those found for the same AED-induced DRESS in the Spanish population. Pharmacol Res 2017;115:168–78.

69. Niihara H, Kaneko S, Ito T, et al. HLA-B*58:01 strongly associates with allopurinol-induced adverse drug reactions in a Japanese sample population. J Dermatol Sci 2013;71(2):150–2.

70. Jarjour S, Barrette M, Normand V, et al. Genetic markers associated with cutaneous adverse drug reactions to allopurinol: a systematic review. Pharmacogenomics 2015;16(7):755–67.

71. Somkrua R, Eickman EE, Saokaew S, et al. Association of HLA-B*5801 allele and allopurinol-induced Stevens Johnson syndrome and toxic epidermal necrolysis: a systematic review and meta-analysis. BMC Med Genet 2011;12:118.

72. Kaniwa N, Saito Y, Aihara M, et al. HLA-B locus in Japanese patients with anti-epileptics and allopurinol-related Stevens-Johnson syndrome and toxic epidermal necrolysis. Pharmacogenomics 2008;9(11):1617–22.

73. Chung WH, Chang WC, Stocker SL, et al. Insights into the poor prognosis of allopurinol-induced severe cutaneous adverse reactions: the impact of renal insufficiency, high plasma levels of oxypurinol and granulysin. Ann Rheum Dis 2015;74(12):2157–64.

74. Carroll MB, Smith DM, Shaak TL. Genomic sequencing of uric acid metabolizing and clearing genes in relationship to xanthine oxidase inhibitor dose. Rheumatol Int 2017;37(3):445–53.

75. Hartmann T, Terao M, Garattini E, et al. The impact of single nucleotide polymorphisms on human aldehyde oxidase. Drug Metab Dispos 2012;40(5):856–64.

76. Wen CC, Yee SW, Liang X, et al. Genome-wide association study identifies ABCG2 (BCRP) as an allopurinol transporter and a determinant of drug response. Clin Pharmacol Ther 2015;97(5):518–25.

77. Roberts RL, Wallace MC, Phipps-Green AJ, et al. ABCG2 loss-of-function polymorphism predicts poor response to allopurinol in patients with gout. Pharmacogenomics J 2017;17(2):201–3.

78. Chung WH, Chang WC, Lee YS, et al. Genetic variants associated with phenytoin-related severe cutaneous adverse reactions. JAMA 2014;312(5):525–34.

79. Tassaneeyakul W, Prabmeechai N, Sukasem C, et al. Associations between HLA class I and cytochrome P450 2C9 genetic polymorphisms and phenytoin-related severe cutaneous adverse reactions in a Thai population. Pharmacogenet Genomics 2016;26(5):225–34.

80. Yampayon K, Sukasem C, Limwongse C, et al. Influence of genetic and non-genetic factors on phenytoin-induced severe cutaneous adverse drug reactions. Eur J Clin Pharmacol 2017;73(7):855–65.

81. Chang CC, Ng CC, Too CL, et al. Association of HLA-B*15:13 and HLA-B*15:02 with phenytoin-induced severe cutaneous adverse reactions in a Malay population. Pharmacogenomics J 2017;17(2):170–3.

82. Kaniwa N, Sugiyama E, Saito Y, et al. Specific HLA types are associated with antiepileptic drug-induced Stevens-Johnson syndrome and toxic epidermal necrolysis in Japanese subjects. Pharmacogenomics 2013;14(15):1821–31.

83. Keane NM, Pavlos RK, McKinnon E, et al. HLA class I restricted CD8+ and class II restricted CD4+ T cells are implicated in the pathogenesis of nevirapine hypersensitivity. AIDS 2014;(13):1891–1901S.

84. Littera R, Carcassi C, Masala A, et al. HLA-dependent hypersensitivity to nevirapine in Sardinian HIV patients. AIDS 2006;20(12):1621–6.

85. Yuan J, Guo S, Hall D, et al. Toxicogenomics of nevirapine-associated cutaneous and hepatic adverse events among populations of African, Asian, and European descent. AIDS 2011;25(10):1271–80.

86. Martin AM, Nolan D, James I, et al. Predisposition to nevirapine hypersensitivity associated with HLA-DRB1*0101 and abrogated by low CD4 T-cell counts. AIDS 2005;19(1):97–9.

87. Chantarangsu S, Mushiroda T, Mahasirimongkol S, et al. HLA-B*3505 allele is a strong predictor for nevirapine-induced skin adverse drug reactions in HIV-infected Thai patients. Pharmacogenet Genomics 2009;19(2):139–46.

88. Carr DF, Chaponda M, Jorgensen AL, et al. Association of human leukocyte antigen alleles and nevirapine hypersensitivity in a Malawian HIV-infected population. Clin Infect Dis 2013;56(9):1330–9.

89. Bertrand J, Chou M, Richardson DM, et al. Multiple genetic variants predict steady-state nevirapine clearance in HIV-infected Cambodians. Pharmacogenet Genomics 2012;22(12):868–76.

90. Ciccacci C, Di Fusco D, Marazzi MC, et al. Association between CYP2B6 polymorphisms and Nevirapine-induced SJS/TEN: a pharmacogenetics study. Eur J Clin Pharmacol 2013;69(11):1909–16.

91. Pichler W, Yawalkar N, Schmid S, et al. Pathogenesis of drug-induced exanthems. Allergy 2002;57(10):884–93.

92. Pichler WJ. Delayed drug hypersensitivity reactions. Ann Intern Med 2003; 139(8):683–93.

93. Pichler WJ, Beeler A, Keller M, et al. Pharmacological interaction of drugs with immune receptors: the p-i concept. Allergol Int 2006;55(1):17–25.

94. Pichler WJ, Watkins S. Interaction of small molecules with specific immune receptors: the p-i concept and its consequences. Curr Immunol Rev 2014;10:7–18.

95. Le Cleach L, Delaire S, Boumsell L, et al. Blister fluid T lymphocytes during toxic epidermal necrolysis are functional cytotoxic cells which express human natural killer (NK) inhibitory receptors. Clin Exp Immunol 2000;119(1):225–30.

96. Leyva L, Torres MJ, Posadas S, et al. Anticonvulsant-induced toxic epidermal necrolysis: monitoring the immunologic response. J Allergy Clin Immunol 2000;105(1 Pt 1):157–65.

97. Nassif A, Bensussan A, Dorothee G, et al. Drug specific cytotoxic T-cells in the skin lesions of a patient with toxic epidermal necrolysis. J Invest Dermatol 2002; 118(4):728–33.

98. Nassif A, Moslehi H, Le Gouvello S, et al. Evaluation of the potential role of cytokines in toxic epidermal necrolysis. J Invest Dermatol 2004;123(5):850–5.

99. Chung WH, Hung SI, Yang JY, et al. Granulysin is a key mediator for disseminated keratinocyte death in Stevens-Johnson syndrome and toxic epidermal necrolysis. Nat Med 2008;14(12):1343–50.

100. Hung S. Pharmaco-immunological synapse of HLA-drug-TCR in SCAR. 7th Drug hypersensitivity meeting. Malaga (Spain), 21-23 April, 2016.

101. Wei CY, Chung WH, Huang HW, et al. Direct interaction between HLA-B and carbamazepine activates T cells in patients with Stevens-Johnson syndrome. J Allergy Clin Immunol 2012;129(6):1562–9.e5.

102. Yun J, Marcaida MJ, Eriksson KK, et al. Oxypurinol directly and immediately activates the drug-specific T cells via the preferential use of HLA-B*58:01. J Immunol 2014;192(7):2984–93.

103. Chung WH, Pan RY, Chu MT, et al. Oxypurinol-specific T cells possess preferential TCR clonotypes and express granulysin in allopurinol-induced severe cutaneous adverse reactions. J Invest Dermatol 2015;135(9):2237–48.

104. Morito H, Ogawa K, Fukumoto T, et al. Increased ratio of FoxP3+ regulatory T cells/CD3+ T cells in skin lesions in drug-induced hypersensitivity syndrome/drug rash with eosinophilia and systemic symptoms. Clin Exp Dermatol 2014;39(3):284–91.

105. Takahashi R, Kano Y, Yamazaki Y, et al. Defective regulatory T cells in patients with severe drug eruptions: timing of the dysfunction is associated with the pathological phenotype and outcome. J Immunol 2009;182(12):8071–9.

106. Shiohara T, Ushigome Y, Kano Y, et al. Crucial role of viral reactivation in the development of severe drug eruptions: a comprehensive review. Clin Rev Allergy Immunol 2015;49(2):192–202.

107. Miyagawa F, Nakamura Y, Miyashita K, et al. Preferential expression of CD134, an HHV-6 cellular receptor, on CD4T cells in drug-induced hypersensitivity syndrome (DIHS)/drug reaction with eosinophilia and systemic symptoms (DRESS). J Dermatol Sci 2016;83(2):151–4.

108. Picard D, Janela B, Descamps V, et al. Drug reaction with eosinophilia and systemic symptoms (DRESS): a multiorgan antiviral T cell response. Sci Transl Med 2010;2(46):46ra62.

109. Kano Y, Hiraharas K, Sakuma K, et al. Several herpesviruses can reactivate in a severe drug-induced multiorgan reaction in the same sequential order as in graft-versus-host disease. Br J Dermatol 2006;155(2):301–6.

110. Funck-Brentano E, Duong T, Family D, et al. Auto-immune thyroiditis and drug reaction with eosinophilia and systemic symptoms (DRESS) associated with HHV-6 viral reactivation. Ann Dermatol Venereol 2011;138(8–9):580–5 [in French].

111. Sato M, Mizuno Y, Matsuyama K, et al. Drug-induced hypersensitivity syndrome followed by subacute thyroiditis. Case Rep Dermatol 2015;7(2):161–5.

112. Ushigome Y, Kano Y, Ishida T, et al. Short- and long-term outcomes of 34 patients with drug-induced hypersensitivity syndrome in a single institution. J Am Acad Dermatol 2013;68(5):721–8.

113. Cookson H, Creamer D, Walsh S. Thyroid dysfunction in drug reaction with eosinophilia and systemic symptoms (DRESS): an unusual manifestation of systemic drug hypersensitivity. Br J Dermatol 2013;168(5):1130–2.

114. Descamps V. Drug reaction with eosinophilia and systemic symptoms and thyroiditis: human herpesvirus-6, the possible common link. Br J Dermatol 2013;169(4):952.

115. Caselli E, D'Accolti M, Soffritti I, et al. HHV-6A in vitro infection of thyrocytes and T cells alters the expression of miRNA associated to autoimmune thyroiditis. Virol J 2017;14(1):3.

116. Caselli E, Zatelli MC, Rizzo R, et al. Virologic and immunologic evidence supporting an association between HHV-6 and Hashimoto's thyroiditis. PLoS Pathog 2012;8(10):e1002951.

117. Sultanova A, Cistjakovs M, Gravelsina S, et al. Association of active human herpesvirus-6 (HHV-6) infection with autoimmune thyroid gland diseases. Clin Microbiol Infect 2017;23(1):50.e1-e5.

118. Broccolo F, Fusetti L, Ceccherini-Nelli L. Possible role of human herpesvirus 6 as a trigger of autoimmune disease. ScientificWorldJournal 2013;2013:867389.

119. Welsh RM, Che JW, Brehm MA, et al. Heterologous immunity between viruses. Immunol Rev 2010;235(1):244–66.

120. Welsh RM, Selin LK. No one is naive: the significance of heterologous T-cell immunity. Nat Rev Immunol 2002;2(6):417–26.

121. van den Heuvel H, Heutinck KM, van der Meer-Prins EM, et al. Allo-HLA cross-reactivities of cytomegalovirus-, influenza-, and varicella zoster virus-specific memory T cells are shared by different individuals. Am J Transplant 2017; 17(8):2033–44.

122. White KD, Chung WH, Hung SI, et al. Evolving models of the immunopathogenesis of T cell-mediated drug allergy: the role of host, pathogens, and drug response. J Allergy Clin Immunol 2015;136(2):219–34 [quiz: 235].

123. Pavlos R, Mallal S, Ostrov D, et al. T cell-mediated hypersensitivity reactions to drugs. Annu Rev Med 2015;66:439–54.

124. Martin MA, Klein TE, Dong BJ, et al. Clinical pharmacogenetics implementation consortium guidelines for HLA-B genotype and abacavir dosing. Clin Pharmacol Ther 2012;91(4):734–8.

125. Gazzard BG, Anderson J, Babiker A, et al. British HIV Association guidelines for the treatment of HIV-1-infected adults with antiretroviral therapy 2008. HIV Med 2008;9(8):563–608.

126. Aberg JA, Kaplan JE, Libman H, et al. Primary care guidelines for the management of persons infected with human immunodeficiency virus: 2009 update by the HIV medicine Association of the Infectious Diseases Society of America. Clin Infect Dis 2009;49(5):651–81.

127. Becquemont L, Alfirevic A, Amstutz U, et al. Practical recommendations for pharmacogenomics-based prescription: 2010 ESF-UB conference on pharmacogenetics and pharmacogenomics. Pharmacogenomics 2011;12(1):113–24.

128. Swen JJ, Nijenhuis M, de Boer A, et al. Pharmacogenetics: from bench to byte–an update of guidelines. Clin Pharmacol Ther 2011;89(5):662–73.

129. Ferrell PB Jr, McLeod HL. Carbamazepine, HLA-B*1502 and risk of Stevens-Johnson syndrome and toxic epidermal necrolysis: US FDA recommendations. Pharmacogenomics 2008;9(10):1543–6.

130. Leckband SG, Kelsoe JR, Dunnenberger HM, et al. Clinical pharmacogenetics implementation consortium guidelines for HLA-B genotype and carbamazepine dosing. Clin Pharmacol Ther 2013;94(3):324–8.

131. Ke CH, Chung WH, Wen YH, et al. Cost-effectiveness analysis for genotyping before allopurinol treatment to prevent severe cutaneous adverse drug reactions. J Rheumatol 2017;44(6):835–43.

132. Wang N, Parimi L, Liu H, et al. A review on dapsone hypersensitivity syndrome among Chinese patients with an emphasis on preventing adverse drug reactions with genetic testing. Am J Trop Med Hyg 2017;96(5):1014–8.

133. Hammond E, Almeida CA, Mamotte C, et al. External quality assessment of HLA-B*5701 reporting: an international multicentre survey. Antivir Ther 2007; 12(7):1027–32.

134. Chen Z, Liew D, Kwan P. Real-world cost-effectiveness of pharmacogenetic screening for epilepsy treatment. Neurology 2016;86(12):1086–94.

135. Chen Z, Liew D, Kwan P. Effects of a HLA-B*15:02 screening policy on antiepileptic drug use and severe skin reactions. Neurology 2014;83(22):2077–84.

136. Saag M, Balu R, Phillips E, et al. High sensitivity of human leukocyte antigen-b*5701 as a marker for immunologically confirmed abacavir hypersensitivity in white and black patients. Clin Infect Dis 2008;46(7):1111–8.

137. Kulkantrakorn K, Tassaneeyakul W, Tiamkao S, et al. HLA-B*1502 strongly predicts carbamazepine-induced Stevens-Johnson syndrome and toxic epidermal necrolysis in Thai patients with neuropathic pain. Pain Pract 2012;12(3):202–8.

138. Man CB, Kwan P, Baum L, et al. Association between HLA-B*1502 allele and antiepileptic drug-induced cutaneous reactions in Han Chinese. Epilepsia 2007;48(5):1015–8.

139. Wang Q, Zhou JQ, Zhou LM, et al. Association between HLA-B*1502 allele and carbamazepine-induced severe cutaneous adverse reactions in Han people of southern China mainland. Seizure 2011;20(6):446–8.

140. Zhang Y, Wang J, Zhao LM, et al. Strong association between HLA-B*1502 and carbamazepine-induced Stevens-Johnson syndrome and toxic epidermal necrolysis in mainland Han Chinese patients. Eur J Clin Pharmacol 2011;67(9): 885–7.

141. Chang CC, Too CL, Murad S, et al. Association of HLA-B*1502 allele with carbamazepine-induced toxic epidermal necrolysis and Stevens-Johnson syndrome in the multi-ethnic Malaysian population. Int J Dermatol 2011;50(2): 221–4.

142. Kim SH, Lee KW, Song WJ, et al. Carbamazepine-induced severe cutaneous adverse reactions and HLA genotypes in Koreans. Epilepsy Res 2011; 97(1–2):190–7.

143. Ikeda H, Takahashi Y, Yamazaki E, et al. HLA class I markers in Japanese patients with carbamazepine-induced cutaneous adverse reactions. Epilepsia 2010;51(2):297–300.

144. Alfirevic A, Jorgensen AL, Williamson PR, et al. HLA-B locus in Caucasian patients with carbamazepine hypersensitivity. Pharmacogenomics 2006;7(6): 813–8.

145. Genin E, Chen DP, Hung SI, et al. HLA-A*31:01 and different types of carbamazepine-induced severe cutaneous adverse reactions: an international study and meta-analysis. Pharmacogenomics J 2014;14(3):281–8.

146. Tassaneeyakul W, Jantararoungtong T, Chen P, et al. Strong association between HLA-B*5801 and allopurinol-induced Stevens-Johnson syndrome and toxic epidermal necrolysis in a Thai population. Pharmacogenet Genomics 2009;19(9):704–9.

147. Kang HR, Jee YK, Kim YS, et al. Positive and negative associations of HLA class I alleles with allopurinol-induced SCARs in Koreans. Pharmacogenet Genomics 2011;21(5):303–7.

148. Lonjou C, Borot N, Sekula P, et al. A European study of HLA-B in Stevens-Johnson syndrome and toxic epidermal necrolysis related to five high-risk drugs. Pharmacogenet Genomics 2008;18(2):99–107.

149. Genin E, Schumacher M, Roujeau JC, et al. Genome-wide association study of Stevens-Johnson syndrome and toxic epidermal necrolysis in Europe. Orphanet J Rare Dis 2011;6:52.

150. Wu R, Cheng YJ, Zhu LL, et al. Impact of HLA-B*58:01 allele and allopurinol-induced cutaneous adverse drug reactions: evidence from 21 pharmacogenetic studies. Oncotarget 2016;7(49):81870–9.

151. Lin LC, Lai PC, Yang SF, et al. Oxcarbazepine-induced Stevens-Johnson syndrome: a case report. Kaohsiung J Med Sci 2009;25(2):82–6.

152. Hu FY, Wu XT, An DM, et al. Pilot association study of oxcarbazepine-induced mild cutaneous adverse reactions with HLA-B*1502 allele in Chinese Han population. Seizure 2011;20(2):160–2.

153. An DM, Wu XT, Hu FY, et al. Association study of lamotrigine-induced cutaneous adverse reactions and HLA-B*1502 in a Han Chinese population. Epilepsy Res 2010;92(2–3):226–30.

154. Shi YW, Min FL, Liu XR, et al. Hla-B alleles and lamotrigine-induced cutaneous adverse drug reactions in the Han Chinese population. Basic Clin Pharmacol Toxicol 2011;109(1):42–6.

155. Kim BK, Jung JW, Kim TB, et al. HLA-A*31:01 and lamotrigine-induced severe cutaneous adverse drug reactions in a Korean population. Ann Allergy Asthma Immunol 2017;118(5):629–30.

156. Manuyakorn W, Mahasirimongkol S, Likkasittipan P, et al. Association of HLA genotypes with phenobarbital hypersensitivity in children. Epilepsia 2016;57(10):1610–6.

157. Manuyakorn W, Siripool K, Kamchaisatian W, et al. Phenobarbital-induced severe cutaneous adverse drug reactions are associated with CYP2C19*2 in Thai children. Pediatr Allergy Immunol 2013;24(3):299–303.

158. Sun D, Yu CH, Liu ZS, et al. Association of HLA-B*1502 and *1511 allele with antiepileptic drug-induced Stevens-Johnson syndrome in central China. J Huazhong Univ Sci Technolog Med Sci 2014;34(1):146–50.

159. Gatanaga H, Yazaki H, Tanuma J, et al. HLA-Cw8 primarily associated with hypersensitivity to nevirapine. AIDS 2007;21(2):264–5.

160. Gao S, Gui XE, Liang K, et al. HLA-dependent hypersensitivity reaction to nevirapine in Chinese Han HIV-infected patients. AIDS Res Hum Retroviruses 2012;28(6):540–3.

161. Vitezica ZG, Milpied B, Lonjou C, et al. HLA-DRB1*01 associated with cutaneous hypersensitivity induced by nevirapine and efavirenz. AIDS 2008;22(4):540–1.

162. Likanonsakul S, Rattanatham T, Feangvad S, et al. HLA-Cw*04 allele associated with nevirapine-induced rash in HIV-infected Thai patients. AIDS Res Ther 2009;6:22.

163. Chantarangsu S, Mushiroda T, Mahasirimongkol S, et al. Genome-wide association study identifies variations in 6p21.3 associated with nevirapine-induced rash. Clin Infect Dis 2011;53(4):341–8.

164. Zhang FR, Liu H, Irwanto A, et al. HLA-B*13:01 and the dapsone hypersensitivity syndrome. N Engl J Med 2013;369(17):1620–8.

165. Kongpan T, Mahasirimongkol S, Konyoung P, et al. Candidate HLA genes for prediction of co-trimoxazole-induced severe cutaneous reactions. Pharmacogenet Genomics 2015;25(8):402–11.

166. Rutkowski K, Taylor C, Wagner A. HLA B62 as a possible risk factor for drug reaction with eosinophilia and systemic symptoms to piperacillin/tazobactam. J Allergy Clin Immunol Pract 2016;5(3):829–30.

167. Lee HY, Shen MX, Lim YL, et al. Increased risk of strontium ranelate-related SJS/TEN is associated with HLA. Osteoporos Int 2016;27(8):2577–83.

168. Hautekeete ML, Horsmans Y, Van Waeyenberge C, et al. HLA association of amoxicillin-clavulanate–induced hepatitis. Gastroenterology 1999;117(5):1181–6.

169. O'Donohue J, Oien KA, Donaldson P, et al. Co-amoxiclav jaundice: clinical and histological features and HLA class II association. Gut 2000;47(5):717–20.

170. Lucena MI, Molokhia M, Shen Y, et al. Susceptibility to amoxicillin-clavulanate-induced liver injury is influenced by multiple HLA class I and II alleles. Gastroenterology 2011;141(1):338–47.

171. Singer JB, Lewitzky S, Leroy E, et al. A genome-wide study identifies HLA alleles associated with lumiracoxib-related liver injury. Nat Genet 2010;42(8):711–4.

172. Kindmark A, Jawaid A, Harbron CG, et al. Genome-wide pharmacogenetic investigation of a hepatic adverse event without clinical signs of immunopathology suggests an underlying immune pathogenesis. Pharmacogenomics J 2008;8(3):186–95.

173. Daly AK, Day CP. Genetic association studies in drug-induced liver injury. Semin Liver Dis 2009;29(4):400–11.

174. Daly AK, Day CP. Genetic association studies in drug-induced liver injury. Drug Metab Rev 2012;44(1):116–26.

175. Daly AK, Aithal GP, Leathart JB, et al. Genetic susceptibility to diclofenac-induced hepatotoxicity: contribution of UGT2B7, CYP2C8, and ABCC2 genotypes. Gastroenterology 2007;132(1):272–81.

176. Daly AK, Donaldson PT, Bhatnagar P, et al. HLA-B*5701 genotype is a major determinant of drug-induced liver injury due to flucloxacillin. Nat Genet 2009;41(7):816–9.

177. Spraggs CF, Budde LR, Briley LP, et al. HLA-DQA1*02:01 is a major risk factor for lapatinib-induced hepatotoxicity in women with advanced breast cancer. J Clin Oncol 2011;29(6):667–73.

178. Urban TJ, Nicoletti P, Chalasani N, et al. Minocycline hepatotoxicity: clinical characterization and identification of HLA-B * 35:02 as a risk factor. J Hepatol 2017;67(1):137–44.

179. Huang CZ, Yang J, Qiao HL, et al. Polymorphisms and haplotype analysis of IL-4Ralpha Q576R and I75V in patients with penicillin allergy. Eur J Clin Pharmacol 2009;65(9):895–902.

180. Huang CZ, Zou D, Yang J, et al. Polymorphisms of STAT6 and specific serum IgE levels in patients with penicillin allergy. Int J Clin Pharmacol Ther 2012;50(7):461–7.

181. Gueant JL, Romano A, Cornejo-Garcia JA, et al. HLA-DRA variants predict penicillin allergy in genome-wide fine-mapping genotyping. J Allergy Clin Immunol 2015;135(1):253–9.

182. Cheung CL, Sing CW, Tang CS, et al. HLA-B*38:02:01 predicts carbimazole/methimazole-induced agranulocytosis. Clin Pharmacol Ther 2016;99(5):555–61.

183. Chen PL, Shih SR, Wang PW, et al. Genetic determinants of antithyroid drug-induced agranulocytosis by human leukocyte antigen genotyping and genome-wide association study. Nat Commun 2015;6:7633.

184. Hallberg P, Eriksson N, Ibanez L, et al. Genetic variants associated with antithyroid drug-induced agranulocytosis: a genome-wide association study in a European population. Lancet Diabetes Endocrinol 2016;4(6):507–16.

185. Sai K, Kajinami K, Akao H, et al. A possible role for HLA-DRB1*04:06 in statin-related myopathy in Japanese patients. Drug Metab Pharmacokinet 2016;31(6): 467–70.

186. Thomas M, Hopkins C, Duffy E, et al. Association of the HLA-B*53:01 allele with drug reaction with eosinophilia and systemic symptoms (DRESS) syndrome during treatment of HIV infection with raltegravir. Clin Infect Dis 2017;64(9): 1198–203.

187. Tohyama M, Hashimoto K, Yasukawa M, et al. Association of human herpesvirus 6 reactivation with the flaring and severity of drug-induced hypersensitivity syndrome. Br J Dermatol 2007;157(5):934–40.

188. Seishima M, Yamanaka S, Fujisawa T, et al. Reactivation of human herpesvirus (HHV) family members other than HHV-6 in drug-induced hypersensitivity syndrome. Br J Dermatol 2006;155(2):344–9.

189. Descamps V, Mahe E, Houhou N, et al. Drug-induced hypersensitivity syndrome associated with Epstein-Barr virus infection. Br J Dermatol 2003;148(5):1032–4.

190. Hamaguchi Y, Fujimoto M, Enokido Y, et al. Intractable genital ulcers from herpes simplex virus reactivation in drug-induced hypersensitivity syndrome caused by allopurinol. Int J Dermatol 2010;49(6):700–4.

191. Mardivirin L, Valeyrie-Allanore L, Branlant-Redon E, et al. Amoxicillin-induced flare in patients with DRESS (Drug Reaction with Eosinophilia and Systemic Symptoms): report of seven cases and demonstration of a direct effect of amoxicillin on human herpesvirus 6 replication in vitro. Eur J Dermatol 2010;20(1): 68–73.

192. Kawakami T, Fujita A, Takeuchi S, et al. Drug-induced hypersensitivity syndrome: drug reaction with eosinophilia and systemic symptoms (DRESS) syndrome induced by aspirin treatment of Kawasaki disease. J Am Acad Dermatol 2009;60(1):146–9.

193. Kano Y, Inaoka M, Shiohara T. Association between anticonvulsant hypersensitivity syndrome and human herpesvirus 6 reactivation and hypogammaglobulinemia. Arch Dermatol 2004;140(2):183–8.

194. Descamps V, Valance A, Edlinger C, et al. Association of human herpesvirus 6 infection with drug reaction with eosinophilia and systemic symptoms. Arch Dermatol 2001;137(3):301–4.

195. Kano Y, Seishima M, Shiohara T. Hypogammaglobulinemia as an early sign of drug-induced hypersensitivity syndrome. J Am Acad Dermatol 2006;55(4): 727–8.

196. Morito H, Kitamura K, Fukumoto T, et al. Drug eruption with eosinophilia and systemic syndrome associated with reactivation of human herpesvirus 7, not human herpesvirus 6. J Dermatol 2012;39(7):669–70.

197. Descamps V, Bouscarat F, Laglenne S, et al. Human herpesvirus 6 infection associated with anticonvulsant hypersensitivity syndrome and reactive haemophagocytic syndrome. Br J Dermatol 1997;137(4):605–8.

198. Coughlin CC, Jen MV, Boos MD. Drug hypersensitivity syndrome with prolonged course complicated by parvovirus infection. Pediatr Dermatol 2016;33(6): e364–5.

199. Hase I, Arakawa H, Sakuma H, et al. Bronchoscopic investigation of atypical drug-induced hypersensitivity syndrome showing viral lung involvement. Intern Med 2016;55(18):2691–6.

200. Ben Fredj N, Aouam K, Chaabane A, et al. Hypersensitivity to amoxicillin after drug rash with eosinophilia and systemic symptoms (DRESS) to carbamazepine

and allopurinol: a possible co-sensitization. Br J Clin Pharmacol 2010;70(2): 273–6.

201. Mine S, Suzuki K, Sato Y, et al. Evidence for human herpesvirus-6B infection of regulatory T-cells in acute systemic lymphadenitis in an immunocompetent adult with the drug reaction with eosinophilia and systemic symptoms syndrome: a case report. J Clin Virol 2014;61(3):448–52.

202. Fujita M, Takahashi A, Imaizumi H, et al. Drug-induced liver injury with HHV-6 re-activation. Intern Med 2015;54(10):1219–22.

203. Draz N, Datta S, Webster DP, et al. Drug reaction with eosinophilia and systemic symptoms (DRESS) syndrome secondary to antituberculosis drugs and associ-ated with human herpes virus-7 (HHV-7). BMJ Case Rep 2013;2013 [pii: bcr2013010348].

204. Ueda T, Oba S, Yoshikawa S. Drug-induced liver injury with human herpesvirus (HHV)-6 reactivation but without exanthema or fever. Intern Med 2016;55(7):853.

205. Tagajdid MR, Doblali T, Elannaz H, et al. Reactivation of cytomegalovirus in a pa-tient with Stevens-Johnson syndrome-toxic epidermal necrolysis. Iran J Med Sci 2013;38(2 Suppl):195–7.

206. Drago F, Cogorno L, Broccolo F, et al. A fatal case of DRESS induced by stron-tium ranelate associated with HHV-7 reactivation. Osteoporos Int 2016;27(3): 1261–4.

207. Michel F, Navellou JC, Ferraud D, et al. DRESS syndrome in a patient on sulfa-salazine for rheumatoid arthritis. Joint Bone Spine 2005;72(1):82–5.

208. Mennicke M, Zawodniak A, Keller M, et al. Fulminant liver failure after vancomy-cin in a sulfasalazine-induced DRESS syndrome: fatal recurrence after liver transplantation. Am J Transplant 2009;9(9):2197–202.

209. Hagiya H, Iwamuro M, Tanaka T, et al. Reactivation of human herpes virus-6 in the renal tissue of a patient with drug-induced hypersensitivity syndrome/drug rash with eosinophilia and systemic symptoms (DIHS/DRESS). Intern Med 2016;55(13):1769–74.

210. Miyashita K, Shobatake C, Miyagawa F, et al. Involvement of human herpesvirus 6 infection in renal dysfunction associated with DIHS/DRESS. Acta Derm Vene-reol 2016;96(1):114–5.

211. Tamagawa-Mineoka R, Katoh N, Nara T, et al. DRESS syndrome caused by tei-coplanin and vancomycin, associated with reactivation of human herpesvirus-6. Int J Dermatol 2007;46(6):654–5.

212. Chen YC, Chiang HH, Cho YT, et al. Human herpes virus reactivations and dy-namic cytokine profiles in patients with cutaneous adverse drug reactions –a prospective comparative study. Allergy 2015;70(5):568–75.

213. Ahluwalia J, Abuabara K, Perman MJ, et al. Human herpesvirus 6 involvement in paediatric drug hypersensitivity syndrome. Br J Dermatol 2015;172(4):1090–5.

214. Funck-Brentano E, Duong TA, Bouvresse S, et al. Therapeutic management of DRESS: a retrospective study of 38 cases. J Am Acad Dermatol 2015;72(2): 246–52.

215. Ishida T, Kano Y, Mizukawa Y, et al. The dynamics of herpesvirus reactivations during and after severe drug eruptions: their relation to the clinical phenotype and therapeutic outcome. Allergy 2014;69(6):798–805.

UNITED STATES POSTAL SERVICE ® Statement of Ownership, Management, and Circulation
(All Periodicals Publications Except Requester Publications)

1. Publication Title	2. Publication Number	3. Filing Date
IMMUNOLOGY AND ALLERGY CLINICS OF NORTH AMERICA	006 – 361	9/18/2017

4. Issue Frequency	5. Number of Issues Published Annually	6. Annual Subscription Price
FEB, MAY, AUG, NOV	4	$320.00

7. Complete Mailing Address of Known Office of Publication (Not printer) (Street, city, county, state, and ZIP+4®)

ELSEVIER INC.
230 Park Avenue, Suite 800
New York, NY 10169

Contact Person
STEPHEN R. BUSHING

Telephone (Include area code)
215-239-3688

8. Complete Mailing Address of Headquarters or General Business Office of Publisher (Not printer)

ELSEVIER INC.
230 Park Avenue, Suite 800
New York, NY 10169

9. Full Names and Complete Mailing Addresses of Publisher, Editor, and Managing Editor (Do not leave blank)

Publisher (Name and complete mailing address)

ADRIANNE BRIGIDO, ELSEVIER INC.
1600 JOHN F KENNEDY BLVD. SUITE 1800
PHILADELPHIA, PA 19103-2899

Editor (Name and complete mailing address)

JESSICA MCCOOL, ELSEVIER INC.
1600 JOHN F KENNEDY BLVD. SUITE 1800
PHILADELPHIA, PA 19103-2899

Managing Editor (Name and complete mailing address)

PATRICK MANLEY, ELSEVIER INC.
1600 JOHN F KENNEDY BLVD. SUITE 1800
PHILADELPHIA, PA 19103-2899

10. Owner (Do not leave blank. If the publication is owned by a corporation, give the name and address of the corporation immediately followed by the names and addresses of all stockholders owning or holding 1 percent or more of the total amount of stock. If not owned by a corporation, give the names and addresses of the individual owners. If owned by a partnership or other unincorporated firm, give its name and address as well as those of each individual owner. If the publication is published by a nonprofit organization, give its name and address.)

Full Name	Complete Mailing Address
WHOLLY OWNED SUBSIDIARY OF REED/ELSEVIER US HOLDINGS	1600 JOHN F KENNEDY BLVD. SUITE 1800 PHILADELPHIA, PA 19103-2899

11. Known Bondholders, Mortgagees, and Other Security Holders Owning or Holding 1 Percent or More of Total Amount of Bonds, Mortgages, or Other Securities. If none, check box ▶ ☐ None

Full Name	Complete Mailing Address
N/A	

12. Tax Status (For completion by nonprofit organizations authorized to mail at nonprofit rates) (Check one)
The purpose, function, and nonprofit status of this organization and the exempt status for federal income tax purposes:
☒ Has Not Changed During Preceding 12 Months
☐ Has Changed During Preceding 12 Months (Publisher must submit explanation of change with this statement)

PS Form **3526**, July 2014 [Page 1 of 4 (see instructions page 4)] PSN 7530-01-000-9931   PRIVACY NOTICE: See our privacy policy on www.usps.com.

13. Publication Title	14. Issue Date for Circulation Data Below
IMMUNOLOGY AND ALLERGY CLINICS OF NORTH AMERICA	MAY 2017

15. Extent and Nature of Circulation			Average No. Copies Each Issue During Preceding 12 Months	No. Copies of Single Issue Published Nearest to Filing Date
a. Total Number of Copies (Net press run)			269	225
b. Paid Circulation (By Mail and Outside the Mail)	(1)	Mailed Outside-County Paid Subscriptions Stated on PS Form 3541 (Include paid distribution above nominal rate, advertiser's proof copies, and exchange copies)	139	126
	(2)	Mailed In-County Paid Subscriptions Stated on PS Form 3541 (Include paid distribution above nominal rate, advertiser's proof copies, and exchange copies)	0	0
	(3)	Paid Distribution Outside the Mails Including Sales Through Dealers and Carriers, Street Vendors, Counter Sales, and Other Paid Distribution Outside USPS®	40	34
	(4)	Paid Distribution by Other Classes of Mail Through the USPS (e.g. First-Class Mail®)	0	0
c. Total Paid Distribution (Sum of 15b (1), (2), (3) and (4))		▶	179	160
d. Free or Nominal Rate Distribution (By Mail and Outside the Mail)	(1)	Free or Nominal Rate Outside-County Copies included on PS Form 3541	41	65
	(2)	Free or Nominal Rate In-County Copies Included on PS Form 3541	0	0
	(3)	Free or Nominal Rate Copies Mailed at Other Classes Through the USPS (e.g. First-Class Mail)	0	0
	(4)	Free or Nominal Rate Distribution Outside the Mail (Carriers or other means)	0	0
e. Total Free or Nominal Rate Distribution (Sum of 15d (1), (2), (3) and (4))		▶	41	65
f. Total Distribution (Sum of 15c and 15e)		▶	220	225
g. Copies not Distributed (See Instructions to Publishers #4 (page #3))		▶	49	0
h. Total (Sum of 15f and g)		▶	269	225
i. Percent Paid (15c divided by 15f times 100)		▶	81.36%	71.11%

* If you are claiming electronic copies, go to line 16 on page 3. If you are not claiming electronic copies, skip to line 17 on page 3.

16. Electronic Copy Circulation		Average No. Copies Each Issue During Preceding 12 Months	No. Copies of Single Issue Published Nearest to Filing Date
a. Paid Electronic Copies	▶	0	0
b. Total Paid Print Copies (Line 15c) + Paid Electronic Copies (Line 16a)	▶	179	160
c. Total Print Distribution (Line 15f) + Paid Electronic Copies (Line 16a)	▶	220	225
d. Percent Paid (Both Print & Electronic Copies) (16b divided by 16c × 100)	▶	81.36%	71.11%

☒ I certify that 50% of all my distributed copies (electronic and print) are paid above a nominal price.

17. Publication of Statement of Ownership
☒ If the publication is a general publication, publication of this statement is required. Will be printed
in the NOVEMBER 2017 issue of this publication. ☐ Publication not required.

18. Signature and Title of Editor, Publisher, Business Manager, or Owner

STEPHEN R. BUSHING - INVENTORY DISTRIBUTION CONTROL MANAGER

Date 9/18/2017

I certify that all information furnished on this form is true and complete. I understand that anyone who furnishes false or misleading information on this form or who omits material or information requested on the form may be subject to criminal sanctions (including fines and imprisonment) and/or civil sanctions (including civil penalties).

PS Form **3526**, July 2014 (Page 3 of 4)   PRIVACY NOTICE: See our privacy policy on www.usps.com

Printed and bound by CPI Group (UK) Ltd, Croydon, CR0 4YY

03/10/2024

01040392-0019